Mammography Wars

Critical Issues in Health and Medicine

Edited by Rima D. Apple, University of Wisconsin–Madison; Janet Golden, Rutgers University–Camden; and Rana A. Hogarth, University of Illinois at Urbana–Champaign

Growing criticism of the U.S. healthcare system is coming from consumers, politicians, the media, activists, and healthcare professionals. Critical Issues in Health and Medicine is a collection of books that explores these contemporary dilemmas from a variety of perspectives, among them political, legal, historical, sociological, and comparative, and with attention to crucial dimensions such as race, gender, ethnicity, sexuality, and culture.

For a list of titles in the series, see the last page of the book.

Mammography Wars

Analyzing Attention in Cultural and Medical Disputes

Asia Friedman

Rutgers University Press
New Brunswick, Camden, and Newark, New Jersey
London and Oxford, UK

Rutgers University Press is a department of Rutgers, The State University of New Jersey, one of the leading public research universities in the nation. By publishing worldwide, it furthers the University's mission of dedication to excellence in teaching, scholarship, research, and clinical care.

978-1-9788-3064-6 (cloth)
978-1-9788-3063-9 (paper)
978-1-9788-3065-3 (epub)

Cataloging-in-publication data is available from the Library of Congress.
LCCN 2022043474

A British Cataloging-in-Publication record for this book is available from the British Library.

Copyright © 2023 by Asia Friedman

All rights reserved

No part of this book may be reproduced or utilized in any form or by any means, electronic or mechanical, or by any information storage and retrieval system, without written permission from the publisher. Please contact Rutgers University Press, 106 Somerset Street, New Brunswick, NJ 08901. The only exception to this prohibition is "fair use" as defined by U.S. copyright law.

References to internet websites (URLs) were accurate at the time of writing. Neither the author nor Rutgers University Press is responsible for URLs that may have expired or changed since the manuscript was prepared.

∞ The paper used in this publication meets the requirements of the American National Standard for Information Sciences—Permanence of Paper for Printed Library Materials, ANSI Z39.48-1992.

rutgersuniversitypress.org

In loving memory of Joe.

Contents

	List of Illustrations	ix
	Introduction: The Mammography Wars	1
Chapter 1	Skepticism and Interventionism as Attentional Types	34
Chapter 2	Attentional Diversity: The Cognitive Structure of Patients' Narratives of Mammography	59
Chapter 3	Attentional Battles over Mammography	92
Chapter 4	Attentional Weight: Relevance, Risk, and Expertise in Mammography	125
Chapter 5	Mammography and Time	163
	Conclusion: Attentional Flexibility	195
	Appendix: Methodological Note	215
	Acknowledgments	229
	Notes	231
	References	233
	Index	253

Illustrations

Figures

1.1.	Skeptic and interventionist beliefs	52
3.1.	Number of publications on mammography, by year (2002–2015) ($N = 589$)	116
3.2.	Number of articles favoring the USPSTF 2009 revision vs. the 2002 guideline ($N = 119$)	117
3.3.	Overall tenor of discussion of mammography by number of articles ($N = 293$)	117
3.4.	Perspective presented on early detection by number of articles ($N = 228$)	119
3.5.	Number of interventionist, neutral, and skeptical articles by year ($N = 293$)	121
3.6.	Percentage of articles mentioning the harms of mammography by year ($N = 340$)	122
3.7.	Number of interventionist, neutral, and skeptical articles by source	123
3.8.	Number of articles mentioning harms of mammography by source	124
3.9.	Number of articles mentioning benefits of mammography by source	124

Tables

I.1.	Summary of conflicting mammography guidelines	6
I.2.	Should women between forty and fifty have mammograms? A history of disagreement over screening guidelines	12
I.3.	Screening recommendations, by country	14
1.1.	Characteristics of skeptics and interventionists	46
1.2.	Early detection filters: comparison of interventionism and skepticism	57
2.1.	Sample characteristics, patients	69

Mammography Wars

Introduction

The Mammography Wars

No medical screening—indeed, perhaps no other medical condition at all—has been more scrutinized than the mammogram. It may be a routine health screening performed some forty million times each year in the United States (Food and Drug Administration 2022), but despite its prevalence, and despite an extensive research program spanning over half a century, breast cancer screening remains one of the most deeply contested topics in medicine. What is more, disagreement has revolved around many of the same ideas and questions for several decades—thus historian of science Robert Aronowitz's (2007, 279) characterization of the conflict as "a long war of attrition along relatively fixed battle lines."

At the heart of the issue lies "mammography's perennial dispute": the question of whether to screen women under age fifty (Reynolds 2012, 2–3). In addition to debates over age guidelines, Aronowitz (2001, 2007) highlights two further historical continuities: a "remarkably stable" belief in the value of early detection (2001, 357), and a pattern of assumptions about the linear and progressive development of breast cancer that underlie that belief. More than a decade has passed since Aronowitz made these observations, yet these same tensions around early detection and the molecular biology of cancer—whether linear and progressive, or idiosyncratic and variable—continue to structure debate and shape the trajectory of research and public discussion. As a result, the question of whether to screen women prior to age fifty is no closer to being resolved.

The mammography conflict is not only stagnant but also notably emotional, with significant judgment directed at each side by the other (Adami et al. 2019;

Carter 2021; Khuri 2015; Reynolds 2012, 4; Welch, Schwartz, and Woloshin 2011, 73). Mammography incites heated exchange in both academic journals and the media. I will highlight just a few examples to provide a sense of the degree of emotional intensity that routinely attends disagreement over the screening. Quanstrum and Hayward (2010, 1076) describe the reaction of one group of stakeholders to new mammography guidelines issued by the U.S. Preventive Services Task Force (USPSTF) in 2009 as follows: "Advocates of breast-cancer screening, particularly breast radiologists, immediately took action [against the USPSTF's 2009 announcement], denouncing the panel's statements as government rationing, suggesting that the panel members had ignored the medical evidence, and even implying that the panel members were guilty of a callous disregard for the life and well-being of women."

A widely publicized 2012 *New England Journal of Medicine* article critical of mammography (Bleyer and Welch 2012) was dismissed in a sharply worded rebuttal (Kopans 2013, 317) as "fundamentally flawed," lacking "scientific rigor," and "just one in a series of methodologically flawed attempts to reduce access to mammography screening."

A 2014 exchange in the journal *Cancer* (Berry 2014; Kopans, Webb, and Cady 2014) similarly included accusations of misleading the public, creating confusion, and imposing the researcher's values on American women, prompting the editor of the journal, Frank Khuri, to publish a follow-up editorial in which he admonished: "Although some are certain, as our dueling protagonists assert, that their view is known, fact-based, and certain ... what we think we know to be facts only occasionally approximate what we really do know" (2015, 5).

Also in 2014, the report on a twenty-five-year follow-up to the Canadian National Breast Screening Study, a major randomized controlled trial of mammography, concluded that mammograms do not reduce breast cancer death rates. In response, proponents of mammography published a storm of angry editorials, including one accusing the Canadian study of attempting to "deny women access to screening based on flawed analyses or rationing in the guise of altruism" (Kopans 2014). This and other similarly dramatic accusations prompted equally angry reactions in the media from experts supportive of the results of the Canadian trial. For example: "Many in the old guard are more likely to attack any suggestion that screening doesn't work as well as advertised, characterizing researchers who raise the possibility as 'malicious' or 'dangerous' and questioning the editorial policies of the journals that publish their work. It's time to stop the unfounded allegations. It might be standard procedure for politics but not for science" (Welch 2014). Welch concludes this editorial by essentially dismissing radiologists from the conversation, stating that it is time to "recognize that mammographers may not be the ideal source for balanced information. It's too much like asking the dentists for balanced information about routine dental x-rays."

The juxtaposition of these three observations—the large amount of research, the lack of evolution of the terms of the debate, the highly charged tone—suggest the need to examine the "mammography wars"[1] as a cultural cognitive conflict: specifically, the constellation of beliefs that underlie and support each viewpoint, how these beliefs rhetorically structure their claims, and the values, attachments, and exclusions that each of the entrenched, polarized perspectives entails. Though studies have focused on the impact of the mammography wars on women's awareness of and adherence to the changing screening guidelines (e.g., Allen et al. 2012; Davidson, Liao, and Magee 2011; Dehkordy et al. 2015; Kiviniemi and Hay 2012; Sprague et al. 2014; Squiers et al. 2011; Wharam et al. 2015), there is surprisingly little academic research that explicitly focuses on the discourse and rhetoric of the conflict itself.

In light of this, in this book I analyze the *cognitive structure* of the mammography wars, drawing on concepts from the sociology of attention to frame the conflict as an *attentional battle* (Zerubavel 2015, 57) rather than a strictly scientific disagreement over the data. Through this analysis, I identify *attentional norms of relevance* and *patterns of attention and inattention* that conceptually and rhetorically organize the debates. I also recast the dominant competing perspectives in the conflict as *attentional types*, which I refer to as *interventionism* and *skepticism*, taking inspiration in part from Georg Simmel's (1908) social types and forms and Max Weber's (1949) ideal types. Through this focus on the *formal organization of attention*, I uncover insights into the entrenched nature of debates about mammography that researchers applying a medical lens have not foregrounded.

My analysis is based on three types of empirical data: interviews with doctors and scientists, interviews with women age forty to fifty, and newspaper coverage of mammography. In 2014 I interviewed twenty-nine clinicians and academic medical researchers representing a range of disciplines including radiology, oncology, public health, and primary care, to better understand: (1) how they make sense of the conflict and, for practicing clinicians, how they communicate the guidelines to their patients; and (2) their understanding of the underlying reasons for the conflicting recommendations. Subsequently, in 2016 and 2017 I interviewed thirty patients between the ages of forty and fifty. These interviews capture patients' knowledge of screening guidelines, experiences with mammograms and follow-up screenings, interactions with doctors about mammography, experiences with friends and family members with breast cancer and/or abnormal mammograms, and feelings about breast cancer risk. Finally, I conducted a content analysis of news reporting on mammography in four prominent, high-circulation newspapers—*The New York Times*, *The Los Angeles Times*, *The Wall Street Journal*, and *USA Today*. This analysis includes all reporting on mammography from the USPSTF guideline announcement in 2002 until the American Cancer Society (ACS) guideline change in 2015. I use these data to discuss how mammography has been presented in the news and whether the news coverage reflects one side of the conflict more than the other. My analysis weaves together these different forms of data to create a multidimensional picture of the two prevailing attentional patterns organizing current cultural and scientific discourses on mammography, interventionism and skepticism.

As a rough characterization, the *interventionist* attention type firmly believes in the benefits of early detection and minimizes any possible harms of screening. They are accordingly critical of any effort to delay the age recommendation for mammograms or reduce the frequency of screening. The *skeptic* attention type is less confident in mammography screening's effectiveness and gives more weight to the harms of screening, which they define more broadly than interventionists. These harms include the psychological stress of repeated inconclusive screenings or false-positive results in addition to physical harms such as overdiagnosis (finding tumors that would not go on to cause harm) and overtreatment (treating all cancers aggressively, even those that would not ultimately cause harm). Skeptics generally advocate delaying the initiation and slowing the frequency of mammography to limit these risks only to those women statistically most likely to benefit from the screening.

The analysis I present both provides a sociological perspective on the mammography conflict, which was previously almost totally absent from the conversation both within and outside of the academy, and offers an empirical case study in the sociology of attention, which to this point has developed predominantly as a theoretical perspective. In this way, I hope to demonstrate the sociology of attention's generative potential as a set of concepts and theories not just for analyzing mammography, but for achieving a deeper understanding of the cognitive structure of cultural conflicts more generally, both within and outside of medicine.

The organization and implications of cultural discourses on mammography are not simply of rhetorical, historical, or sociological interest, of course. Breast cancer remains one of the most common cancers among women. In 2019 an estimated 268,600 new cases of invasive breast cancer were diagnosed in women in the United States, along with 62,930 new cases of noninvasive (in situ) breast cancer. Roughly 41,760 U.S. women die of the disease each year ("U.S. Breast Cancer Statistics" 2019). At this point, given that the different positions in the mammography wars are so entrenched, more scientific knowledge alone seems unlikely to meaningfully advance the debate. As Rogers (2019, 134) stated, "breast cancer screening researchers continue to argue past each other by producing contradictory reviews based upon different trials and using different assumptions." My aim is to identify these assumptions, mapping the cognitive frameworks and cultural beliefs about breast cancer that provide preexisting filters for how any new research is received and interpreted.

A Brief History of the Mammography "Age Wars"

Prior works have thoroughly documented the history of mammography (Aronowitz 2007; Lerner 2003; Reynolds 2012), so I limit my treatment here to illustrating two key points: First, since the 1970s, official recommendations have flipped back and forth on the question of whether to screen women under fifty. Second, intense emotion and discord have accompanied every swing of this pendulum.

The question of whether women under fifty should be screened first became a point of debate in 1976, only three years after mammography's introduction (Reynolds 2012, 2–3), yet institutionalized, public disagreement among expert organizations persists to this day. Currently, the USPSTF, a national independent panel tasked with making evidence-based recommendations about clinical preventive services, recommends biennial mammograms for women at average risk for breast cancer beginning at age fifty (Siu and U.S. Preventive Services Task Force 2016). This represents a change from their prior recommendation of annual mammograms beginning at age forty, in place from 2002 to 2009 (U.S. Preventive Services Task Force 2009).[2] The American College of Radiology (ACR) rejects this revised recommendation, continuing to recommend annual screening beginning at age forty (American College of Radiology 2021). In 2015 the ACS released a third guideline, recommending the initiation of annual mammography at the age of forty-five and continuing until age fifty-five, when biennial screening is recommended (Oeffinger et al. 2015). In the period since 2015, multiple organizations, including the American College of Obstetricians and Gynecologists and the American College of Physicians, have shifted to recommending informed decision-making rather than purely age-based screening guidelines for women in their forties. (Table I.1 compares the guidelines of six leading organizations.) While this may appear to reflect an emerging consensus, even if the consensus is to not provide any specific recommendation for the forty- to fifty-year age group—and it certainly represents a growing

Table I.1
Summary of conflicting mammography guidelines (verified as of November 2021)

Organization	Recommendation
American Academy of Family Physicians (American Academy of Family Physicians 2017)	Biennial screening with mammography age 50–74. Informed decision-making with a healthcare provider age 40–49.
American Cancer Society (Oeffinger et al. 2015)	Women should have the option to begin screening at age 40 if they wish. Annual screening age 45–54 is recommended, followed by biennial screening from 55 until 10 years of life expectancy.
American College of Obstetricians and Gynecologists (Committee on Practice Bulletins—Gynecology 2017)	Mammography should be offered starting at age 40 and initiated if the patient desires. Recommendation is to commence either annual or biennial screening no later than age 50 and continue until at least age 75.
American College of Physicians (Qaseem et al. 2019)	Biennial screening with mammography age 50–74. Informed decision-making with a healthcare provider age 40–49 with mammography every 2 years if a woman requests it.
American College of Radiology (American College of Radiology 2021; Lee et al. 2010)	Annual screening age 40 until life expectancy is less than 5–7 years.
United States Preventive Services Task Force (Siu and U.S. Preventive Services Task Force 2016)	Biennial screening age 50–74. Informed decision-making with a health care provider age 40–49.

public acknowledgment of the potential harms of screening—deeper divisions remain over how best to define and measure the harms and benefits of mammography, and the fundamental validity of the very idea of early detection.

The 1962 mammography trial initiated by radiologist Phillip Strax in collaboration with the Health Insurance Plan of Greater New York provided the first scientific validation of the concept of breast screening and remains to this day the only randomized controlled trial of mammography performed in the United States. The results demonstrated a significant benefit from mammography for women age fifty to fifty-nine (Shapiro, Strax, and Venet 1971). Women over fifty-nine also benefited from screening, but, likely due to a low sample size, these results did not reach statistical significance. Women under fifty, however, did not benefit from screening (Klawiter 2008, 88; Reynolds 2012, 18).

Despite this, the Breast Cancer Detection Demonstration Project (BCDDP), initiated shortly after in 1973, initially included women age thirty-five to forty-nine in its participant pool (Aronowitz 2007, 238; Klawiter 2008, 89–90; Reynolds 2012, 20–29). Cosponsored by the National Cancer Institute (NCI) and the ACS, the BCDDP was a large project in terms of the number of participants, the number of participating centers, and the screening period, and it was this program that really made mammography "a mainstream, widely accepted, and heavily promoted public health technology" (Klawiter 2008, 89). Of the 245,000 women who participated in the project in the first year, approximately half were under fifty (Aronowitz 2007, 239). Eventually, due to criticisms of the lack of scientific support for screening women under fifty combined with additional concerns about radiation risk (Bailar 1976; Greenberg and Randal 1977; Reynolds 2012, 24), the BCDDP issued a new guideline that women under fifty should only be enrolled if they had a high risk of breast cancer (Aronowitz 2007, 241–242). This revised guideline was affirmed at the first-ever National Institutes of Health (NIH) Consensus Development Conference, held in 1977, and it remained the official policy of the BCDDP through the remaining years of the program (Aronowitz 2007, 248; Klawiter 2008, 94; Reynolds 2012, 26).

The NIH Consensus Guideline notwithstanding, throughout the 1980s and 1990s, national medical organizations continued to revisit and revise their mammography guidelines, remaining deeply divided over the forty- to forty-nine-year-old age group. There have been three national institutional attempts to come to consensus on screening women in their forties in the United States: the 1977 Consensus Development Conference, the National Medical Roundtable on Mammography in 1989, and a second NIH Consensus Development Conference in 1997. At each, the existing recommendation on screening women in their forties was overturned. As mentioned already, the 1977 conference affirmed the BCDDP's decision to exclude women under fifty from mammography screening. The 1989 roundtable meeting, however, reversed this position, recommending in favor of screening women in their forties (Reynolds 2012, 34–35). The official statement of the 1997 conference panel upended the roundtable's recommendation, concluding once again that the evidence did not warrant universal mammography screening for women in their forties (National Institutes of Health Consensus Development Panel 1997; see also, Reynolds 2012, 59).

These three formal attempts to come to scientific consensus resulted in twenty years of shifting guidelines on the question of screening women under fifty. They also failed to reflect actual consensus among participating organizations or to result in any significant alignment of those organizations' guidelines. For example, while eleven major medical organizations, including the NCI and the American Medical Association, supported the new recommendation to screen women from age forty to forty-nine following the Medical Roundtable in 1989 (Reynolds 2012, 34), several other important groups did not, including the USPSTF and the American College of Physicians. The USPSTF, which is charged with periodically reviewing evidence on clinical preventive services (and which would ultimately become a major focus of the debate), cited high costs and high rates of false positives as reasons for opposing screening women under fifty in its 1989 *Clinical Guide to Preventive Services* (U.S. Preventive Services Task Force 1989). The American College of Physicians, the largest medical specialty society, also opted to retain its prior guideline excluding women under fifty from screening in the absence of high risk. Similarly, following the 1997 Consensus Development Conference's recommendation not to screen women under fifty, it quickly emerged that several members of the conference committee felt uncomfortable with this change. Two resigned in protest, and two others issued a minority report (Reynolds 2012, 60). Notably, in the previous 102 Consensus Development Conferences hosted by the NIH since 1977, unanimous consent had been achieved in all but two (Reynolds 2012, 60).

The difficulty coming to consensus on mammography has been compounded by contradictions in the scientific data. Specifically, in the 1990s, two important studies from Canada and Sweden brought new data to the debate about women in their forties, but their results did not correspond. The Canadian National Breast Screening Study was the first randomized controlled trial specifically designed to study the effectiveness of mammography in women under fifty. I have mentioned already how inciting the twenty-five-year follow-up to this trial was when it was published in 2014; the initial results, published in 1992, were equally controversial. The Canadian trial data showed that, after eight years, mammography did not reduce the death rate from breast cancer. The study was immediately and harshly criticized by mammography proponents. These groups, led by the ACS and the ACR, "denounced the study as so deeply flawed that its results were untrustworthy and should be ignored" (Reynolds 2012, 51–52).

Nevertheless, by the mid-1990s, eight randomized controlled trials of mammography had included women under fifty. Whereas none of them showed a statistically significant reduction in mortality in this age group within the first decade of screening, all but one showed a statistically significant mortality benefit for women over fifty. The 1996 Swedish Overview, however, combined the results of five Swedish trials and found a demonstrable benefit for women between forty and forty-nine (Reynolds 2012, 57; "Breast Cancer Screening with Mammography in Women Aged 40–49 Years" 1996). At the second NIH Consensus Development Conference in 1997, the Swedish and other data were combined and, together, again showed a statistically significant 23 percent reduction in mortality for women under fifty (Klawiter 2008, 94; Reynolds 2012, 55–59). The Swedish data were so strong, in fact, that even when combined with the Canadian trial data, they showed a statistically significant 16 percent mortality reduction (Reynolds 2012, 58–59). It was despite this favorable new data, then, that the 1997 conference panel did not find the evidence to warrant universal mammography screening for women in their forties (National Institutes of Health Consensus Development Panel 1997). A vocal minority of the committee published a dissenting report expressing their reservations with the panel's conclusion.

The competing reports and lack of true consensus coming out of the 1997 Consensus Development Conference also drew considerable attention and pressure in the political arena around the issue of mammography. A nonbinding resolution proposed by Senator Olympia Snowe with fifty-two cosponsors called for the reestablishment of screening recommendations including women in their forties. Following this political pressure, in March 1997 the ACS and ACR came out with their most aggressive screening guideline yet—annual screening beginning at forty (both groups had previously recommended screening every one to two years). The NCI's advisory committee, the National Cancer Advisory Board, also soon voted seventeen to one in favor of reinstituting their pre-1993 guideline that advised women over forty to undergo mammography screening every one to two years (Reynolds 2012, 59–61).

The USPSTF, the organization at the heart of the conflict over screening in the current era, did not recommend annual mammography for women under fifty until 2002. Its recommendations, which are updated every five years, are not official government policy, but they can play an important role in policymaking. Recall that in 1989, the USPSTF split with eleven other organizations, including the NCI and the American Medical Association, by rejecting new guidelines to begin screening women in their forties that were generated at the National Medical Roundtable on Mammography. It therefore likely came as a surprise to many when, in 2002, the Task Force announced a new recommendation supporting the initiation of mammography screening at age forty (Stolberg 2002). This is an interesting moment in the history of mammography not only because it marks the establishment of the guideline whose repeal in 2009 would set off arguably the most incendiary moment in the current period of conflict but also because it aligned the USPSTF with supporters of more aggressive screening and earned them the favor of specialist organizations—the very same groups that would be fervently opposed to the positions they would hold just seven years later.

The USPSTF announcement in 2002 expanding their recommendation to include all women over forty followed yet another period in which mammography's value was in vigorous debate. In 2000 *The Lancet* published a divisive meta-analysis of clinical trials that concluded there was no convincing evidence that mammography reduced the risk of dying from breast cancer for women in *any* age group (Gøtzsche and Olsen 2000). Klawiter describes the debates that followed this publication as particularly intense:

> Over the course of the next few months *The New York Times* published more than a dozen articles, editorials, and letters debating the conclusions and implications of the latest study. Public agencies, expert advisory panels, professional associations, cancer charities, and research foundations issued press releases and formal statements in support of mammographic screening. . . . An alliance of public service agencies and private organizations (including the ACS, the American Society of Clinical Oncology, and the American Academy of Family Physicians) even placed a full-page advertisement in the *New York Times* reassuring the public of the life-saving benefits of mammographic screening. (Klawiter 2008, 259)

In this context, the USPSTF's screen-at-forty guideline, which went against the grain of this wave of criticism of mammography, feels very pro-screening. This highlights the remarkable contrast between the Task Force's 2002 decision and its current views, which are more closely aligned with mammography critics. Even more notable are the responses by proponents of screening to the 2002 USPSTF guideline, which praised the panel as independent and evidence-based (in contrast with mammography critics). One example is the following comment from an ACS board member, reported in *The New York Times*: "'I'm very happy,' said Dr. Carolyn Runowicz, a gynecologist-oncologist and breast cancer survivor who serves on the board of the American Cancer Society. 'It's a very well-respected group,' Dr. Runowicz said, referring to the committee. 'They examine data very carefully and they come up with what they feel is good evidence-based medicine, and they are politically independent'" (Stolberg 2002).

Seven years later, using the exact same methodological rigor, the USPSTF reversed their position on mammography under age fifty (U.S. Preventive Services Task Force 2009). While it may not be surprising that their 2009 reversal drew criticism from the same groups that praised them in 2002, the reasons those groups cited in their criticisms are worthy of note. Ironically, the USPSTF was criticized in 2009 for what had earlier earned them accolades—basing their decisions purely on scientific evidence. The Task Force's purely evidence-based approach, previously hailed for independence and lack of bias, was now framed as a limiting exclusion that prevented their research from accounting for the human face of the clinical encounter.

The 2009 USPSTF guideline not only rescinded their prior recommendation to begin screening at age forty but also recommended only biennial rather than annual mammography, even for women over fifty. Mammography has always been a politicized screening, but the 2009 USPSTF change of recommendation was particularly so, arriving as it did during debates about the Affordable Care Act. The Task Force's recommendation was actually finalized in 2008, but due to journal publication timetables, it was not published until 2009, when debates about the Affordable Care Act were under way and fears of "death panels" and "rationing" dominated public discourse. Perhaps in part because of this context, but also not entirely out of keeping with the history of mammography I have just reviewed, the guideline change was met with unprecedented media attention and public criticism. As Reynolds describes, "In its twenty-five-year existence, the USPSTF had issued hundreds of guidelines on scores of subjects. Most had received no media attention whatsoever. None had ever received this type of public denunciation" (Reynolds 2012, 67).

Part of the USPSTF's charge is to re-review available evidence and update their position every five years. Their next review was completed in 2015, and in response to that reanalysis, they upheld their 2009 recommendation (Siu and U.S. Preventive Services Task Force 2016). That same year, the ACS changed their guideline to recommend that screening remain annual but that it be initiated not at forty or fifty, but at forty-five (Oeffinger et al. 2015). (See Table I.2 for a summary of key events in the history of mammography age recommendations.)

The United States, it is also important to note in terms of sociohistorical context, is virtually alone internationally in the degree of its support for mammography in women under fifty (Ebell, Thai, and Royalty 2018; Reynolds 2012, 50). Although similar debates have taken place elsewhere, most comparable nations have backed off from mammography much more aggressively than the United States, and many have never considered annual screening beginning at forty (Aschwanden 2015; Ebell, Thai, and Royalty 2018). See Table I.3 for a snapshot of some of these different recommendations.

As I write this in early 2022, major U.S. medical institutions appear no closer to the consensus on mammography that experts have sought since the

Table I.2
Should women between forty and fifty have mammograms? A history of disagreement over screening guidelines

1962	Health Insurance Plan of New York (HIP) begins first mammography trial.
1971	HIP reports that mammography reduces breast cancer deaths for women age 50–59 (but not under 50) (Shapiro, Strax, and Venet 1971).
1973	Breast Cancer Detection Demonstration Project (BCDDP) begins, enrolling women age 35–49 despite the lack of demonstrated benefit for this age group in HIP data.
1976	John Bailar publishes "Mammography: A Contrary View," in which he raises concerns about radiation risk. BCDDP publishes new guidelines recommending the inclusion of women under 50 only if they have an elevated risk of breast cancer.
1977	The first National Institutes of Health (NIH) Consensus Development Conference affirms the BCDDP recommendation not to screen women under 50 (see Reynolds 2012, 26).
1981	BCDDP ends, with just over 280,000 participants and 1,481 tumors detected by mammography. Of these, 42% were found in women age 50–59 (compared with 41% among participants in the HIP study), and 35% were found in women age 40–49 (compared with 19% for HIP) (Reynolds 2012, 28).
1983	American Cancer Society (ACS) issues guidelines recommending screening women age 40–49, citing BCDDP results as a rationale (see Reynolds 2012, 34).
1989	National Medical Roundtable: Eleven health care organizations recommend mammograms every one to two years for women over 40. The United States Preventive Services Task Force (USPSTF) is one of the organizations that does not support the recommendation (U.S. Preventive Services Task Force 1989; see also Reynolds 2012, 34–35).
1992	Results of Canadian Trials trials show no mortality benefit for women age 40–49 (Reynolds 2012, 51).
1993	Citing growing evidence from randomized trials, the NCI drops its recommendation for screening women in their 40s (Reynolds 2012, 57).
1996	The results of the Swedish Overview, which combined the results of five Swedish trials, indicates a benefit for women age 40–49 ("Breast Cancer Screening with Mammography in Women Aged 40–49 Years" 1996).
1997	A second NIH Consensus Development Conference concludes there is not enough evidence to recommend routine screening for women in their 40s (National Institutes of Health Consensus Development Panel 1997). However, the Senate votes to encourage the NCI advisory board to reject this conclusion, and the NCI recommends beginning mammography in the 40s and continuing every one to two years. ACS and the American College of Radiology recommend annual mammography for all women over 40. (See Reynolds 2012, 61)

Table I.2 (cont.)

2000	Meta-analysis of randomized controlled trials published in *The Lancet* concludes that there is no convincing evidence that mammography reduces breast cancer mortality risk in any age group (Gøtzsche and Olsen 2000).
2002	The USPSTF issues new guidelines recommending mammography begin at age 40 (Stolberg 2002).
2009	USPSTF rescinds 2002 recommendation. New guidelines recommend that most women start regular breast cancer screening at age 50, not 40, and that women age 50 to 74 should have mammograms less frequently—every two years, rather than every year (U.S. Preventive Services Task Force 2009).
2015	USPSTF reviews the evidence again and upholds its 2009 recommendation of biennial screening beginning at 50 (Siu and U.S. Preventive Services Task Force 2016). ACS issues a new guideline recommending women initiate annual mammography at age 45 rather than 40 (Oeffinger et al. 2015).

1970s. There are currently at least three different official recommendations, and with each new announcement the debate is inflamed once more. Yet the discussions both in medical journals and the lay media appear to circulate around the same themes that have defined the discourse and culture of mammography since the beginning. The conflict between interventionists and skeptics in the current period thus has the same basic shape and rhetoric it has all along. It is also notable that the "controversial" 2009 USPSTF guideline change to age fifty rather than forty was nothing new. It was identical to the position the USPSTF held in the 1990s. Taking this longer view of mammography's history, age forty was only their recommendation for seven years.

The United States is an outlier not just with respect to breast cancer screening but in terms of the aggressiveness of other screening recommendations—for example, lung cancer screening (Ebell et al. 2018). This is not simply a reflection of higher U.S. healthcare spending overall, as I explore further in the next section, but is associated with other institutional features of the U.S. system. For example, in their analysis of cancer screening recommendations in the twenty-one countries with the highest per capita spending on health care, Ebell et al. (2018) found that more aggressive screening guidelines were not associated with higher spending but with the prominence of specialty organizations. As mentioned already, the USPSTF recommendation for breast screening is actually consistent with most other countries, whereas the more intensive recommendations from specialty societies such as the ACR are unique to the United States. In addition to

Table I.3
Screening recommendations, by country

Country	Recommendation	Year of recommendation or most recent update	Reference
Austria	Age 45–69, every two years	2014	https://www.frueh-erkennen.at/en
Australia	Age 50–74, every two years	2018	https://www.health.gov.au/initiatives-and-programs/breastscreen-australia-program/having-a-breast-screen/who-should-have-a-breast-screen
Canada	Age 50–74, every two to three years	2018	https://canadiantaskforce.ca/guidelines/published-guidelines/breast-cancer-update/
France	Age 50–75, every two years	2015[a]	https://www.e-cancer.fr/Comprendre-prevenir-depister/Se-faire-depister/Depistage-du-cancer-du-sein; https://institut-curie.org/dossier-pedagogique/breast-cancer-france-screening-program-women-between-50-and-74-years-age
Germany	Age 50–69, every two years	2017	https://www.g-ba.de/richtlinien/17/ https://www.ncbi.nlm.nih.gov/books/NBK361021/
Italy	Age 50–69, every two years	2015	http://www.osservatorionazionalescreening.it/sites/default/files/allegati/ONS_2015_full.pdf
Netherlands	Age 50–75, every two years	2017[a]	https://www.rivm.nl/en/breast-cancer-screening-programme
Norway	Age 50–69, every two years	2010[a]	https://www.kreftregisteret.no/screening/mammografiprogrammet/; https://www.kreftregisteret.no/screening/mammografiprogrammet/Aldersgruppen/
United Kingdom	Age 50–71, every three years	2019	https://legacyscreening.phe.org.uk/breastcancer; https://www.nhs.uk/conditions/breast-screening-mammogram/when-youll-be-invited-and-who-should-go/

Note: All guidelines and links accessed on October 1, 2021. See Ebell, Thai, and Royalty 2018 for a more extensive comparison of international guidelines.

[a] Source: Ebell, Thai, and Royalty, 2018.

being an outlier in terms of offering inconsistent, more aggressive screening recommendations than other comparable nations, Howard, Richardson, and Thorpe (2009, 1846) found that U.S. cancer screening *rates* are significantly higher than Europe, which they similarly attribute in part to "system and cultural differences" rather than just higher spending: "Many features of the U.S. health-care system—fee-for-service reimbursement, the malpractice system, insurers' programs to measure quality, and pay-for-performance initiatives—promote screening."

The Mammography Wars in Broader Context: The U.S. Healthcare System

Medical sociologists and other experts have identified a number of shared global pressures that one might expect to lead to the convergence of healthcare systems with regard to their approaches to screening. These include rising costs (Mechanic and McAlpine 2010; Quadagno 2010; Timmermans and Oh 2010); the rapid development of new medical technologies (Conrad 2005; Casper and Morrison 2010); changing definitions of disease (Moynihan, Henry, and Moons 2014; Welch, Schwartz, and Woloshin 2011); and, increasingly, concerns about overuse, overdiagnosis, and overtreatment (Hicks 2015; Moynihan, Doust, and Henry 2012; Moynihan, Henry, and Moons 2014; Reibling, Ariaans, and Wendt 2019; Welch, Schwartz, and Woloshin 2011). Instead, most comparative analyses have found that the embeddedness of healthcare systems within specific cultural and institutional contexts creates contingency and path dependence rather than convergence, even though they are faced with similar pressures (Beckfield, Olafsdottir, and Sosnaud 2013; Kikuzawa, Olafsdottir, and Pescosolido 2008; Mechanic and Rochefort 1996). It is therefore important for any discussion of the U.S. healthcare system to consider its unique cultural and structural context. The full body of research on the U.S. healthcare system is wide ranging, deep, and interdisciplinary. In this brief treatment I establish a broader context for the mammography wars and the divergent and comparatively more intensive screening recommendations in the United States.

The United States spends more than other comparable nations on health care, but for worse, less equitable outcomes (Hejduková and Kureková 2017; Light 2004; Mechanic and McAlpine 2010; Timmermans and Oh 2010). It is broadly recognized that higher spending and higher-intensity care do not necessarily equate to better health outcomes (Hejduková and Kureková 2017; Mechanic 2004; Reibling, Ariaans, and Wendt 2019). Most analysts likewise agree that the U.S. healthcare system is characterized by a culture of overuse, suffering from "too much medicine" (Pathirana, Clark, and Moynihan 2017), "runaway medicalization" (Hankin and Wright 2010), and an "epidemic of diagnosis" (Welch, Schwartz, and Woloshin 2011). An important qualification, however, is that the United States also has significant disparities of care, where too much care for some is often coupled with too little for others (Hankin and Wright 2010; Rosich and Hankin 2010). Many have written about the drivers of the U.S. healthcare system's culture of overuse (Armstrong 2021; Conrad 2005; Hicks 2015; Moynihan, Doust, and Henry 2012; Moynihan, Henry, and Moons 2014; Welch, Schwartz, and Woloshin 2011), which include sensitive new medical technologies; broadened definitions of disease; direct-to-consumer advertising of pharmaceutical drugs and other medical services; growing public awareness of health, treatable health conditions, and the value of medical care; a culture of fear (both fear of illness and death and legal fears among practitioners); and a managed care system that rewards diagnosis and treatment and provokes resistance to utilization-management strategies among practitioners and patients alike.

There is also growing awareness of overdiagnosis as a specific concern within the culture of overuse in the U.S. healthcare system (Adami et al. 2019; Welch, Schwartz, and Woloshin 2011). Overdiagnosis is a key point of contention in disagreement over mammography, making some additional explanation of the idea necessary. Moynihan, Henry, and Moons (2014, 10) define overdiagnosis in the following way: "Overdiagnosis occurs when increasingly sensitive tests identify abnormalities that are indolent, non-progressive, or regressive and that, if left untreated, will not cause symptoms or shorten an individual's life. Such overdiagnosis leads to overtreatment when these 'pseudo-diseases' are conventionally managed and treated as if they were real abnormalities; because these findings have a benign prognosis, treatment can only do harm. More broadly defined, overdiagnosis happens when a diagnostic label is applied to people with mild symptoms or at very low risk of future illness, for whom the label and subsequent treatment may do more harm than good."

The concept of overdiagnosis was largely unknown until the 1990s and is still not fully acknowledged as a clinical problem despite the growing understanding that it is one of the overarching concerns in cancer screening (Adami et al. 2019). Indeed, the very idea remains conceptually challenging, and disagreement persists about the best way to conceptualize overdiagnosis (Harris et al. 2011; Hofmann 2014). This is because overdiagnosis is both *counterintuitive* in the context of the cultural promotion of early detection and *counterfactual* in the sense that it presupposes that one is able to know what would happen if a condition diagnosed as a disease had not been detected. It is also counterfactual because it is not clinically observable. "A current diagnosis can never be characterized as an overdiagnosis, and hence . . . overdiagnosis does not exist (in presence)" (Hofmann 2014, 599). Put simply, no individual overdiagnosed patient can be identified and studied; the concept can only be explored hypothetically or as a population-level phenomenon (Hofmann 2014; Rogers 2019; Rogers, Entwistle, and Carter 2019).

Although breast cancer is arguably the most prominent case of overdiagnosis, other examples include thyroid cancer, gestational diabetes, chronic kidney disease, asthma, pulmonary embolism, and Attention Deficit Hyperactivity Disorder (ADHD), illustrating the relevance of concern about overdiagnosis to the healthcare system more broadly. While often treated in the medical literature as a problem of individual decision-making, leading to inadequate "informed choice" solutions (Rogers 2019), overdiagnosis must be understood sociologically—as the result of the healthcare system and dominant beliefs and values in U.S. culture—and thus as driven by many of the same forces that result in the broader culture of overuse (Armstrong 2021; Moynihan, Doust, and Henry 1012; Moynihan, Henry, and Moons 2014; Pathirana, Clark, and Moynihan 2017; Rogers 2019; Rogers, Entwistle, and Carter 2019). These forces include frequent screening; increasingly sensitive technologies that identify indolent, nonprogressive, or regressive abnormalities; expanding definitions of disease; cultural faith in early diagnosis and enthusiasm for screening and testing without a balanced understanding of the risks of early detection; and health system incentives favoring more tests and treatments, including legal fears, fear of missing a diagnosis, and financial incentives.

Somewhat counterintuitively, given that they are most commonly perceived as a form of care rationing, some analysts implicate evidence-based population guidelines (i.e., those based on generalizable scientific evidence, ideally meta-analyses of randomized clinical trials [Timmermans and Berg 2003, 3]), including mammography recommendations, in the culture of overuse and the problem of overdiagnosis in U.S. medicine. For example, in a discussion of the harms of overuse in health care, Hicks (2015) points out that population guidelines and other quality improvement measures can have an unintended effect of contributing to overuse when physicians feel compelled to follow them for all patients. Armstrong (2021, 60) similarly points out that evidence-based medicine and movements to improve care quality can result in more treatment than necessary, especially in an "audit society" (Power 1999) in which quality control instruments and performance standards are used to regulate professionals' work. Doctors often resist such measures to preserve professional autonomy and may also order more tests and treatments "just to be safe." At the same time, current quality improvement measures lack adequate guidance on preventing overdiagnosis and overuse (Pathirana, Clark, and Moynihan 2017). Health disparities create additional complexity here, as Hankin and Wright

(2010, s12) point out; since the impact of evidence-based guidelines may be different for those who already overuse versus underuse medicine, such measures can deepen existing inequalities. Beckfield, Olafsdottir, and Sosnaud (2013, 135) similarly highlight the way that a population approach does not always reduce inequities in health. This is in part because of a lack of nuanced understanding of how to interpret and apply population data to specific groups of patients (Moynihan et al. 2014).

The managed care system, and the larger field of for-profit medicine of which it is a product, is of course the institutional context, and in some cases arguably the very cause, of many drivers of both overuse/overdiagnosis and healthcare disparities. Managed care, the use of which has escalated since the 1990s (Mechanic 2004, 81), has changed the way physicians practice medicine by centering cost and attempting to standardize care (Wright and Perry 2010). This has raised concerns about the impact of third-party payers and "rationing" of care on both care quality and equitable access (Light 2004; Mechanic 2001, 2004). Managed care also creates different interest groups within the healthcare system—for example, insurers, general practitioners, specialist organizations—that compete for resources and resist various reforms (Quadagno 2010). I already mentioned the finding that more aggressive screening guidelines are associated with specialty organizations (Ebell et al. 2018). Physicians likewise often resist evidence-based clinical guideline changes, movements toward standardization, and other measures aimed at quality improvement and utilization-management, particularly when they are perceived as overregulating medicine, a critique sometimes called "McDonaldization" or "cookbook medicine" (Genuis and Genuis 2004; Knaapen 2014; Light 2004; Mechanic 2001, 2004; Timmermans and Oh 2010, s98).

Although some of the physician backlash against managed care is likely more about a perception of lost professional autonomy and care rationing than any impact on actual care provision (Mechanic 2001, 2004), research does show that managed care has changed the way doctors actually practice medicine. For example, managed care increases the use of primary care, preventive medicine, and outpatient treatment but reduces hospitalizations, visits to specialists, and more intensive, costly procedures (Wholey and Burns 2000; Wright and Perry 2010). As mentioned previously, there is also evidence that population guidelines, although intended to curb spending and limit care to those patients most likely to benefit, can in some cases actually contribute to overuse, particularly when physicians feel compelled to practice "defensively," following them in every case (Hicks 2015). This is exacerbated by what Heath (2014) describes as a "terrible synergy" of fear and uncertainty that plays a substantial role in the healthcare crisis and in overdiagnosis. This complex of fear includes patients' fears about their health, which are exacerbated by screening and preventive medicine rhetoric, as well doctors' fear of legal action in a system of asymmetrical legal risk where there are "legal penalties for underdiagnosis (failure to diagnose) and no corresponding penalties for overdiagnosis" (Welch, Schwartz, and Woloshin 2011, 161). Fear thus drives both patients and practitioners to want more care rather than less, further contributing both to resistance to evidence-based guidelines and standardization and to overuse and overdiagnosis.

In addition to shaping the way doctors provide care, the institutional and national context I have just described also influences laypeople's perspectives and beliefs about health care. The type of healthcare system in a country creates expectations that shape citizens' attitudes toward spending and government regulation in a way that is separate from other kinds of pressures at the international level, such as demographic trends, economic pressures, or technological development. For example, citizens in centralized or National Health Service-type systems are more supportive of government regulation and standardization than those in insurance model countries (Kikuzawa, Olafsdottir, and Pescosolido 2008). More generally, the meanings assigned to health are forged and reproduced in social groups and within group norms (Umberson and Karas Montez 2010). In the United States we see a culture of heightened concern about health with growing fear and perception of risk. In addition, some find that with biomedicalization and consumers' increasing ability to access information about health, the U.S. public's expectations for health and health care are changing, with the "threshold of health" rising (Schnittker 2009). That is, even if health is objectively increasing, consumer perceptions of health are decreasing, and the level of symptoms that people interpret as poor health is lower.

These changing expectations and growing fears both derive from and contribute to a culture of early detection and overuse. U.S. screening rates are significantly higher than in Europe, for example, which Howard, Richardson, and Thorpe (2009, 1845–1846) tie to both the "system differences" that promote screening as well as to associated "cultural differences" in the U.S. public's beliefs about screening: "Culturally, U.S. patients and providers may be more favorably disposed to screening than their European counterparts and have greater faith in the ability of medical technology to cure and prevent disease. Compared with women in the United Kingdom, Italy, and Switzerland, American women are more likely to overestimate the number of deaths prevented because of mammography."

Schwartz et al. (2004, 73–74) similarly find very high "enthusiasm" for screening and a strong belief that it is an unambiguous positive among U.S.

patients. Their telephone interview study of a nationally representative sample of five hundred Americans (in which mammography is a featured example) found that most believe cancer screening is always beneficial, even when it leads to false positives, and even when presented with a hypothetical scenario of finding "pseudodisease," or overdiagnosis. On the other hand, there is very little public resonance for the harms of screening, despite growing awareness in medicine that screening is a double-edged sword. This hegemonic, deeply rooted "true belief" (Welch, Schwartz, and Woloshin 2011, 151) in the benefits of early detection, undampened by balanced consideration of the potential harms, including overdiagnosis, is widely documented in the literature (Carter 2021, 31; Harris et al. 2011, 33; He et al. 2018; Hoffmann and Del Mar 2015; Hofmann 2014; Moynihan, Doust, and Henry 2012; Rozbroj et al. 2021; Stefanek 2011, 1823; Welch, Schwartz, and Woloshin 2011, 22). Faith in early detection has become the conventional wisdom—a default, intuitive cultural logic—in large part because of long-standing, prominent public health messages that have emphasized the benefits and ignored the harms of early diagnosis for many diseases (Adami et al. 2019, 4; Carter 2021, 31; He et al. 2018, 1905; Hoffmann and Del Mar 2015; Hofmann 2014; Rogers 2019, 132; Stefanek 2011, 1823; Welch, Schwartz, and Woloshin 2011). Indeed, Welch and his colleagues (2011, 25) argue that the dominant logic of medicine may be organized around an asymmetrical focus on benefits over harms: "The conventional ethos of medicine has been to focus on the potential benefit for the few and to downplay the rest." In short, the United States is characterized by a hegemonic cultural belief in early detection and screening, which is likely encouraged by the institutional structure of the U.S. healthcare system.

The debates over mammography that are the focus of this book offer a fruitful case to bring balanced attention to both the benefits and the harms of screening—and thus to challenge the ingrained cultural belief in early detection (Moynihan et al. 2012). Although the mammography wars clearly reflect a dominant, deeply rooted faith in early detection and screening, they also illustrate a still much less prominent but increasingly consistent discursive countercurrent of skepticism of the culture of "too much medicine" (Pathirana, Clark, and Moynihan 2017). Many analysts have argued that sociologists are uniquely well positioned to reveal the definitions and systems of meaning and classification that underlie the healthcare system and our cultural beliefs about health and their consequences, including the construction of beliefs about mammography (Beckfield, Olafsdottir, and Sosnaud 2013; Broom and Kenny 2021; Casper and Morrison 2010; Conrad 2005; Conrad and Barker 2010; Fosket 2004; Rosich and Hankin 2010). Some have specifically pointed to the need to apply social theory and concepts from cultural cognitive sociology to the healthcare system (Beckfield, Olafsdottir, and Sosnaud 2013, 138; see also Martinelli and Veltri 2021; Pescosolido and Kronenfeld 1995; Ward and Peretti-Watel 2020).

In this book, I analyze both doctors' and patients' beliefs about mammography from a cognitive sociological perspective, specifically using the sociology of attention to map the patterns of attention and inattention underlying various perspectives in and on the debate. By examining the debate outside of just the scientific evidence, and instead examining how and why the debate exists sociologically and the specific attentional and cognitive form it takes, I hope to offer new ways of understanding what it is that really divides thought on this issue. Parker, Rychetnik, and Carter (2015, 6) point out that the beliefs underlying disagreement over mammography are not usually explicitly recognized, leading to experts "speaking at crosspurposes about what is important in breast screening, despite using similar terminology." As I describe in the next section, the sociology of attention offers a unique set of concepts that make these structuring beliefs explicit. In addition to driving analytic focus to the meaning structures and sociomental processes of attending and inattending underlying cultural conflicts and taken-for-granted ideas, the sociology of attention also reveals attentional alternatives that are inevitably left out in any given interpretation. Importantly, mapping these attentional alternatives illuminates the set of excluded ideas upon which any interpretation is constructed—moving beyond what Timmermans and Berg (2003, 201) call "the illusion of unequivocal evidence." Analyzing the cognitive structure of a debate can also reveal attentional commonalities among seemingly opposed perspectives, identifying potential ideas upon which, despite "speaking at crosspurposes" (Parker, Rychetnik, and Carter 2015, 6), it may be possible to build greater mutual understanding. An evenhanded mapping of the attention patterns structuring each side of a disagreement is particularly powerful in situations of epistemological, political, or social asymmetry, when one set of ideas, such as early detection in the case of mammography, has the status of "truth" or "reality."

The Sociology of Attention

Social psychologists Arien Mack and Irvin Rock (1998, 25–26) define attention as "the process that brings a stimulus to consciousness." Attention processes, or the *selection* of certain features or details among those technically available to us, including both perceptual attention and processes of selection in cognition, have been a consistent topic of interest in cognitive sociology, which aims as a field to identify those aspects of thinking attributable to membership in one or more "thought collectives" (Fleck 1979, 38–51). Although attention was a significant thematic focus of his prior work (Zerubavel 1991, 1993, 1997), it was only with Eviatar Zerubavel's *Hidden in Plain Sight* (2015) that sociology as a discipline can claim an explicit and sustained theory of attention. Zerubavel argues that attention, like cognition more generally, must be understood as the product of our membership in "attentional communities" defined by distinct "styles of attending" (Zerubavel 2015, 10). Schroer (2019, 427) points out that it is precisely in the process of selection that the social nature of attention resides, since "there is no general answer to the question of why one possibility takes precedence over the other," and "societies, when compared both diachronically and synchronically, can be shown to vary . . . in their respective foci of attention." The central task of a sociology of attention, therefore, is to examine these variations, which Zerubavel calls "socio-attentional patterns" (Zerubavel 2015, 53).

In addition to "attentional communities" and "socio-attentional patterns," the concept of "attentional relevance" is essential to capturing the connection between our sense of what is "relevant" or "irrelevant" and our attentional socialization into socially shared attentional norms, traditions, and habits (Zerubavel 2015, 52–53). As Schutz (1962, 227) describes it, our perceptions are structured by "systems of relevances": "We are not equally interested in all the strata of [reality]. The selective function of our interest organizes the world in both . . . space and time in strata of major and minor relevance. . . . Those objects are selected as primarily important which are . . . ends or means . . . or . . . dangerous or enjoyable or otherwise relevant to me." While such patterns of "major and minor relevance" are sometimes totally individual and idiosyncratic and can also be influenced by human biological universals, they are often the result of the attentional traditions and conventions of our social groups. This is evident in accounts of cross-cultural differences in attention (Masuda and Nisbett 2001; Nisbett 2003; Zerubavel 2015, 54–55). It is also exemplified in Goffman's descriptions of interactional "rules of irrelevance" and attention (Goffman 1961, 19–21; 1963; 1974) as well as studies on cultural norms of marking (Brekhus 1998, 2003; Zerubavel 2018, 21–26), which define some things as marked as relevant for our focus and others as the taken-for-granted background—things that are socially appropriate, even necessary, to ignore. Thus distinguishing the relevant from the irrelevant—learning what to notice and what to ignore—is something we learn through our socialization as members of attentional communities (Zerubavel 1997, 32–33, 46–51; 2015, 63).

Importantly, this attentional socialization includes not only norms of attention—indications of what types of information we should positively select for sensory or cognitive focus—but also norms of inattention, or notions of what is irrelevant and need not—in fact, often must not—be selected. Goffman (1961, 19–20) described such social "rules of irrelevance" as follows: "The character of an encounter is based in part upon rulings as to properties of the situation that should be considered irrelevant, out of frame, or not happening. . . . Irrelevant visible events will be disattended; irrelevant private concerns will be kept out of mind. An effortless unawareness will be involved, and if this is not possible then an active turning away or suppression will occur." Further, according to Goffman, those details we must ignore because they are irrelevant to the "definition of the situation" are equally significant to our sense of reality as those to which we do pay attention. In his words, "the set of rules which tell us what should not be given relevance tells us also what we are to treat as real" (Goffman 1961, 20). In this way, the sociology of attention explicitly highlights the existence of aspects of reality that are necessarily not selected when focusing attention elsewhere. Underlying selective attention, in other words, is always also selective inattention, which is why Zerubavel (2015, 2) refers to attention's "inherently exclusionary nature." One important contribution of the sociology of attention is thus to emphasize the importance of *collective forms of unawareness and inattention* to understand the constitution of any belief, perception, or experience.

Given that different attentional communities have different *relevance structures*, and thus different patterns of attention and inattention, attention is often contested, and "attentional battles" (Zerubavel 2015, 57) can ensue. When relevance is in dispute, comparatively analyzing conflicting attentional patterns from a sociological perspective offers the potential to bring the normatively inattended aspects of each into the foreground, opening up attentional alternatives and revealing backgrounded or unselected, attentionally excluded information. This work of comparing—and thereby dereifying—differing patterns of attention can thus help alleviate the inherent narrowing of our perceptions and cognition due to attention's "exclusionary nature" (Zerubavel 2015, 2).

The epistemological and ontological significance of engaging these *attentional exclusions* cannot be overstated. That which is excluded is always integrally constitutive of an idea or phenomena (Barad 2007, 57). In addition, "exclusions foreclose the possibility of determinism, providing the condition of an open future" (Barad 2007, 214). A sincere engagement with exclusions across differences of perspective, allowing them to, as Haraway put it, "interrupt each other productively" (as quoted in Schneider 2005, 149), heightens our humility and awareness of our own patterns of inattention, and makes us more accountable for them. This is what Barad (2007, 205) calls "the political potential of deconstructive analysis": "insisting on accountability for the particular exclusions that are enacted and . . . taking up the responsibility to perpetually contest and rework the boundaries." It also increases our *attentional flexibility*—the ability to perceive more than one possible interpretation simultaneously, recognizing that different, even contradictory, perceptions are simultaneously possible, and possibly even equally valid. Further, in conditions of epistemological, political, or social asymmetry or inequality, some interpretations or exclusions—and thus some meanings—can seem to take on a status of truth or reality, making a symmetrical treatment of attentional differences and exclusions even more important. This is best accomplished by approaching attentional conflicts through what Haraway (1992) termed "diffractive" analysis. Barad (2007, 30) describes diffraction as a method of "reading insights through one another in ways that help illuminate . . . how different differences get made, what gets excluded, and how those exclusions matter." Further, as Meißner (2016, 44) explains, diffractive analysis "implies a generosity in the reading of different perspectives; it is not a critique that dismisses one theory from the standpoint of another. . . . It is a respectful engagement attempting to carefully read the questions being asked and the arguments being made while at the same time being attentive to their (necessary) presuppositions and limitations as well as to their possibly universalizing presumptions." The sociology of attention approaches attentional conflicts in this spirit of generous accountability for differences and patterns of inattention and exclusion, reading contradictory or otherwise divergent lines of thought "through one another for the patterns of resonance and dissonance that illuminate new possibilities for understanding and for being" (Barad 2007, 142).

In prior research, I have worked to develop two additional concepts directly intended to facilitate such a dereifying, diffractive analysis of irrelevance and inattention—*filter analysis* (DeGloma and Friedman 2005; Friedman 2013) and *cultural blind spots* (Friedman 2019). The filter as a metaphor for attention is based on the image of a mental "strainer" through which information passes before it is consciously perceived. The function of a filter in general is to allow selected elements to pass through a set of holes while blocking others. Thinking in terms of filters thus analytically directs focus to questions about which features or details pass through and are attended and, arguably more importantly, which are blocked out by our mental filters and thus remain unnoticed. The related concept of cultural blind spots captures social influences on the structure of attention, specifically what is considered irrelevant and therefore not perceived or acknowledged (Friedman 2019).

While sociologists have begun to develop a powerful analytic vocabulary for studying attention, we have not yet fully demonstrated the insights possible through the application of these ideas in empirical research. As Schroer (2019, 444) argues, the concept of attention has "tremendous heuristic value for examining current developments and changes in contemporary society," yet "its theoretical potential remains yet untapped." He further suggests that science is a field where attention may be particularly salient for our sociological understanding (441).

Prior Research on the Mammography Conflict

As my earlier discussion of the history of the mammography age debates indicates, medical researchers have studied mammography for decades—primarily its risks and benefits at different ages, participation rates, and barriers and facilitators to adherence to recommendations—but the disagreement itself has received very little direct attention. Exceptions include a small body of research on how the conflict has affected women's participation (Dehkordy et al. 2015; Sprague et al. 2014; Wharam et al. 2015) and what guideline doctors follow in practice (Anderson et al. 2014; Corbelli et al. 2014; Hinz et al. 2011; Kadivar et al. 2012, 2014). Another small set of studies examines women's awareness of and reaction to the guideline changes, primarily finding that women's knowledge of the guidelines is low and that they are confused by the debates and resistant to delaying screening (Allen et al. 2012; Davidson, Liao, and Magee 2011; Kiviniemi and Hay 2012; Squiers et al. 2011).

There is, however, a significant body of medical literature that debates the benefits and harms of mammography screening (Bleyer 2015; Bleyer and Welch 2012; Keen 2010; Kopans 2010; Lewin et al. 2018; Raftery and Chorozoglou 2011). A large subset of this work studies the effect of reducing screening frequency (largely moving the age recommendation later, but also spacing screening out) on the stage or size of tumors at diagnosis and/or compares mortality estimates for the different screening recommendations (Arleo et al. 2017; Carter, Castro, and Morcos 2018; Kalager et al. 2010; Keating and Pace 2015; Patel 2018; Ray et al. 2018). When examining the risks and benefits of screening, however, again none of these studies takes the conflict itself as an object of analysis—whether in general or specifically in terms of attention, cognition, or narrative structure.

In the more limited body of social science research touching on disagreements over mammography, here again none has looked at the cognitive organization of the conflict. Steele et al. (2005) analyzed newspaper coverage of debates about mammography, but this research was conducted prior to the 2009 USPSTF change of guidelines, which significantly intensified the conflict. Barker and Galardi's (2011) study directly addresses the conflict by examining internet postings responding to the 2009 USPSTF guideline change. Their content analysis reveals posters' belief in their own "lay expertise" and resistance to the scientific expertise represented by the USPSTF (1353). These two studies notwithstanding, like the medical literature, most prior sociological and broader social science literature on mammography focuses on barriers and facilitators to screening (usually with the seemingly unquestioned underlying assumption that participating in mammography is desirable), rather than making the conflict itself a central focus (e.g., Arana-Chicas et al. 2020; Dean et al. 2014; Eibich and Goldzahl 2020; Farr et al. 2020; Goldzahl 2017; Miller et al. 2019; Mishra et al. 2012; Missinne, Neels, and Bracke 2014; Moudatsou et al. 2014; Solazzo, Gorman, and Denney 2017).

At the same time, social scientists have made important contributions to our understanding of other aspects of breast cancer culture, among them Klawiter's (2008) analysis of breast cancer activism and the evolution of the breast cancer movement, and Sharlene Hesse-Biber's (2014) examination of the experiences of women who learn they have an elevated genetic risk for breast and ovarian cancer, which highlights social influences on their understandings of and decisions about the risk they face. There is also a growing body of work examining "pink ribbon culture," or the intersection of hegemonic gender ideologies with breast cancer discourse, diagnosis, funding, and treatment (e.g., King 2008; Sledge 2021; Sulik 2010). In addition, several social histories of breast cancer and mammography (Aronowitz 2007; Lerner 2003; Reynolds 2012) touch on the conflict and are especially useful for tracing historical continuities of the contemporary debates.

Further, on a more general level, several foundational literatures in medical sociology can support an analysis of the social discord surrounding mammography guidelines. Research addressing the social construction of medical knowledge, including medical diagnosis and decision-making, is particularly useful here, as well as work on the sociology of medical screening. For example, it is well established in the field that medical knowledge and the science that underlies it are imbued with biases reflecting cultural norms and traditions. This point has been particularly well documented in studies of obstetric knowledge and practice related to cesarean sections (De Vries and Lemmens 2006; Wendland 2007). This literature also documents a general bias in medical diagnosis toward the creation of illness and overtreatment relative to nontreatment. Perhaps most well known is Thomas Scheff's (1963, 99) application of the distinction between Type 1 and Type 2 errors to argue that Type 1 errors—not detecting a patient's illness, or underdiagnosis—are considered far less acceptable in medicine than Type 2 errors—diagnosing an illness that is not actually present, or overdiagnosis. This normative bias in medicine in favor of Type 2 errors contributes to the prevailing culture of overuse. It is also directly relevant to debates about mammography because overdiagnosis and overtreatment are considered by skeptics to be the most significant harms of mammography and are the primary reasons some argue that screening should be less frequent and start later in life. Interventionists, on the other hand, in keeping with Scheff's (1963) argument, find underdiagnosis more problematic than overdiagnosis. I will suggest that it is in part the attentional norms of each group that make Type 1 vs. Type 2 errors more or less acceptable.

As this example of normative bias favoring diagnosis illustrates, the literature on the social construction of medical knowledge, diagnosis, and decision-making shares the focus of the sociology of attention and the broader field of cognitive sociology on the important role of cognition, specifically socially shared patterns of thought, in shaping medical knowledge. For example, Wendland (2007, 277) engages Haraway's (1988) concept of *situated knowledge* to show that empirical data never speaks for itself but is always interpreted, including some degree of "partial perspective." Others rely on Fleck's (1979) concepts of *thought collectives* and *thought styles* to highlight the construction of medical knowledge: for example, to explain the incommensurate thought styles between different medical specialties (Arksey 1994). Similarly, Berg (1992) and Hunter (1991) apply Kuhn's (1962) concept of *scientific paradigms of thought* to demonstrate that what is perceived in the process of medical diagnosis depends on what is expected, portraying medicine as an interpretive, narrative activity. While it is generally assumed that physicians are simply "using" biomedical knowledge, implying that the cognitive domain of medicine is self-evident and not in need of sociological scrutiny, such research points to the importance of sociocognitive practices of selection and interpretation in shaping that knowledge. I likewise take a cognitive approach to analyzing medical discourse, specifically focusing on the role played by norms of attention and relevance in structuring interpretations of mammography. Despite these overlapping concerns, cognitive sociology is not a broadly recognized theoretical perspective in medical sociology, one notable exception being a very small handful of recent work on the topic of vaccine hesitancy (Martinelli and Veltri 2021; Ward and Peretti-Watel 2020).

In addition to the social construction of medical knowledge and the importance of attending to the role of cognition in its construction, sociologists have previously studied various other forms of medical screening, with conclusions relevant to understanding the meanings attributed to mammography. Among the other types of screening previously studied from a sociological perspective are prostate-specific antigen (PSA), cholesterol, cervical cancer, and various forms of genetic screening, including pregnancy and newborn screenings. The sociology of screening also overlaps with the emerging body of work in the sociology of overdiagnosis, mentioned previously. In addition to overdiagnosis, other cross-cutting themes within the sociology of screening relevant to mammography screening and the current conflict surrounding it include new forms of identity that can result from screening, the social meaning of risk, and the impact of the uncertainty inherent in any population screening. Modern medical technologies, including screening technologies, can create new categories and forms of identity that Sulik (2009) calls *technoscientific identities*. In the case of screening technologies, patients often learn they are at elevated *risk* of a disease that they do not yet actually have, which Willis (1998) describes as the "asymptomatic ill" (178) or "people living with future genetic disease" (179), and Gillespie (2015) captures using the concept of a *proto illness*. Both Gifford (1986) and Hesse-Biber (2014) document the creation of such "at-risk" identities for breast cancer, which motivate some women to seek surgical intervention in their otherwise healthy bodies. Faulkner's (2012) work on PSA testing further suggests that uncertainty can persist even after normal results of a screening test, leading to the creation of identities based on uncertainty.

Research in the sociology of screening also demonstrates the cultural and autobiographical meanings that shape risk perceptions and thus the necessity of analyzing how actors interpretively integrate the social into their understandings of the risks and benefits of screening. Risk must be understood in the context of everyday routine life, not just what is defined scientifically or numerically (Bloor 1995). Biomarkers, for example, which are often numerical, have "meanings for patients that are quite different from their biological meanings" (Gillespie 2015, 974). In presenting his "phenomenological alternative" to prior models of thinking about risk, emphasizing the everyday, routine world, Bloor (1995, 25–28) further points out that we must not assume risk is hugely relevant but *investigate* what it means to be at risk, including the culturally available frameworks people adapt and modify to interpret risk in an intersubjectively meaningful way. One of these cultural frameworks used to interpret risk is gender, specifically gendered ideologies of responsibility for health rooted in narratives of family, work, and caring, as well as the medicalization of women's bodies (Green, Thompson, and Griffiths 2002; Lupton 1994; Moore 2010). The broader cultural context of overuse and faith in early detection also contribute to increasing perceptions of risk. The concept of the *screening paradox* is sometimes used to illustrate such social influences on risk. As I discuss in greater detail in later chapters, in the case of mammography the screening paradox refers to the social influence on women's perceived risk of breast cancer of the growing number of women who have had a breast cancer diagnosis and understand themselves as survivors. This is paradoxical, according to skeptics, because many of these women were likely overdiagnosed, distorting any resulting sense of elevated risk. I also introduce the concept of *attentional alignment* in chapter 2 to capture how patients' perceptions of the risks and benefits of mammography emerge from the interplay between their autobiographical experiences and hegemonic cultural ideas such as early detection.

Another point of emphasis in sociological research on screening is the uncertainty produced by screening tests. Uncertainty is created when population screening alters concepts of disease previously taken as given, or produces unexpected results (Timmermans and Buchbinder 2010). This is equally true of genetic screening, even though genetic testing is assumed to be highly accurate (Davison, Macintyre, and Smith 1994; Timmermans and Buchbinder 2010, 215): Applications of genetic risk information to any individual is "inherently probabilistic" (Davison, Macintyre, and Smith 1994, 343), since not all who have an allelic pattern or chromosomal abnormality go on to develop the disease. Even beyond genetics, however, there is an inherent tension, rooted in this uncertainty, between population data and the application to any individual patient (Griffiths, Green, and Bendelow 2006; Willis 1998). Attending to population health needs inevitably causes disruption for some individuals. Likewise, attending to individual needs may use resources that could have been used for the needs of the population. For example, in the case of mammography, most individuals see no benefit from it, and some arguably face a significant and physical detriment: for example, if they are subjected to interventions following a false-positive result.

The uncertainty generated by screening is further increased with the introduction of new temporal meanings into medicine, fragmenting a previously unilinear temporal space of disease and medicine based on a model of progressive decay. Such temporal challenges can be seen both in the notion of *risk factors*, which are nonlinear, multidimensional causes of disease (Armstrong and Eborall 2012, 185), as well as the way screening shifts the temporal framework of doctor's work with patients from present disease to future disease (Griffiths, Green, and Bendelow 2006, 1079). As I explore in chapter 5, which focuses on temporality, skeptics argue that mammography is not effective because the unilinear model of disease underlying early detection frameworks does not reflect the biotemporal complexity of tumor growth. Such misalignments between biotemporality and the sociotemporal order of screening, Armstrong and Eborall (2012) argue, are one reason screening tests for diseases with more of a risk factor profile have had less success and longevity than those for diseases with a linear biological history. Armstrong actually characterizes breast cancer as one of these linear diseases for which it is possible to screen successfully, but more recently mammography skeptics have challenged such linear, progressive conceptions of breast cancer, raising questions about the value of mammographic screening and early detection more broadly.

My analytic approach throughout the book also draws from several methodological implications explored in the sociology of screening literature. Here the pertinent question is how to best focus and conduct a sociological analysis of screening. I have touched upon some of these lessons already, including the importance of attending to the everyday contexts and taken-for-granted ideas that shape the meanings we apply to screening (Bloor 1995; Cox and McKellin 1999). Related to this, a number of works emphasize the importance of attending to the *epistemological aspects* of screening, arguing that they are underemphasized relative to research on barriers or adherence rates. To get at these "tacit dimensions" "requires paying particular attention to their discursive repertoires" (Lehoux et al. 2010, 123). An epistemological approach to screening thus involves examining the structure of people's narratives, particularly their patterns of relevance and inattention. Such an emphasis does not have to be evaluative but can be beneficially focused instead on methods and strategies (Martin 2004, 714; Sarda 2009). This puts less emphasis on which side of a disagreement is correct and more emphasis on how claims are constructed rhetorically and epistemologically. Another term used in this context is "symmetrical analysis" (Martin 2004), or the suspension of judgments regarding which arguments are right or wrong. Applied to attentional battles, I suggest that a symmetrical analysis demands not only avoiding taking an evaluative stance but also providing comparable analysis of the attention patterns of both sides of a conflict, including both attention and inattention. This analytic symmetry is also an essential aspect of "diffractive" reading, particularly the focus on "respectful engagement that attends to detailed patterns of thinking of each" side of a conflict and reads these "patterns of difference" through one another (Barad 2007, 90, 29).

Overview of the Book

In summary, while many prior works touch on disagreements over mammography, none have focused on the rhetorical, conceptual, and cognitive structure of the conflict. In light of this, my analysis of skepticism and interventionism as attentional types maps the structure of beliefs and concepts that form the competing narratives in disputes over mammography, emphasizing attention, inattention, meaning, and interpretation. Through this focus on the *attentional organization* of the conflict, I offer insights into the entrenched nature of debates over mammography that researchers applying a medical lens have not emphasized.

Tracking patterns of attention and inattention in discourses on mammography allows me to address such questions as: What are the exclusions of dominant cultural discourses about mammography? What are the salient beliefs different actors attach to mammography? How do these beliefs shape how they think about breast cancer, and make it hard to think differently about screening, early detection, and the natural history of breast cancer? How are these cognitive biases and nodes of inattention borne out in the ongoing debates? And how might thinking about the different perspectives in the debate as conflicting attentional patterns provide insight into the perennial standoff over whether to screen women in their forties, and the relative risks and benefits of doing so?

While the empirical focus of my analysis is mammography screening, I also highlight several more generalizable concepts and methodological implications. For example, I frame my analysis using the concept of an "attentional battle" (Zerubavel 2015, 57), which I argue allows me to draw out normally unrecognized patterns of inattention through comparative analysis of the two Simmelian *attentional types* dominating the mammography wars, *interventionism* and *skepticism*. Comparing attentional types also analytically cultivates mental and attentional flexibility through recognizing multiple attentional possibilities, thereby dereifying any singular attentional pattern. These methodological and analytical benefits of mapping the attentional structure of the mammography conflict apply equally to other cultural and political conflicts, both within medicine and more generally. Thus, while I am focused on mammography and specifically interested in intervening in this case, I am also making a broader claim that it is beneficial to analyze patterns of attention to more fully understand the cognitive basis for cultural and political battles, including why they can be so intractable.

Beyond advocating for the generic method of comparatively analyzing attention types to chart the cognitive patterns of cultural conflicts, on another level I also recognize that the specific attention types I present—interventionism and skepticism—are themselves applicable beyond the case of mammography as formal structures of attention. The most obvious parallel is to prostate cancer. As Aronowitz (2021, 42) describes, "there is little consensus about whether efforts to prevent and treat prostate cancer have caused more harm than good." While skeptics emphasize that "American men have been experiencing a problematic epidemic of invasive treatments triggered by prostate cancer screening"

(Aronowitz 2021, 42), there is little consensus on the disease's clinical course in the absence of interventions to diagnose and treat it. Aronowitz further argues that, as with breast cancer, one's position in the debate has mostly to do with what one believes about early detection and the biological progression of prostate cancer. Other cases one might point to within medicine where interventionists battle with skeptics include medical versus midwifery approaches to pregnancy and childbirth, naturopathic versus pharmaceutical approaches to addressing illness, and pro- and anti-vaccination perspectives. Outside of medicine, one might further draw connections to social conflicts as seemingly far afield from mammography as penal reform (where the relevant contrast could be between prison expansion and the abolitionist movement) or disagreements in economics over government regulation versus free-market approaches. While each of these cases is obviously substantively quite different, and they do not necessarily "align" politically in the sense that interventionism is not always politically liberal or conservative, by connecting them analytically as common attention types it becomes possible to identify formal similarities in patterns of attention and relevance that their very different substantive content and political alignment would normally obscure.

In order to signal these broader implications, while only directly analyzing mammography, I have organized each chapter around a generic attention concept. In chapter 1, I introduce the two *attentional types* that broadly organize the conflict over mammography, interventionism and skepticism, drawing on the concepts of attentional collectives, attentional norms, and attentional socialization. Chapter 2 addresses *attentional diversity* through a focus on whether and how the patients I interviewed fit into the attentional types of interventionism and skepticism, or whether they present distinct attentional patterns. In chapter 3 I recast the mammography conflict as an *attentional battle* between interventionists and skeptics, highlighting each side's efforts at polarization, discrediting, and marginalization using claims of "incorrect" attention. This focus on attentional battle also illuminates the attentional roots of some of the elevated emotions of the conflict. Further, analytically, examining something as a battle over the organization of attention drives focus to a level of analysis that is normally not foregrounded when examining cultural conflicts. Specifically, the focus becomes the attentional structure of the dispute as a whole, with the aim of understanding how the different viewpoints are connected conceptually. Chapters 4 and 5 each look in greater depth at one attentional strategy being used in the attentional battle over mammography. Focusing on *attentional weighing*, chapter 4 explores how both interventionists and skeptics define relevance, risk, and expertise in mammography, and use these value weightings to discredit the other. Chapter 5 considers disputes over mammography as a *temporal conflict*, highlighting the centrality of temporal themes and strategies in the attentional battle over mammography, illustrating how temporal norms are fundamentally attentional norms and, further, how both skeptics and interventionists use temporal narratives to frame the other as temporally deviant. The book concludes with a reflection on why it is valuable to apply the sociology of attention to the data-driven realm of population science and medical guidelines. Social actors do not simply perceive scientific data; they attend and inattend data through frameworks of meaning that function to narrow the information they are able to perceive. I argue that the sociology of attention as a perspective is uniquely positioned to overcome such mental constriction by promoting mental flexibility through symmetrically drawing awareness to attentional alternatives and "diffractively" juxtaposing them to explicitly consider their exclusions. Cultivating cognitive flexibility through comparative analysis of attention types is equally beneficial for understanding cultural and political conflicts beyond mammography, and even beyond medicine.

Chapter 1

Skepticism and Interventionism as Attentional Types

Disputes over mammography are constructed around contrasting patterns of underlying meaning and belief about breast cancer, early detection, and screening. This chapter draws from the field of cognitive sociology, specifically theories and concepts relating to the sociology of attention, to recast these contrasting perspectives as *attentional types*. After introducing this theoretical framework, I use original data culled from twenty-nine interviews with doctors and scientists to empirically illustrate two ideal-typical patterns of attention, *interventionism* and *skepticism*, that overwhelmingly define the mammography conflict. In addition to providing a broad overview of these two attentional types, I use the issue of early detection to provide a deeper examination of the contrasting attentional patterns that organize both the medical professional participants' narratives and broader cultural discourse on mammography.

Thinking and Perceiving as Sociocultural Processes

The sociology of attention is embedded in the broader field of cognitive sociology, which seeks to illuminate the ways that thinking and sensory perception are both social phenomena, bearing the mark of our memberships in different cultures and subcultures. Cognitive sociologists have demonstrated this point by analyzing variations and patterns in thought and linking them to social norms. From a sociological perspective, although our thoughts often feel very private and idiosyncratic, they are similar in key respects to those of the people who surround us. Yet we should not conclude based on this commonality that thinking is a human universal deriving from biology. Rather, in addition to being on some level a biological process, and at times reflecting our individual idiosyncrasies, thinking is fundamentally culturally patterned (Brekhus 2015; Cerulo 2002; DiMaggio 1997; Zerubavel 1991, 1997). This is the essential point of both Tamotsu Shibutani's (1955) concept of *reference groups* and Thomas Kuhn's (1962) *scientific paradigms*. Basic cognitive processes such as *categorization* (Zerubavel 1991), *backgrounding* (Zerubavel 2015), and *metaphorical thinking* (Lakoff and Johnson 1980) can all vary across cultures and subcultures. The *cultural patterning of thought* has also been illustrated through examinations of variations in groups' reckonings of time and history (Fine 2012; Zerubavel 2003), genealogy (Zerubavel 2011), purity and pollution (Douglas 1966), and safety and danger (Simpson 1996). Others have exemplified *cultural cognitive patterns* using concepts of sexuality and sexual identity (Brekhus 2003; Davis 1983), race (Banaji and Greenwald 2013; Brekhus et al. 2010; Feagin 2010; Friedman 2016; Omi and Winant 1986; Schwalbe et al. 2000), and sex and gender (Friedman 2013; Kessler and McKenna 1978; Ridgeway and Correll 2004).

Attentional Groups

Recognizing *attention* as a process is essential for understanding such variations in cognition, as well as cognition and perception as sociocultural processes in general. Attention can be defined as the selection of certain features or details among those technically available to us. This includes both perceptual attention and processes of selection in cognition. This is in contrast to a passive view of perception as "something that happens to us, or in us" (Noe 2004, 1). Rather, for perception to be experienced, to have representational content, requires that we select and organize the features of the world that are relevant to us. This process of attentional selection is what "brings a stimulus to consciousness. It is, in other words, the process that permits us to notice something" (Mack and Rock 1998, 25–26). The sociology of attention analytically centers cross-contextual differences in patterns of relevance and awareness (Zerubavel 2015, 49). Zerubavel's body of work as a whole provides an essential foundation for the development of the sociology of attention, but his contributions are perhaps most crystallized in his books *Hidden in Plain Sight* (2015), an examination of irrelevance and backgrounding, and *Taken for Granted* (2018), which focuses on the unmarked, the default, and the taken for granted. Social norms of attending and ignoring are also central to Brekhus's work on sexual identity (2003) and the sociology of the unmarked (1998) as well as my own analysis of the visual classification of bodies as male and female (Friedman 2013).

At the core of any sociological understanding of attention is some concept of an attentional collective, group, or subculture, all of which drive analytic focus to meso-level influences on our attention, that is, patterns of attention that, because they are neither unique to us as individuals nor universal to all human beings, are therefore connected to our cultures and social groups. Zerubavel (2015, 53) describes this focus as follows: "The most visible manifestation of the social underpinnings of human attention are attentional patterns that are shared by some individuals (and therefore evidently not entirely idiosyncratic), yet nevertheless not by others (and thus also far from universal).... Although the way we focus our attention often resembles the way some others do, it is at the same time also quite different from the way still others focus theirs." Given that the organization of our attention reflects the norms and conventions of our social groups, we can speak of attentional socialization into distinctly social *attentional norms and conventions* (Zerubavel 2015, 59–63). Through this socialization process, we learn not only what we should pay attention to but what we should ignore. Thus, our sense of what is "relevant" and "irrelevant" is a key part of attentional socialization. As Zerubavel (2015, 63) describes, "separating the relevant from the irrelevant is a sociomental act performed by members of particular attentional communities who *learn* to focus their attention on certain parts of their phenomenal world while systematically inattending or even disattending others in accordance with their community's distinctive attentional traditions, conventions, biases, and habits. As members of such communities, we thus essentially learn what to notice and what to ignore as part of our *attentional socialization*." Such collective notions of relevance largely underlie the patterns of attention and inattention that we share with the members of our attentional groups.

The related concept of an *attentional type* conceptually distills these collective norms of attention into ideal-typical patterns for analytic purposes. Drawing on the Weberian tradition of *ideal types* (Weber 1949) and Simmel's concepts of *social types* and *social forms* (Simmel 1908), attentional types extract the features most salient to illustrating attentional variations or disputes between different attentional collectives and highlight the way that attentional norms function as generic, transposable frameworks of interpretation at a supraindividual level. As broad attentional worldviews that adherents apply cross-contextually, attentional types emphasize attentional form or structure over the content of what is perceived. For example, Murray Davis (1983) contrasts the attentional types of "Jehovanism" and "Naturalism" to illustrate that one's experience of sex depends largely on one's attention filter (or, in Davis's words, "worldview, paradigm, belief system, ideology or ethos" [166]). Each sexual attentional type filters the world through a different "cognitive-normative grid" (165–172), causing different body parts and behaviors to be marked as highly relevant and attended to and others to recede into the irrelevant. Similarly, as

Ruth Simpson (1996) demonstrates, perceptions of safety and danger largely depend on whether one filters the world through a cautious, confident, or neutral attentional type. Each results in an ideal-typical pattern of attention that, like Davis's sexual filters, marks some information as relevant and thus meaningful to attend to, while leaving other information unmarked and thus ignored as relatively mundane. A cautious framework involves heightened attention to items that are marked safe (assuming, by default, all else to be dangerous). Alternatively, a confident framework involves heightened attention to all that is marked dangerous (assuming all else to be safe by default). Analyzing such formal, cross-contextual patterns of attention further allows for a distinction between the attentional type (e.g., skepti*cism* and intervention*ism* as generic attentional forms that can be applied across many contexts) and actual individual adherents of a particular attentional worldview (e.g., skept*ics* and traditional*ists*), who will likely embody some but not all of the ideal type's defining features.

Attentional Filters in Science and Medicine

Professions are excellent examples of attentional groups, as "attentional patterns . . . often vary from one profession to another" (Zerubavel 2015, 66) and professional socialization frequently involves attentional socialization through which "members come to acquire its [their profession's] distinctive attentional habits" (67). That professions have distinct attentional norms, traditions, and habits that shape what members are able to notice is precisely the insight of such concepts as scientific "thought collectives" (Fleck 1979) and "paradigms of thought" (Kuhn 1962). As Zerubavel (1997, 48) describes,

> The considerable extent to which thought communities' specific cognitive "biases" affect what their members come to notice is quite evident in science. After all, only after having been "optically" socialized in a particular way do physicists, for example, come to notice certain objects, structures, and patterns which only other physicists can "see." . . . The facts observed by scientists are not available to just anyone who happens to look at the world. Rather, they are a product of the particular way in which observers' attention is directed as a result of specific cognitive "intentions" they acquire during their professional "optical" socialization.

Within medicine, different subspecialties have different thought styles (Arksey 1994; Bosk 1979). For example, part of medical education for clinicians is the refinement of "clinical judgment," which is distinct from strictly scientific reasoning as it is classically conceived in that it must adjust "scientific abstractions to the individual case" (Hunter 1991, xvii). As a result, clinicians have different attentional norms from research scientists, for example. As Hunter describes, clinical judgment is rarely based only on "the hard scientific facts"; it must also consider how to best apply scientific knowledge to the specific circumstances of the individual patient. This requires "sensing when to act and when to subject received knowledge to skeptical scrutiny. On those occasions when clinicians are in full possession of the necessary information, the hard scientific facts, they still must allow for their own subjectivity, the fallibility of the tests' technology, and the uncontrolled, uncontrollable variable that is the patient" (40).

In terms of conventions of attention and relevance, Hunter further observes that in the clinical encounter, the "expected" is treated as "irrelevant"; anticipated or "normal" data, symptoms, and reactions are neither recorded nor noted. Only anomalies, surprises, and variants are attended to as "noteworthy occurrences" (Hunter 1991, 69). In addition, what the clinician considers relevant is largely determined by preestablished ideas about which aspects of patients' reported symptoms fit with the available diagnostic possibilities (Berg 1992, 157–158). Attentional socialization also varies across the spectrum of clinical specialties. Consider, for example, the training involved in radiologists learning to interpret an MRI (or a mammogram) (see Alac 2008; Dumit 2004; Joyce 2008; Prasad 2005) compared with the attentional and visual socialization of an ear, nose, and throat specialist or that of a dermatologist. Similarly, one might expect that the clinical generalist's (e.g., family medicine or general practitioner) concern with a broad spectrum of diseases as well as with community health promotion would result in attentional norms that differ significantly from the more narrowly specialized attention filters used by anesthesiologists or podiatrists.

Attentional variation in the medical encounter extends beyond professional socialization processes across medical specialties to differences in what is relevant to the patient—and therefore a focus of their attention—and what is relevant to the physician. For example, Silverman et al. (2001) describe the ways that patients' "mental models" of cancer differ from those of physicians. Timmermans and Berg (2003, 71) likewise describe the very different perspectives patients and providers bring to research protocols for treating life-threatening illnesses; in this case, Hodgkin's disease:

Patients bring their own goals and hopes to the research protocol. . . . They rarely care about the research goals of the protocol (although sometimes they do); all they care about is preserving life and having a possible future. Drawing on the protocol in this way, patients will often negotiate their eligibility for a protocol, try to adjust the times of the chemotherapy courses for their convenience, or skip courses when they no longer see a meaningful link between their own future and the protocol's trajectory. . . . In their turn, many health-care workers evaluate . . . research protocols in light of their own personal research interests.

Hunter (1991, 127) similarly describes aspects of the patient's illness experience that are "irrelevant" from the perspective of the provider: "For most physicians . . . the details of the patient's story that are not perceived as medically problematic are not medically narratable. This irrelevance includes much of the subjective experience of illness: suffering, uncertainty, helplessness, fear of death, anxiety over loss of control. These are matters about which medicine in general and physicians in particular customarily have little to say." The subjective experience of illness, however, is of course centrally relevant to the patient, and this gap between patients' and doctors' frameworks of relevance can be a source of dissatisfaction or discomfort, particularly if patients feel that their perspective is being ignored or invalidated when it is incommensurable with clinical definitions and norms of relevance (131).

From this perspective, we can think of patients and physicians as different attentional groups, with different frameworks of relevance, "constructed from different points of view with different motives and themes" (Hunter 1991, 14). This dissonance between patients' and physicians' frameworks of attention has been identified as essential to address for improving patient care and doctor-patient interaction but is rarely directly acknowledged or studied (14). When we ignore the gap between patients' and providers' narratives or dismiss it as simply a question of patients' incorrect understanding, however, we "contribute to the widespread dissatisfaction with contemporary medicine" (Hunter 1991, 123) and miss an opportunity to engage patients' lived experience and thus more effectively shape their understanding (Hesse-Biber 2014, 118). This dissatisfaction is evident in the case of patients' understanding of breast cancer and mammography, as I will discuss in chapter 2. Here the point is that the sociology of attention provides a perspective and a set of concepts to engage these differences in attention productively, rather than judgmentally. The more typical approach, which uses a "deficit model" to understand how and why patients' understandings differ from those of providers, is aimed at better informing patients for the purpose of attentionally aligning them more closely with the experts. A cognitive sociological approach, on the other hand, links cognitive processing to social group membership and symmetrically analyzes differences in patterns of meaning and categorization (Ward and Peretti-Watel 2020). In this case, the goal is to identify and explore the structure of both lay and expert understanding rather than to align them behind the one that is predetermined to be "correct."

Occupational attention norms, like all attentional conventions, always include some aspect of inattention, as exemplified by physicians' inattention to the expected and to features of the illness experience central to their patients' attention. Such norms of inattention are equally if not more sociologically important to examine than what is positively selected for attention. This is in part because of our *attentional asymmetry*—that is, the fact that what we do *not* attend is proportionately much greater than what we *do* attend and therefore essential to understanding the meanings we ultimately generate. Such attentional exclusions are also what make all perceptions partial; they are what cannot be perceived or recognized from within any given framework of thought. As such, they are the key to a fuller understanding through increasing *attentional flexibility*—awareness of epistemological and ontological alternatives to what was previously taken for granted—as well as *accountability* for the particular exclusions of one's own attentional filters.

The Sociology of Inattention

One key benefit of the sociology of attention as a theoretical framework is that it intentionally facilitates symmetrical analysis of both attention and inattention. As a process of selection, attention always implies reciprocal forms of inattention that are equally socially normative—and equally important in the process of reality construction—yet are less recognized, whether in everyday life or sociological analysis. Goffman (1961, 20) refers to these as social "rules of irrelevance" that designate those aspects of any situation socially defined as irrelevant, and which therefore must be ignored. This social expectation that we adhere to collective norms of inattention is just as influential in "defining the situation" as our selective attention to what is deemed relevant and actively attended.

Further, as I alluded to already, human attention is actually asymmetrical in that the number of details we actively and clearly attend is far smaller than the number of details we do not perceive. As Schutz (1970, 74) put it, "there is a relatively small kernel of knowledge that is clear, distinct, and consistent in itself. This kernel is surrounded by zones of various gradations of vagueness, obscurity, and ambiguity." The conceptual distinction between "figure" and "background" conveys the fundamentally asymmetrical nature of our attention; that is, we are typically aware of only a small number of well-defined features of our perceptual field (the "figure"), while most of the technically available sensory information is in the "background" and therefore indistinct and unnoticed—yet it is not for this reason any less influential in shaping the meanings we apply (Schutz 1970, 72–73). This attentional asymmetry is also reflected in the concept of "unmarkedness." In his call for sociologists to analytically foreground the unmarked, Brekhus (1998, 35) defines "social markedness" as "the ways social actors actively perceive one side of a contrast while ignoring the other side as epistemologically unproblematic." In other words, we "observe the world in an uneven fashion, cognitively attending to socially marked features, while virtually ignoring and taking for granted unmarked features" (Brekhus 2015, 25). Using the figure/ground distinction, and again invoking the asymmetry between the attended and the inattended, Brekhus (1998, 35) further points out that "*most* of our social landscape blends into the unmarked background." Thus, studying inattention is sociologically essential, not only because it is constitutive of any thought or perception, arguably with more influence over our perception and cognition than attention, but also because we tend not to be consciously aware of it. Yet, if we can access and engage patterns of inattention with intellectual generosity across differences of perspective, such exclusions create a deep form of accountability for the limits of our own perspective and thus forestall determinism (Barad 2007, 205, 214). This results in greater *attentional flexibility*, or the ability to recognize the different, even contradictory, perceptions that are simultaneously possible.

Despite its sociological importance, analytically recognizing and capturing the inattended poses a challenge. As Zerubavel (2018, 14) has put it, "unlike the marked, the unmarked is methodologically elusive, as absence is much more difficult to observe than presence." Considering this, lacking positive evidence for those things we do not perceive is the first obstacle to studying the inattended (2015, 7), and any effective analytic strategy must therefore focus on providing access to this information. Despite these challenges, it is possible to cultivate a mindset of "observing the absences" (2018, 14). Both Garfinkel (1967) and Schutz (1970), for example, argued that recognizing background expectancies and the taken for granted requires adopting a specific mental perspective. For Garfinkel, this is the mindset of a "stranger to the 'life as usual' character of everyday scenes" (37). Schutz similarly discusses a "special motive" required to make the taken for granted into the problematic, one that questions received notions of relevance (116). Schutz further argues that only a "shock" can lead us to abandon the cognitive style of the paramount reality (254), and it was precisely the point of Garfinkel's breaching experiments to generate this kind of mental shock.

Zerubavel (1991, 115–122) identifies a number of additional mental stances helpful for recognizing the backgrounded, the unmarked, and the inattended. He argues for instance that both "fuzzy"- and "flexible"-minded perspectives can help us to "unlump" and "unsplit" culturally taken-for-granted categories, which requires recognizing normally unnoticed cross-category similarities and within-category differences. In other work, he suggests that "multifocal attention," "open awareness," and "mindfulness" can cultivate awareness of absences (Zerubavel 2015, 75–79). Taking a slightly different emphasis, Brekhus (1998, 47) suggests adopting an "analytically nomadic" perspective so that "in place of observing issues from a single fixed cultural viewpoint we can observe them from multiple perspectives, combining elements from each." Note that one key reason all of these proposed mental stances help reveal cultural nodes of inattention is that they explicitly define attention and relevance as social and selective rather than logical or natural.

Another key analytic strategy for studying the inattended is *reversing* or *inverting* the normative structure of attention. Other terms for the strategy of reversing include "foregrounding," "marking the unmarked" (Zerubavel 2018, 87–123), "figure-ground reversal" (Zerubavel 2015), and "reverse marking" (Brekhus 1998, 43). The analytic power of reversing is to expand the boundaries of perception by effectively shifting our attention from the marked to the unmarked. Reversing in this manner challenges conventions of attention by bringing focus to the normally backgrounded, unmarked—and thus unseen—information. In expanding our attention to the unmarked, reversing also performs "semiotic subversion," eliminating "the semiotic asymmetry between the marked and the unmarked" (Zerubavel 2018, 87).

In prior work I have proposed using the metaphor of a *perceptual filter* as an orienting guide to analytically track both attention and inattention (DeGloma and Friedman 2005; Friedman 2013). The term "filter" invokes a mental "strainer" or "sieve" through which stimuli pass before they are consciously perceived, letting in culturally meaningful details while sifting out the culturally irrelevant. Thinking in terms of filters thus specifically directs us to examine the question of which features or details pass through and are attended and, arguably more significantly given the importance yet elusiveness of what we do not attend, those that are blocked by the filter and thus remain unnoticed. Comparative analysis of different filters thus emerges as a very effective means by which to bring such attentional exclusions to the fore. In light of this,

I will spend the remainder of this chapter conceptualizing disputes over mammography as a conflict between attentional filters. As part of this discussion, I empirically introduce the two primary attentional types in the disagreement, interventionism and skepticism, focusing symmetrically on their patterns of attention and inattention.

First, however, a brief note on the *skeptic* and *interventionist* terminology I use throughout the book. These terms are similar to others used in prior research on mammography: Reynolds (2012, 1) refers to the opposing sides in the mammography conflict as "skeptics" and "true believers," and Aronowitz (2007, 245) uses the terms "skeptics" and "boosters," for example. Some of the names my interview participants used to describe the two sides are "true believers," "screening proponents," "the screening establishment," "screening zealots," as well as "skeptics," "detractors," and "anti-screening researchers." At times these terms are used as self-identification. For example, one participant, Dr. Franklin,[1] a primary care physician and academic researcher, describes the typical skeptic as follows: "The detractors or skeptics, you know, these are people such as myself who are in general a little bit skeptical about the value of medical care in people who are well. You know, we see the strong thing and the good things that medical care can do for the acutely ill and injured. Uh, but worry about the spreading of medical care into well populations with its mixtures of effect—and its very misleading feedback. I mean, we tend to be sort of schooled in epidemiology, thinking about populations and thinking about measurements of outcomes."

At other times, such labels are applied judgmentally. Dr. Cashman, a radiologist, refers to these same skeptics as holding views that are consistently "against all screening for any disease," for example, and Dr. Adams, also a radiologist, similarly describes them as an "anti-screening group," who try to "reduce access to screening." Judgmental labels are also applied in the other direction, as when Dr. France, a surgeon and specialist in breast cancer and breast cancer screening, refers to those who favor earlier and more frequent mammography as "screening zealots": "I think people who are screening zealots cannot, simply cannot, come to terms with the fact that catching it early isn't a good thing." Later, he adds, "they simply cannot see—think outside the box." Many of these descriptions are clearly rhetorically charged, reflecting the emotional and dichotomized nature of the conflict. In order to capture the terminology used in prior research—as well as by the interview participants themselves—but also remain as neutral as possible in my analysis, I refer to the two camps as "interventionists" and "skeptics." Below I summarize the disciplines, professional roles, and other demographic characteristics of the participants in each group, then I outline the basic patterns of focus defining these two attentional types. I also begin to suggest ways that each perspective's patterns of inattention and exclusion can be revealed by contrasting their different relevance structures.

Skepticism and Interventionism as Attentional Types

In very broad strokes, interventionists are critical of the USPSTF recommendation to delay mammograms until age fifty and to reduce the frequency of screening from once a year to once every two years. They firmly believe in early detection and minimize any possible harms of screening. Skeptics, on the other hand, are basically supportive of the USPSTF recommendation, are less persuaded of mammography screening's overall effectiveness, and are more concerned about the risks of screening. There is significant resonance between these two attention types and the "traditionalist" and "evidence-based" models of thinking described by Timmermans and Berg (2003, 87–88), particularly with respect to their different evaluations of evidence and concepts of expertise and authority. They characterize the traditional model as prioritizing individual-level clinical and diagnostic experiences over population-based guidelines, whereas the evidence-based model subordinates such clinical experiences to what has been demonstrated in systematic, generalizable empirical studies.

Like the traditionalist model, the interventionist attention type places considerable value on clinical experience while also selectively emphasizing empirical studies when they bolster arguments for early detection and screening. Also in keeping with the individualist clinical orientation of the traditionalist model of thought, interventionists are primarily concerned with not missing any individual woman who could benefit from mammography, which leads them to support being as expansive as possible with screening guidelines, on the basis that population evidence-based standards "over-regulate" (Timmermans and Berg 2003, 20). They couple this expansion of the pool of patients who should be screened with an attentional narrowing of the definition of screening's harms (e.g., by excluding "theoretical" harms such as overdiagnosis or "insignificant" harms such as anxiety).

The skeptic attention type, in contrast, reflects the evidence-based model in that they tend to be mistrustful and dismissive of individual-level information or experience, accepting only population-based evidence as valid. Timmermans and Berg (2003, 215) evoke both a key attentional exclusion of the skeptic attention type and the associated emotional dynamics when they describe evidence-based medicine as an "overall *attitude*, scorning experience-based knowledge and demanding hard (meaning: randomized, clinical trial-based) evidence." Skeptics are concerned with the negative byproducts of broadening the population for screening, namely more overdiagnosis and overtreatment, and thus advocate contracting screening guidelines to include only those women most likely to benefit. At the same time, skeptics attentionally expand the definition of screening's harms beyond direct physical harms by including emotional impacts and harms based on population-based estimates (of overdiagnosis, for example). As critics of evidence-based approaches point out, however, in excluding from consideration the unique circumstances of individual patients, skeptics fail to acknowledge that there is no such thing as an average patient in reality. As Timmermans and Berg describe, there are only specific patients, and there is an "inevitable gap between clean, universal research, and a messy, localized clinical practice" (142).

Interventionism and skepticism are clearly attentional ideal types, and as with all ideal types, there is more nuance and complexity present in individual cases. As Weber (1949, 101–102) described them, as opposed to descriptive types, ideal types conceptually isolate the elements that the analyst identifies as of particular importance in relation to their question. Their value is not in their comprehensiveness, then, but in how well they help explain a concrete problem or empirical case. It is in this spirit that I construct and explore the contrast between interventionism and skepticism; it is my contention that these two categories capture the most salient elements of medical and cultural disagreement over mammography, providing deeper insight into the attentional organization of the conflict.

Only three of the doctors and scientists I interviewed were difficult to categorize using this typology; the remaining twenty-six were relatively easy to label as fundamentally "skeptics" ($N = 16$) or "interventionists" ($N = 10$). It may initially appear contradictory that I have more skeptical than interventionist participants in light of my claim that early detection remains a widely accepted cultural norm. However, my sense is that more skeptics were drawn to the study precisely because they view themselves as attentional deviants. This motivated them to participate in the interviews as an opportunity to generate more cultural recognition of the harms of early detection. In terms of discipline and professional role, the skeptics in the sample include more people trained in epidemiology or public health ($N = 8$ vs. 0) and more academic researchers ($N = 9$ vs. 0), whereas the interventionist group is primarily made up of clinicians (nine of ten total participants classified as interventionists). The three participants who are not easily categorizable using this typology because their views include elements of each can be exemplified by Dr. Brown, a breast surgeon, who describes the data on routine screening between forty and fifty as a "grey zone" and admits that "the biology of cancer is unclear" but still supports annual screening beginning at age forty because it is "best to be cautious." (See table 1.1

Table 1.1
Characteristics of skeptics and interventionists

	Skeptics ($N = 16$)	Interventionists ($N = 10$)
Discipline	8 Internal medicine/family medicine 8 Public health/epidemiology 1 Radiology 1 Oncology 3 Surgery	4 Internal medicine/family medicine 3 Radiology 1 Ob/Gyn 1 Oncology 1 Surgery
Professional role	8 Clinician and/or medical school faculty 9 Academic researcher 2 Leader of government or medical organization	9 Clinician and/or medical school faculty 1 Leader of government or medical organization

Note: Total counts for discipline and role do not match the number (N) of respondents because several respondents were trained in more than one discipline or work in more than one professional role. In addition, although twenty-nine participants were interviewed, the three who could not be categorized as either "interventionists" or "skeptics" are not included here.

for sample characteristics. More details on the recruitment and interview process are available in the appendix.) To empirically introduce the attentional patterns of skeptics and interventionists, I profile a few representative examples from each group, beginning with the skeptics.

Three Skeptics: Doctors Franklin, France, and Jackson

Dr. Franklin is a primary care physician and academic. He describes himself as generally "a little bit skeptical about the value of medical care in people who are well," which he ties to his discipline. As a general practitioner, he says, he is no more concerned about breast cancer than other forms of cancer, chronic diseases, health promotion, and the healthcare system as a whole. He uses the terms "proponents" and "true believers" contrasted with "detractors" or "skeptics" to describe the two sides of the conflict, and he emphasizes that breast screening was originally undertaken with "the absolute best of intentions": to bring attention to the disease and—on the assumed logic of early detection—to bring women in earlier for screening to improve their chances of survival. However, he now feels strongly that the early detection paradigm and the associated idea that we should be trying to find as many cancers as possible, as early as possible, has led to overdiagnosis and harm. As I described in the introduction, overdiagnosis, also known as a Type 2 error (Scheff 1963, 99), refers to the idea that there are tumors found through screening that may not cause harm during the person's lifetime. They may remain stable or, some claim, may at times even reduce in size. Or they may just be so slow growing that they will not cause symptoms before the person dies of another cause. Overdiagnosis is arguably a direct consequence of our efforts at early diagnosis, as we are increasingly looking for abnormalities in people without symptoms. As Dr. Franklin explains, "We're trying to find as many cancers as possible. And that's a recipe for a lot of false alarms and a lot of overdiagnosis." He also emphasizes that we have created a cultural "climate of fear" as part of the promotion of screening, adding that he finds it "egregious that we have a population-based screening program that roughly alarms half of women over a 10-year period of annual screening.... I mean we have made a breast cancer scare almost a rite of passage for middle-aged American women."

Dr. France is a surgeon with expertise in breast cancer and screening who has published papers on the harms of screening. Like Dr. Franklin, he uses the term "skeptical" to describe his current views: "As more and more data has appeared, I have become more and more skeptical about the value of screening." Referring derisively to the other side of the conflict as "the screening establishment" and "screening zealots," he emphasizes that it is essential to consider which side of the debate has the greater conflict of interest. "Being a skeptic does me no favors," he says. "It has been against my best interest to take this position. So there is no conflict of interest on my side. I am just a clinical scientist who goes where the data leads." When describing "screening zealots," in contrast, he argues that they do have conflicts of interest, both financial and in terms of reputation. Financially, they are "earning their living from screening." They are also seeking to protect their self-image and professional reputation: "There are those whose career was built on screening and they don't want to lose face, which is another conflict of interest." Highlighting the cognitive dimension of the conflict, and specifically pointing out norms of inattention, he further argues that the "screening zealots" suffer from what he calls a "conceptual problem, a paradigmatic problem," which is that they are "locked into a conceptual model of the disease" that is incorrect because it is linear. As a result, "they simply can't see beyond that conceptual model of the disease that you've got to catch it early." Those on the skeptical side, he says, are trying to understand why screening is not successful. "To me the most interesting thing about screening is that it fails, because the reason it fails is that the conceptual model is wrong, and breast cancer does not obey the simple rules of the linear dynamic."

Dr. Jackson is an epidemiologist and family medicine doctor in a community practice. He supports the USPSTF guideline change and refers to it as the "national evidence-based guideline," which he contrasts with the "consensus-based guidelines" of organizations favoring earlier screening guidelines. He also feels that, although the change caused quite an uproar, it was actually very benign—about as uncontroversial as one could expect in the face of complex evidence. He describes the USPSTF's position as essentially this: "the evidence is ambiguous, and uncertainty is even more pronounced for women in their 40s, so we think they need to consult their doctor on an individual basis." "Mammogram advocates," he claims, twisted the revised guidelines into something like "don't screen." He contrasts the USPSTF's "pretty benign recommendation . . . to . . . talk to your doctor" with the recommendation of "reflexive routine screening" promoted by other organizations, which he believes is equivalent to screening without deliberation or discussion. Dr. Jackson also strongly emphasizes the point that breast cancer screening is extremely well studied, so it is not the case that there is not enough research. Rather, the problem is that the data are being weighed selectively. The USPSTF, in his view, has "no bias coming in whatsoever. They are not an interested party. They do not benefit from doing mammograms; they do not benefit from not doing mammograms. They just completely look at the evidence and say, you know, 'Where is the weight of the evidence?'" On the other side are "the radiology groups who obviously benefit from more mammograms, the surgical groups that benefit from more women getting diagnosed because they do more surgery, and the oncology groups who obviously benefit because, you know, more women get diagnosed and they do more treatment." He finds it problematic that he sees little popular skepticism of the clear conflicts of interest of these groups. In addition to their conflicts of interest, such groups are often insulated from criticism because of their claims to "expertise." He finds these claims of expertise limited, however, because they are based on clinical experience rather than population data, which is what he feels is really needed to assess the studies and data. Although Dr. Jackson is a clinician, he also has a graduate degree in public health, and in his experience his clinical training was of no use in understanding population health. "That's why I think the American College of Radiology or whatever should really get out of the business of making guidelines because they don't have any expertise and they have a conflict of interest."

Three Interventionists: Doctors Adams, Jones, and Kramer

Dr. Adams is a radiologist whom many consider a national expert and key spokesperson for the pro-screening perspective. The words he chooses to refer to his role in the landscape of the mammography debates imply an awareness of this vaunted status: "I am one of the champions supporting screening." When describing the current guidelines, he emphasizes that more expert organizations support retaining the prior guideline than support the USPSTF revision and further adds that these groups all use "science-based" guidelines (implying that the USPSTF guidelines are "unscientific"): "Most groups that have science-based guidelines, such as the American Cancer Society, advise women to have a mammogram every year beginning at the age of 40."[2] He also heavily stresses the point that breast cancer *experts* oppose the USPSTF change: "None of the *major cancer organizations* and *experts who actually care for women with breast cancer* support the USPSTF" (emphasis added). These "experts," he says, know that early detection is paramount; none oppose screening from age forty to fifty. On the other hand, "The opposition to screening is coming, primarily, from doctors who do not actually care for women with breast cancer. They either do not practice medicine or are primary care doctors who see very few cases of breast cancer." He at one point refers to this group as "those whose goal is to reduce or eliminate access to screening." Continuing to emphasize the importance of direct clinical expertise, he states that in their efforts to eliminate all conflicts of interest in composing the panel, the USPSTF also eliminated all expertise. "This has become a major problem, because if you have no COI [conflict of interest], you likely have no expertise on the topic." Reflecting on the harms of screening, for Dr. Adams it comes down to mental weighing. He feels that "opponents of screening" have "exaggerated the negative aspects of screening." He characterizes the harms of screening as minimal—the "anxiety and inconvenience of being recalled," which "most women and supporters of screening" agree are "certainly not equivalent to dying from breast cancer." Despite this, "screening opponents" have managed to get papers published in academic journals that he feels should never have passed peer review. At the same time, he claims, refutations of these papers have been "prevented from being published," leading to a bias in the available research, and a situation where "women and physicians are confused," "the public is unaware they are being misled," and "misinformation is taken as fact."

Dr. Jones, also a radiologist as well as a director of breast imaging at a health network, similarly stresses that proportionately more organizations support earlier and more frequent screening, including "the American College of Radiology, the American Cancer Society, American College of Surgeons, Society of Breast Imaging, and on and on I could go." Like Dr. Adams, she points to the importance of specific expertise in breast cancer diagnosis and treatment, saying that these organizations align with her "professional opinion," "what [she's] been practicing for 20 years," and what "those of us in breast imaging know." This expert knowledge, she explains, was not represented on the USPSTF, which "did not have anybody who specialized in breast cancer detection or treatment" and "created a lot of confusion." She further believes there were cost-cutting motives behind the Task Force's "attacks on mammography." In addition, even beyond the USPSTF, her feeling is that mammography is unfairly singled out as a medical test: "There is no other screening test that has been scrutinized as much as mammography... It's sad to me that this continues to be a debate. I don't think we see any other medical test that is consistently in the news and attacked the way mammography is." Yet critical perspectives continue to "get a lot of media attention." This is, in part, she argues, because mammography skeptics are trying to advance their careers—"trying to advance themselves, advance their CVs"—by publishing new and exciting, but controversial, findings. She summarizes the conflicts of interest of skeptics as follows: "I think it's ego driven, I think it's financially driven, and I think it's academically driven."

Dr. Kramer, a family medicine doctor and director of a cancer center, echoes the other interventionists' characterization of the USPSTF as standing basically alone in its recommendation, with many more organizations supporting more frequent screening: "The U.S. Preventive Services Task Force is to my knowledge the only one that really has differing recommendations. Everyone else recommends—and that's the American Cancer Society, and National Comprehensive Cancer Network... all recommend annual mammograms beginning at age 40." She argues that this is a question of values and emphasis, or how each side mentally "weighs" things differently; the Task Force is focused on the harms, while all others are focused on the benefits. She says the harms are "a feather" on one side of a scale in her view, weighed against a one-hundred-pound brick of benefits. The USPSTF, in contrast, is weighing the harms much more heavily. From her perspective, getting a false-positive mammogram is "not a pleasant consequence, but I think it's more reasonable than having women die." She attributes this difference in value weightings to her experience as a clinician: "I see the devastation." "That's why I think a lot of clinicians have a different value weighting" than people who are "just looking at the numbers" and taking the values deriving from clinical experience out of their recommendations.

Early Detection as an Attentional Filter

As can be seen already in these six case profiles, in addition to the appropriate starting point and interval for mammography, interventionists and skeptics have very different perspectives on a number of arguably more significant related ideas, including the importance of early detection, the possible harms of screening, and the most relevant sources of medical authority. In this manner, their different views on the proper guideline for mammography are connected with a constellation of other ideas and beliefs, some of which are highlighted in figure 1.1.

Most of these beliefs will be treated in greater depth in later chapters. At this point, I am mainly concerned with providing an initial introduction to the formal patterns of each attentional type and demonstrating some of the benefits of analyzing the mammography conflict in terms of attention. I therefore proceed, at least initially, by focusing on just one element of skeptic and interventionist beliefs: early detection. While only one piece of the conflict's attentional puzzle, early detection is centrally important to the patterns of focus defining each side. As discussed in the introduction, early detection is a hegemonic, deeply ingrained cultural belief, and interventionism is essentially an attentional manifestation of that belief. On the other hand, skepticism as a system of attention is oriented by challenging the taken-for-grantedness of early detection. Thus, early detection is not just a hegemonic cultural belief but a *foundational filter* (DeGloma and Friedman 2005) and *attentional anchor* (connecting attention to mental weight or the application of significance) for both interventionism and skepticism.

This highlights an additional contribution of attention as an analytic focus, which is that it can reveal the *attentional relationships* among different aspects of a narrative. For example, one can identify beliefs and concepts that are particularly foundational or structuring, functioning as *attentional weights* or *anchors* that dictate how one attends or frames other ideas. My analysis suggests that early detection functions in this case to organize the attentional filters that shape interventionists' and skeptics' overall patterns of attention. This also resonates with Aronowitz's (2021, 42) observation about the foundational role of early detection in organizing similar conflicts over prostate cancer screening: "Where one stands on this controversy seems to depend on what one believes about the natural history of prostate cancer—the disease's clinical course in the absence of intervention. How likely is untreated, screening-detected cancer to progress and do harm?"

The following pair of contrasting quotes from Dr. Cohen and Dr. Price illustrates how it is fundamentally two different perspectives on early detection that organize the mammography conflict. Dr. Cohen, a general internist and medical expert, feels "there is no way for us to escape what we intuitively believe and we know to be true, which is that if you find a cancer at stage 1, you can resect it and out it goes, and life goes on. I think that part that's been ingrained is true. But I think the part that we're having a difficulty trying to figure out is that the modality with which we screen, does it actually help us find it early enough?"

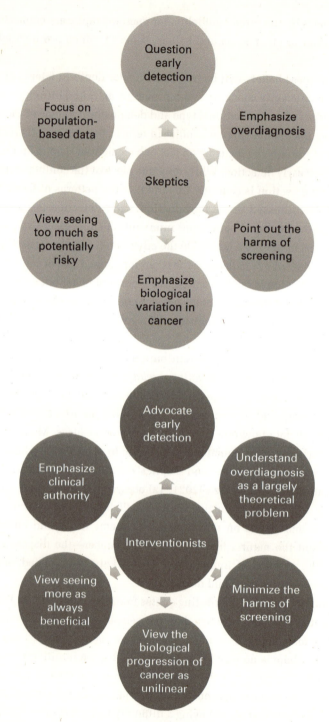

Figure 1.1. Skeptic and interventionist beliefs.

Dr. Cohen clearly takes for granted the importance of early detection—which he calls "what we intuitively believe and we know to be true"—and feels that, if anything, the medical profession should be seeking ways to find abnormalities even earlier. Compare this with the skeptical view of early detection of Dr. Price, a clinical oncologist and public health expert: "I think it's been oversimplified and the—the medical profession has in essence gotten across messages that are quite strong. One is that cancer is a death sentence unless you are detected early, and that's not true. . . . And that screening is, early detection is always beneficial. And again, we have learned that that's not true. So I think that in part, the reason why the recent evidence is so counterintuitive is that the messages have been so consistent and so strong in one direction and have been so simplified." One of the key claims made by skeptics such as Dr. Price is that a taken-for-granted belief in early detection has created patterns of irrelevance and inattention that make it difficult for interventionists to perceive and accept a number of ideas that skeptics consider critically important to attend and weigh.

Another skeptic, Dr. Light, a radiologist, explicitly uses the term "overbelief" to describe what he views as a limiting assumption that "early detection is essential." It is an *over*belief for him because it exceeds what is scientifically supported and produces *cognitive resistance* and *inattention*: "To some extent there is also a genuine overbelief, like overdiagnosis, an overbelief that any time you can detect cancer early, you have to be doing good. You just have to be. That's the principle of early detection, early diagnosis, early treatment, being able to give less treatment because you detected something early. That drives a lot of the emotion. There is a real belief in that principle. It has to be true. It just has to be! It's—it's an obvious, logical point. And it's very hard to overcome that belief."

Dr. France, the surgeon and specialist in breast cancer and breast cancer screening profiled earlier, similarly highlights the cognitive exclusions produced by what he calls the "mantra" of early detection:

> There is this mantra that one of the best ways of improving the cure for cancer is catch it early. And they can't seem to—there's a conceptual problem, a paradigmatic problem. They simply can't see beyond that conceptual model of the disease that you've got to catch it early. So you've got two types of academics: those who are locked in a conceptual model of the disease which is linear, and then there are those who can look at the evidence and start explaining the failure of screening.

Here Dr. Light and Dr. France both highlight what gets inattended—left out of one's understanding—when one reflexively applies the attentional logic of early detection. Dr. France identifies what for him is the most important oversight of early detection, which is that, as he puts it, "the conceptual model is wrong and breast cancer does not obey the simple rules of the linear dynamic." This idea arises most often during discussions of the concept of "overdiagnosis," which, as previously noted, signifies that some tumors found through mammography might never have progressed to cause harm if left unfound and untreated. From the skeptics' perspective, in excluding overdiagnosis, interventionism ignores a critical paradigm shift in thinking about cancer that is currently under way. Welch, Schwartz, and Woloshin (2011, 53) describe this changing concept of cancer as follows: "It used to be assumed that all cancers relentlessly progressed. If they weren't treated, they would invariably grow, metastasize, and ultimately lead to death. But we are learning that assumption is wrong." Thus, fundamentally, the idea of overdiagnosis is that there are "some cancers that don't matter" (Welch, Schwartz, and Woloshin 2011, 53) because they are "pseudodisease"—literally a "false disease" in that they will not make a person ill (Moynihan, Doust, and Henry 2012; Welch et al. 2011, 54).

In attention terms, these criticisms of both overbelief and overdiagnosis by skeptical participants can be understood as claims of *overattention*. In both cases, what skeptics object to is what they perceive as interventionists' excessive focus on and application of unwarranted significance to the detection of tumors as early as possible, regardless of their biological danger. In this same sense, *overattention* can be seen as the "error" in Type 2 errors more broadly, as what is false in a false positive is the attention given to something that is in fact benign or nonexistent. This criticism of overattention also implies an attentional bias and resulting asymmetry in which some things, in this case the danger of early tumors, are given too much attention, while others are not attended to adequately—in this case, overdiagnosis. In contrast, interventionists object to skeptics' *underattention* to the potential dangers of allowing tumors to progress and their corresponding overattention to overdiagnosis. If overattention is the basis for Type 2 errors, underattention is the attentional structure of a Type 1 error, or false negative, in which the error is in not giving adequate attention to something that turns out to be dangerous. Like Simpson's (1996) cautious attentional type, interventionists apply a default norm of danger to all tumors, understanding anything less as a form of risky underattention. Skeptics are more similar to Simpson's neutral mindset, in which risk is viewed as undeterminable without further information as to safety or danger.

Another way skeptics highlight interventionists' underattention to overdiagnosis is by framing it as "counterintuitive," or difficult to consider within the framework of a belief in early detection and associated assumptions about the unilinear, progressive nature of cancer. Dr. Price, who is a clinical oncologist, for example, refers to overdiagnosis as "very hard to communicate" and "counterintuitive even to most physicians."

> Overdiagnosis in my opinion is the rule rather than the exception in any screening test.... The problem is, number one, it's very hard to, uh, communicate the issue surrounding overdiagnosis since at the individual level no one knows whether they have been overdiagnosed or not.... And the other problem is it's so counterintuitive.... So we have grown up to learn or to think that all cancer is bad and a cancer is a cancer and all cancers progress. And so it's highly counterintuitive even to most physicians that there could be overdiagnosis.

In short, what Dr. Price is pointing out is that early detection as a framework of attention creates an inability to perceive (or underattention to) overdiagnosis. Overdiagnosis is "counterintuitive" (Rogers, Entwistle, and Carter 2019) and even "medical heresy" (Welch, Schwartz, and Woloshin 2011, 45), however, only in the light of the assumed benefits of early detection. Overdiagnosis "upends these assumptions as there are more harms than benefits from the diagnosis, often because the detected condition would not have progressed to advanced disease, thus there is no benefit to detection" (Rogers, Entwistle, and Carter 2019, 237–238). Stated another way, to accept overdiagnosis in effect requires cognitively shifting away from early detection as centrally "relevant" to addressing cancer. This is an example of analytically reversing the structure of attention to access the previously excluded, in that it demonstrates that when we attend to overdiagnosis, early detection must be defined as of no or limited relevance. For early detection to be defined as relevant, in turn, overdiagnosis must be defined as invalid or irrelevant and ignored. In fact, when interventionists discuss overdiagnosis, they often explicitly define it as only "academic" or "theoretical" and thus not important to attend (i.e., overattended), thereby defending the validity of early detection. They also make their own claims about the problematic exclusions of skeptics, most consistently pointing out that a belief in overdiagnosis leads skeptics to be inattentive to what they call the "real" harm of breast cancer, which is the possibility that a patient could die.

On the topic of overdiagnosis, interventionists' primary argument is that because we do not have the ability to apply overdiagnosis clinically to individual patients—since we do not yet know which specific tumors will grow quickly or slowly—it is "just theoretical" or "counterfactual" and ought not be given much relevance in cancer detection and treatment (again, in terms of attention, it is "overattended"). The following comments from Dr. Andrews, an ob-gyn and breast health specialist, serve as an illustration: "I feel like it's—the overdiagnosis thing right now I feel is somewhat academic.... We don't have the knowledge. We know that some DCIS [ductal carcinoma in situ][3] will progress. It doesn't all regress obviously. And so we don't know . . . And until we do, to me, it's slightly irrelevant."

This is sometimes described in the literature as the "epistemic challenge" of demonstrating some of the most significant harms of screening, particularly overdiagnosis. As a counterfactual, overdiagnosis can almost never be directly observed (a research scenario known as the "non-identifiability problem"). This is because people diagnosed with cancer generally receive treatment. "Once diagnosis and treatment occur, it is not possible to know what would have occurred 'without' diagnosis and treatment. Thus helpfully diagnosed individuals cannot be distinguished from overdiagnosed individuals, and overdiagnosis cannot be observed and counted" (Carter 2021, 33). We can only estimate this information at the level of population statistics (Carter 2021; Rogers 2019; Rogers, Entwistle, and Carter 2019; Welch 2011, 55). Given this counterfactuality and non-identifiability, interventionists argue, overdiagnosis is "just academic" or "theoretical"—not a "real harm" that actual women experience—and therefore "irrelevant."

Interventionists also reverse the focus of attention to argue that, rather than the harms of overdiagnosis, what is "relevant" to focus on is the risk of *under*diagnosis, which would be a Type 1 error, or a failure to detect a patient's illness (Scheff 1963, 99). To convey this, they often reframe discussions of the harms of screening using an emotionally powerful rhetorical substitution. The harm that interventionists argue is most relevant to them, and that they see skeptics as underattending, is the harm of dying from cancer. Dr. Kramer, a family medicine doctor, describes this as follows: "I do realize more women are going to be called back for what turns out to be a false positive. And that's not a pleasant experience, but seeing on the other side women who die from breast cancer, I think it's a more acceptable consequence than having more women die." Note that, rhetorically, such statements shift focus from the harms of *screening* to the harms of *breast cancer*. In doing so, they add to the fear and emotion of the debates in a manner that both minimizes the claims of skeptics as irrelevant and reinforces the logic of early detection.

In summary, I find that participants' differing beliefs about early detection organize the information they consider relevant and attend with respect to a series of "sub-beliefs." These include questions about overdiagnosis versus underdiagnosis, as we have seen. There is also a related disagreement over the relationship between improved therapies and the importance of early detection,

Table 1.2
Early detection filters: comparison of interventionism and skepticism

Interventionist view of early detection: *Early detection saves lives*	Skeptical view of early detection: *The cultural "overbelief" in early detection needs to be questioned*
The earlier the better.	Earlier is not always better.
In screening, seeing more is always better than seeing less.	Greater sensitivity in screening tests leads to overdiagnosis.
Overdiagnosis is merely theoretical.	Overdiagnosis is documented at the population level and is not debatable.
Treatment works, but only with early detection.	Improvement in treatment is responsible for mortality improvements in breast cancer, not screening.
Cancer is progressive.	Cancer is not always progressive.

which I discuss in greater depth as an illustration of attentional weighing in chapter 4. Finally, there are differing views on whether it is ever possible to see too much via a screening test, or if seeing more is always better. To capture the way a participant's position on early detection sets their pattern of attention and inattention for these other questions, I conceptualize early detection as a *foundational attentional filter*. The metaphor of a filter is based on blockages and holes, which here represent attention and inattention. Thus, a participant's position on early detection provides the shape of the filter and the number, arrangement, and size of the holes, organizing what details they select (and the details to which they are inattentive) with respect to other points of disagreement, and also what they perceive others as either over- or underattending. The result is a web of interlinked beliefs and perceptions created through attention that is logically coherent with respect to one's view of early detection. (See table 1.2 for a selection of these ideas interconnected via early detection.)

Critically, conceptualizing early detection as an attention filter allows us not only simply to trace the additional "positively" held beliefs associated with each perspective but also to identify what each inattends or treats as irrelevant. Analytically, this requires symmetrical analyses of both sides of the conflict as well as of both attention and inattention. The goal is to read the two attention patterns both generously, in the sense that the aim is not to prove or disprove either, and "diffractively," allowing their differences to create productive tensions (Barad 2007, 142).

In the example of early detection and overdiagnosis, I pointed out some key nodes of inattention of both sides of the debate. To briefly recap, a belief in early detection may limit interventionists' ability to acknowledge overdiagnosis and to think in new ways about breast cancer diagnosis and treatment beyond a relentless search for more and smaller cancers. At the same time, resistance to early detection can restrict skeptics' ability to fully acknowledge other important aspects of breast cancer diagnosis and treatment. The most notable example is the point made by interventionists that, even if documented at a population level, overdiagnosis cannot yet be applied to any individual patient, because we do not know whether any specific tumor will grow or not.

Having introduced interventionism and skepticism as attentional types through the example of early detection, in chapter 2, I add further attentional diversity to the analysis, complicating the attentional binary between skepticism and interventionism by reading it through the arrangements of attention and relevance emerging from interviews with thirty patients ages forty to fifty. There I introduce the concept of autobiographical alignment and the attentional distinctions among default interventionists, conscious interventionists, conflicted skeptics, and conscious skeptics.

Chapter 2

Attentional Diversity

The Cognitive Structure of Patients' Narratives of Mammography

Attentional diversity is fundamental to the sociology of attention. From a sociological perspective, analyzing attentional alternatives is essential both to demonstrate that attention is neither biological nor universal and to challenge presumed notions of relevance and irrelevance. In this chapter I examine the patterns of attention and relevance present in patients' narratives of mammography, drawing on interviews with a sample of thirty women ages forty to fifty. The interviews address their beliefs and experiences relating to mammography and their awareness of the conflict among experts, focusing specifically on how patients' attention patterns reflect and diverge from interventionism and skepticism. Although interventionism and skepticism are the two dominant attentional types organizing medical and scientific debates, they certainly do not exhaust the attentional possibilities. Further, while the conflict over mammography is supposedly about women, I take as an open question whether interventionism and skepticism also reflect women's patterns of attention. This focus on capturing attentional diversity allows me to move beyond a binary conception in which two polarized positions offer the only attentional alternatives, as well as to better understand the broader attentional influence of culturally hegemonic ideas like early detection. Explicitly rejecting a "deficit model" of the public understanding of science, which posits a lack of knowledge among laypeople (Ward and Peretti-Watel 2020), and emphasizing instead the cultural influences on all cognition, I further foreground differences in attention as a way to drive analytic focus to normally unrecognized alternative meanings residing in the constitutive exclusions of dominant or expert patterns of attention.

Before directly analyzing the patterns of attention present in patients' narratives about mammography, however, I contextualize them in two ways. First, I explore how the doctors and scientists I introduced in chapter 1 characterized women's behavior around mammography and reactions to the conflict. As I will demonstrate, skeptics and interventionists offer very different accounts of what women believe and how they behave in relation to breast screening. These characterizations seem to be driven substantially by their prior attentional commitments and intention to discredit the other point of view. Following that discussion, I summarize the existing research on patient reactions to the mammography conflict.

I identified four dominant themes in doctors' and scientists' characterizations of patients, the first two of which have two contrasting subtypes associated with either skepticism or interventionism:

Theme 1. *Women "just want their screening."* The skeptic version of this narrative emphasizes the *cultural hegemony of early detection* and women's lack of agency, that is, that the dominant cultural logic of early detection is so strong that women cannot think outside of it and ultimately come to feel it is their moral duty to get screened. The traditionalist version (*skeptical paternalism*), in contrast, presents skeptics as the ones attempting to limit women's agency. They suggest that women are being paternalistically restricted from getting screening tests that they feel are valuable by anti-screening champions who seek to control their individual choices based on abstract, population-data-based ideas like overdiagnosis that have no practical application to any particular woman's life. They also connect the skeptic perspective to healthcare rationing and the practice of "cookie cutter" medicine, rather than patient-centered care.

Theme 2. *Women are terrified of breast cancer.* One prominent argument made by skeptic doctors and researchers was that patients are overly fearful of or "misfear" (Rosenbaum 2014) breast cancer because of both cultural messaging and what is sometimes called the "screening paradox" or the "popularity paradox of screening" (Welch, Schwartz, and Woloshin 2011, 187–188), which refers to the increasing number of women who have had a breast cancer diagnosis and understand themselves as survivors even when the mortality rate from breast cancer is technically unchanged. This creates a "looping effect," a concept Aronowitz (2021, 43) borrows from Ian Hacking to describe the way prostate cancer screening creates its own demand through overdiagnosis. Regardless of whether many of these diagnoses were overdiagnoses, as skeptics claim, the increase in "survivors" results in more visibility and awareness of breast cancer in our lives—most often in the form of compelling emotional stories of family, friends, and celebrities who were diagnosed with, and often survived, breast cancer, and thus feel they "owe their lives" to screening. This paradox simultaneously creates a climate of fear (*misfearing*) and reinforces the idea that "early detection saves lives." Interventionists, on the other hand, use fear to again invoke women's agency and right to be screened, arguing that women want the *reassurance* of screening to assuage their (valid) fear of breast cancer.

In these first two themes, interventionists and skeptics actually agree on the fundamental point that women want and seek screening, but they differ in how they understand why this is the case and whether it is a problem. The third and fourth themes, however, cut directly against this idea and were only expressed by interventionists:

Theme 3. *Women are always already "looking for any reason to avoid getting a mammogram."*

Theme 4. *Women are confused by the conflict among experts and simply shut down.* Interventionists used both of these narratives to highlight the negative ramifications of skeptics' attempts to challenge ingrained wisdom about early detection and alter screening schedules.

Skeptics: The Screening Paradox, the Cultural Hegemony of Early Detection, and Fear—Women "Just Want Their Screening"

Mammography-skeptical doctors and scientists frequently emphasize women's fear of cancer in the interviews. They point to dominant cultural messages that reinforce these fears (e.g., about the high prevalence of breast cancer and the necessity of early detection) and drive women to seek mammograms and to resist the change in recommendation to begin screening at age fifty rather than forty. Dr. Blakely, a primary care physician, connects women's fear with resistance to the change in guidelines this way: "Women are terrified that their breast cancers will be missed because of all the statistics about 1 in 9 women and all the breast cancer walks and all the people they know who have breast cancer. So there is sort of a terror of changing something that's been a given that from 40 on, you're going to get a mammogram every year and if you don't, you're messing up." Dr. Blakely illustrates with the final words, "if you don't, you're messing up," the way skeptical participants also emphasize that messages women receive about early detection have a moral dimension that suggests it is women's responsibility to get screened, and if they do not, they are at fault for risking their own lives.

Dr. Freeman, a breast surgeon and former leader of a cancer screening program, also discusses this moral dimension of screening in connection with women's fear of breast cancer: "I think that most of our choices are not based on reasoning. It's based on emotion and—and something else. And we can scare people easily by saying that, you know, 'You might be—it might be your fault that you are dying from breast cancer because you didn't go to mammography screening.'" This view is consistent with literature on the gendered construction of health in general, and prevention specifically, as women's responsibility (Green, Thompson, and Griffiths 2002; Howson 1999; Raspberry and Skinner 2011; Reed 2009). Directly with respect to mammography, prior research finds that the promotion of early detection has been emotionally intensified by these gender ideologies connecting women, family, and personal responsibility for health (Aronowitz 2007; Lerner 2003, 60; Moore 2010, 112).

Skeptic doctors and researchers further argue that this sense of moral obligation to be screened, particularly in a cultural context that is overwhelmingly in favor of screening, combines with women's fear of breast cancer to create a dynamic wherein patients are actually driving demand for mammograms—in some cases, more so than their doctors. Dr. Markman, a professor of medicine and epidemiology, brings together the themes of fear, social pressure, and a sense of moral duty in the following comments, in which he argues that even if patients are made aware of the new USPSTF guidelines and the scientific research supporting that change, social and emotional influences will still drive them to want more frequent mammograms:

> Knowledge is not sufficient. So you can have women pass all the exams you want about screening, but a bunch of them are still going to want to get mammograms every year or if—probably if we offered them, they'd get them every six months. . . . I think that there are many other factors that, um, influence our decision-making about things like this and not just scientific evidence and the—and the tradeoffs and the numbers that I was just talking about. . . . But also a matter of "What is it your friends think? What is it that society as a whole thinks?" There are lots of feelings about breast cancer especially more than other conditions, but especially about breast cancer in which it's kind of your moral duty to get a mammogram.

Some skeptical participants argue that, in addition to making women feel it is their moral duty to protect themselves from breast cancer through regular screening, the prominence of pro-mammography cultural messages makes it difficult for women to cognitively reconcile the idea that screening could be negative.

Mammography skeptic doctors and researchers perceive cultural discourses about mammography as having been so strongly supportive of early detection, and for so long, that "cognitive dissonance" ensued when the discourse shifted and patients started being told that screening can be harmful. They believe such messaging continues to make it very difficult for patients to understand the skeptical viewpoint and concepts like overdiagnosis. Dr. Price, who is a clinical oncologist, describes the creation of this cognitive dissonance: "In part, it might have been because the messages were so strong, so consistent, and so simple. . . . Their guideline may have created cognitive dissonance. That is, if you carry around in your head a belief that's been reinforced for decades and then all of a sudden someone comes out against it . . . or not against it, comes out with a nuance, um, sometimes because of cognitive dissonance . . . there is a tendency to go with your preexisting construct of the issues." While skeptics emphasize the consistency of pro-mammography cultural messages and patients' fear of cancer—and the way that these both drive women to seek mammography and create mental resistance to critical ideas such as overdiagnosis or the harms of screening—interventionists offer an entirely different characterization of women's mammography beliefs and behaviors.

Interventionists: Paternalism, Avoidance, and Confusion— Do Women "Just Want Their Screening"?

Interventionist doctors and researchers primarily argue that patients typically avoid getting a mammogram if they can, and therefore any information critical of mammography, as Dr. Jones, a radiologist, puts it, "is easily embraced," and patients quickly "jump on that bandwagon":

> I think that how it has impacted on patients is that patients are always looking for a reason not to have a mammogram. Um, so anything that's presented in the—in the media that's against mammography is easily embraced by women. Um, look, the vast majority of mammograms are normal and so a lot of women may feel, "Well, why am I even getting this test? It never shows cancer." You know, very few—there are very few screening-detected cancers if we look at the numbers. So I think for the women who don't like to go or the women who have had scares

or the women whose cancers weren't detected on mammography, it's easy to jump on that bandwagon.

An alternative framing of patients' avoidance by interventionist doctors portrays them as confused by the inconsistent information to the point where they "shut down" and avoid taking action on mammography: "There is a lot of confusion. And the resultant confusion is—well, that in some cases women just become kind of stymied and—and then just shut down. 'I don't know what to do, so I'm not doing anything.' . . . Uh, I think that's an unintended, but a real consequence of that. And—and I think it's just that women go, 'I don't know what to do and the experts can't agree. I—I don't know. I'm just not going to do anything'" (Dr. Kramer, family medicine doctor and head of a cancer center). Another example of this interventionist emphasis of patients' confusion comes from Dr. Cohen, a general internist: "I am sure it's equally challenging and daunting for patients. Uh, I can only imagine that if you're not even in the field and you find these conflicting guidelines, then you're left wondering, um, which of the ones that you give more weight to. Right? . . . I can only imagine if you're a patient and you see conflicting information like this, trying to sort it out on your own cannot be an easy—cannot be an easy thing to do. I mean, heck, it's not easy for doctors, right?"

Such arguments that the recent circulation of messages critical of mammography leaves patients confused, conflicted, and avoidant are quite different from the claims made by skeptics that information about the harms of screening is cognitively resisted due to patients' deeply held preexisting mental framework of early detection. In these examples, then, interventionist and skeptic doctors and researchers present rhetorically polarized accounts of patients' dispositions and reactions to the conflict over mammography. Skeptics describe patients as so deeply cognitively embedded in a culture of early detection and routine mammograms that they cannot even take in the critical perspectives emerging in the scientific research. Interventionists, on the other hand, portray patients as very tenuous in their commitment to mammography and therefore easily pushed away by any criticisms.

While some interventionist doctors and researchers describe patients as seeking to avoid screening and problematize the conflict over guidelines on the basis that it contributes to this tendency, and others argue that the existence of conflicting information and the resulting confusion can make patients shut down and avoid taking action on their preventive care, a third, totally different—even contradictory—viewpoint offered by interventionists emphasizes that patients "just want their screening" (as characterized by the skeptics). When expressing this view, however, interventionists are actually taking critical aim at the skeptical perspective as out of alignment with patients' wishes, and even paternalistically limiting their choices. Dr. Hodges, a general internist, exemplifies this perspective: "Well, I have a broad spectrum of patients, um, from [different] socioeconomic levels and educational [levels] and, they for the most part, they are aware of confusion and a lack of consensus. And most women just want their screening."

For others I spoke with, although the underlying message is similar—patients just want to be screened—more emphasis is placed on patients' willingness to endure the harms of screening because they want the peace of mind that they feel it brings. Dr. Kramer provides an example of this view that patients are willing to "take on" the harms of screening for the benefits they perceive it as offering: "Um, you know, the woman in her forties, she goes, 'You know, I'll go through a lot—a lot of call backs if it means that the one time it's real, I've caught it early so I'm going to be there for my kids and my husband and my parents, who I'm taking care of.' . . . That they're willing to take that on so that they, um, if that makes sense, I guess." Dr. Cashman, a radiologist, similarly argues that even patients who have to endure repeat screenings are more than willing to do so—and risk the stress and potential physical discomfort of call backs and other follow-up procedures—for the solace it brings: "My experience in seventeen years of doing this is I have never had a woman be so traumatized psychologically or otherwise by a call back where they have to come in for some additional imaging or for a biopsy that ends up not being cancerous. In fact, they are extremely relieved that a) they don't have cancer of course, but b) that we are thorough to make sure."

Thus, while some interventionist doctors and researchers present an image of patients as avoidant, and the conflict as exacerbating their tendency to skip recommended screenings, others present patients as happy to be screened and accordingly criticize skeptics as not supporting patients or honoring their wishes. Ironically, the latter perspective is basically aligned with the skeptics' characterization of patients as motivated to seek screening by fear and dominant cultural messages about the necessity of early detection, even though when expressed by interventionists it is intended as a criticism.

It is unsurprising that skeptics and interventionists present opposing rhetorical characterizations of the notable tendencies in patient behavior given that they are seeking to support very different claims about mammography and early detection. Yet, as seen in the example of narratives about patients seeking screening, at times the two groups draw on the same set of ideas about patients for the opposite ends. Further, even within interventionism, the doctors and scientists

I spoke with presented multiple narratives, at times making totally different claims about patients' behavior; patients are on the one hand avoidant and confused, using the conflict as an excuse not to get screened, and yet are also so clear in their desire for mammography that they are willing to deal with any unpleasant consequences relating to follow-up appointments, or additional screenings or procedures. With these flexible uses of narratives about patient behavior and their shifting points of emphasis, interventionists are strategically using logically contradictory narratives about "how patients behave" as a rhetorical tool to support their viewpoints in favor of mammography and early detection.

Fundamentally, how the doctors and researchers describe patients' views and behavior directly reflects the attention type—interventionism or skepticism—they apply. The very different accounts each present about what patients believe and how they behave when it comes to mammography—particularly given the way the different narratives are filtered through, and used strategically to prop up, each side of the conflict—beg for a more direct examination of what patients actually know about mammography and how they think about the conflicting guidelines.

Prior Research on Patient Reactions to the Mammography Conflict

Barker and Galardi's (2011) analysis of internet postings reacting to the USPSTF 2009 guideline change is to my knowledge the only direct sociological analysis of patients' awareness of and response to the mammography conflict. They find that the posts illustrate patients' resistance to the change and the scientific expertise represented by the USPSTF and a strong belief in their own "lay expertise." The medical literature addressing patients' knowledge about and reactions to the guideline changes primarily focuses on the effects of the guideline change on frequency of screening. Some studies report decreases in screening (Finney Rutten et al. 2014; Jiang, Hughes, and Duszak 2015; Sharpe et al. 2013; Sprague et al. 2014), while others find screening behavior unchanged (Block et al. 2013; Dehkordy et al. 2015; Howard and Adams 2012), and at least one study finds an increase in screening (Pace, He, and Keating 2013). Others find differential results in specific groups, for example, decreases among high-income or younger women (Block et al. 2013; Dehkordy et al. 2015; Howard and Adams 2012). Wharam et al. (2015) find a decrease in screening among all groups except Black women ages fifty to sixty-four. Other subgroups examined include women with prior false-positive mammograms, who are not found to be less likely to be screened following the guideline change (Brewer, Salz, and Lillie

2007; Hardesty, Lind, and Gutierrez 2016), and women with disabilities (Xu, Mann, et al. 2017; Xu, McDermott, et al. 2017), who are found to face disparities in receipt of mammography recommendations and are less likely to be fully adherent. Taken as a whole, this work, which focuses on determining the conflict's influence on screening rates, is based on an underlying assumption that early detection is valid, regular mammography is desirable, even between forty and fifty years of age, and skepticism of screening, whether due to false-positive results or the debates themselves, is something to avoid. (In fact, in many cases, the authors state explicitly that their goal is to promote screening.) It also does not seek to examine how patients *understand* mammography guidelines or the disagreement, *why* they understand them as they do (including their patterns of attention), or *how* these beliefs and attentional patterns may relate to any changes in screening behaviors.

There is a smaller body of medical research that delves into patients' understanding of and reactions to the conflict. This research is consistent in finding that patients' knowledge of the conflict and specific guidelines is quite low, and their response to the USPSTF guideline change is negative (Allen et al. 2012; Davidson, Liao, and Magee 2011; Friedman et al. 2013; Hersch et al. 2013; Kiviniemi and Hay 2012; Squiers et al. 2011). For example, Kiviniemi and Hay (2012) used a telephone survey of 508 women to examine awareness of and reaction to the current guidelines, finding that less than half of women were aware of the change, and only 12 percent of those who were aware could correctly report the change in both the age and frequency of screening. Consistent with Barker and Galardi (2011), the authors further report that most respondents across demographic categories had a negative reaction to the change in recommendations. Davidson, Liao, and Magee (2011) also found that women responded negatively to the change of recommendation. In a survey of 249 women, 89 percent of participants reported that they wanted yearly mammograms, and 84 percent said they would not delay until age fifty. The change of guideline by the USPSTF was viewed as unsafe by 86 percent of participants, even when recommended by a doctor. A separate web-based survey of 1,221 women similarly found that the majority of participants were unsupportive of the new recommendation, and less than 25 percent could correctly identify the different guidelines for ages forty to forty-nine and fifty to seventy-four (Squiers et al. 2011).

With the exception of a handful that used focus-groups (e.g., Allen et al. 2012; Friedman et al. 2013; Hersch et al. 2013), the medical literature on patients' reactions to the mammography conflict is largely based on survey research, which can provide a broad sense of the basic contours of patients' beliefs but limits our depth of understanding. *Why*, for example, are many patients unsupportive of the change of guideline? How do they understand the motivations and meanings behind the change? In the remainder of this chapter, I draw on thirty in-depth interviews to explore the frameworks of belief and attention structuring patients' response to the mammography conflict in greater detail.

What Patients Attend

The thirty patients I interviewed about mammography were all women between ages forty and fifty. I selected this age range because it roughly captures the group about which the guidelines are inconsistent.[1] Of the interview participants, 63 percent (N = 19 out of 30) self-identified as white, 33 percent (N = 10 out of 30) as Black, and one as Hispanic/Latina. In terms of education, twenty-three (77 percent) participants had college degrees and thirteen (43 percent) had obtained additional graduate degrees. Five participants had a high school diploma only, and two completed some high school but did not graduate. (See table 2.1 for the sample characteristics. More detailed information about recruitment and analysis are available in the appendix.)

Out of the thirty patients I interviewed, seven (23 percent) had never had a mammogram. Of these, four are of high socioeconomic status (SES), defined as employed and having either an undergraduate or graduate degree, while three are low SES (unemployed, no college degree). On the other end of the spectrum, thirteen participants (43 percent) had had more than four mammograms, with seven of these (23 percent) having had more than six. Recall that all interview participants were between forty and fifty years old, so at least based on the USPSTF guidelines, it would not necessarily be recommended that they have even one mammogram yet. Of those participants who had had a prior mammogram, 70 percent (sixteen out of twenty-three), or 53 percent of the total sample, had been recalled for one or more additional diagnostic mammograms or for another form of follow-up such as an ultrasound or biopsy. None of the participants were diagnosed with breast cancer. Estimates of the rate of false-positive mammograms in other research varies, but this figure is within the range reported in other sources. Farr et al. (2020, 581) cite a 20 to 65 percent lifetime risk of receiving a false-positive result, for example, while Schwartz et al. (2004) report that 35 percent of their respondents had had at least one false-positive mammogram.

On the whole, reflecting the findings of prior research, the patients I interviewed were not particularly well informed about the specifics of the medical disputes or mammography recommendations more generally. Allison, a fifty-year-old white professor who has had two or three mammograms, described the general state of the sample's knowledge well when she said there is high

Table 2.1
Sample characteristics, patients

Characteristic	N
Age of respondent	
40–43	7
44–47	15
48–50	8
Employed for wages	80% (24 of 30)
Highest level of education	
Graduate school	13
College	10
High school graduate	5
Some high school	2
Race/ethnicity	
White	19
Black	10
Hispanic/Latina	1
Number of mammograms	
0	7
1	4
2–3	6
4–5	6
6 or more	7
Follow-up required?	70% (16 out of 23 screened)

awareness—"breast cancer and pink ribbons everywhere"—but "actually information is probably pretty low." Very few of the patients I spoke with had been made aware by their doctors that there is any conflict over the recommended age or frequency of breast screening.[2] In fact, only two patients out of thirty report having had any conversation with their doctor that referred to the mammography conflict, and even in these two cases they recall the discussions being brief and not very informative or emphasized. On the other hand, nineteen participants (63 percent) report that their doctors had *never* presented information about the disagreement. For example:

> I saw her last April and she, you know, had this paper like, "Here, you know the script or whatever to have one done." And so I did. But yeah, I don't really recall them getting into, either of those two doctors, getting into like the confusion around it or when you go or don't go, or how often you have one and that kind of thing. (Nancy, forty-six-year-old white counselor who has had four or five mammograms)

I have not had that conversation. I mean usually they just look into the system and see what else I have had done. . . . But there is not a lot of conversation about any sort of controversy about guidelines and things like that. (Lauren, forty-four-year-old white professor who has had two or three mammograms)

Well, according to my doctor, I think it's just yearly from forty up. And I told him I'm not really any risk, and he said, "Well, you might as well just to get a baseline." (Sarah, forty-four-year-old white contingent university faculty who has had one mammogram)

For at least two participants (Abby and Ruby), their interview with me was the first time they were hearing about the conflict. Others had some degree of awareness, but not of the specifics, and had never brought it up to their doctors or had it brought up to them. However, a few told me they had raised the issue with their doctors and felt dismissed: "In fact, they all—when I suggest there is [disagreement], they all get kind of defensive. . . . The last gynecologist I saw got really defensive and she said . . . something about morbidity, 'We're helping with morbidity,' or something like that. . . . Um, but, yeah no, no doctor has really sort of admitted it to me" said Eva, a forty-three-year-old white editor who has never had a mammogram. Eva is actively seeking a new provider who follows the USPSTF recommendations, but she has had trouble finding one.

Kelly and Jocelyn also initiated conversations with their doctors about the conflict and felt their providers had been dismissive: "So since I turned forty, I would say my primary care doctor has been like, 'You should go get a mammogram.' And then I pushed back and I said, 'Well, the United States Preventive Services Task Force says that it's not really necessary in your forties. And I'm going to follow their recommendations.' And she was sort of like, 'Well, you know, that's your choice,'" said Kelly, a forty-six-year-old white journalist who has had two or three mammograms. Kelly continued, "It's because I brought it up that it was even acknowledged." Jocelyn, who has had three mammograms, is a forty-seven-year-old researcher and instructor in a medical school. She initially hoped not to get another mammogram after learning about the change of guidelines but feels her doctor was unreceptive when she brought it up: "It was in my regular annual. It was probably just about a year ago now. . . . It was I think right after this had been in the news last spring. She told me to go get a mammogram, and me not wanting to get a mammogram, said, 'I thought that the guidelines had changed.' . . . Um, and she basically said that she counseled her patients to get mammograms if they're nervous. And that since I had already had a mammogram, I should get another mammogram."

Remarkably, although still a small number, twice as many participants—four versus two—mentioned that their doctors had brought up the recent change in recommendations for cervical cancer screening but not mammograms. This is notable because the change in recommendation for pap smears similarly makes screening less frequent—cervical cancer screenings were reduced from annual to every five years. In the following comments, Samantha and Nancy both explicitly point out that their doctors told them about the change in cervical screening but did not mention that there was disagreement about mammography:

> The disagreement, that he didn't discuss. I don't think he discussed. I mean the only thing that he was discussing to me was . . . about how often I should do pap smears. That is the conversation. That's the controversy he brought up. That I shouldn't do them every year. I had some HPV in the past, but once I was cleared, he wanted to make it very clear to me that I should come every five years and not, you know, and so that he made very clear and in fact was insistent. But in terms of mammography, he [said], you know, every year. (Samantha, forty-seven-year-old white professor who has had four or five mammograms)

> I know my doctor did about pap smears. . . . And so it seemed like there was a change with those at some point where you don't need that actual—she'll still do like an exam, but they don't do like a pap. . . . And so that was more clear and consistent but the—the mammogram thing really hasn't been, I don't think. Yeah, that I recall. (Nancy, forty-six-year-old white counselor who has had four or five mammograms)

Without exception, then, the patients I interviewed were not receiving information about the USPSTF change in mammography recommendations—or even that there is any disagreement about mammography screening—from their doctors. In this sense, they also appear to be interacting primarily with interventionist practitioners who do not find the possible harms of mammography relevant to attend or acknowledge. It is further notable in this context that the emphasis of the USPSTF change, and many other organizations' current guidelines, is that patients in their forties should be having a conversation with their doctors about the risks and benefits of mammography rather than relying on a blanket recommendation to screen them by default. At least based on the experiences of the thirty patients I interviewed, this conversation does not appear to be happening. This finding is consistent with prior research that finds that most doctors are not actively talking to patients about the risks of screening. For example, Wegwarth and Gigerenzer (2013) report in a study of three hundred

U.S. patients that only 8.4 percent of women recommended to undergo cancer screening by their physicians (largely mammography) reported that their doctors told them about overdiagnosis or overtreatment, yet 80 percent of participants stated that they would want information about such potential risks prior to undergoing any screening.

It is important also to note relating to women's knowledge that whether someone was aware of the specifics of the dispute did not correlate directly with SES or education. While the four most knowledgeable interview participants all had college degrees, and three of the four had graduate degrees, more participants with graduate degrees, for example, were not particularly conversant in the specifics of the guidelines and debate. Since knowledge of the debate was so limited, I summarized the conflicting guidelines for each participant and asked for their reaction during the interview. In what follows, I describe these responses, analyze whether they reflect doctors' characterizations and/or the findings of prior research, and identify several additional attentional foci and patterns of relevance not captured by skepticism and interventionism.

Skepticism and Interventionism among Patients

While specific knowledge of the conflict and recommendations was overall very low among the women I interviewed, several defining ideas of the skeptic/interventionist typology structure their narratives in a more general sense. Roughly speaking, the most well-informed participants are also the least convinced of mammography's benefits, aligning them more with the skeptical viewpoint as established among the doctors and medical researchers. I refer to this group as *conscious skeptics* because of their heightened knowledge of the conflict. Less well-informed participants, who make up the majority of the sample, are more likely to rely loosely on long-standing cultural narratives about the benefits of early detection. For example, eighteen of the thirty participants told me they either stick to the guideline of annual screening starting at age forty or they believe the "earlier the better," with some expressing the belief that forty is actually too late.

However, there is notable variation in how informed these eighteen participants are in terms of the specifics of the guidelines and debates. Some are quite knowledgeable and conversant with this information, while others are totally unaware of the disagreement and are just following ingrained wisdom or prior medical recommendations, which is why I differentiate between *conscious interventionism* and *default interventionism*. As discussed in the introduction, the broader research on screening overwhelmingly concludes that there exists a hegemonic, deeply rooted "true belief" in the benefits of early detection (Welch, Schwartz, and Woloshin 2011, 151), coupled with a lack of knowledge of the potential harms of screening, including overdiagnosis and overtreatment (Carter 2021, 31; Harris et al. 2011, 33; He et al. 2018; Hoffmann and Del Mar 2015; Hofmann 2014; Moynihan, Doust, and Henry 2012; Rozbroj et al. 2021; Schwartz et al. 2004; Silverman et al. 2001; Stefanek 2011, 1823; Welch, Schwartz, and Woloshin 2011, 22).

Most participants, then, having been socialized in this cultural context of faith in early detection, begin from a default position of interventionism. For some, that default belief in screening and early detection becomes a more conscious, informed, active interventionism due to life experiences with screening and breast cancer. I refer to this process as *autobiographical alignment*, building on DeGloma's (2015, 160) concept of "mnemonic alignment," which usefully highlights the process of reconciling autobiographical experiences with collective discourses. In comparison, I characterize five participants as *conscious skeptics*. Skeptics are almost always at odds with friends and family in their attention to the risks of early detection, and they report difficulty finding doctors that support the significance they attribute to the risks of mammography and their decision to abstain from it until at least age fifty. In this way, skeptics are conscious *by default*; in other words, given the hegemony of early detection, being a skeptic requires intentionality and some degree of attentional deviance by definition, and thus there is no "default skeptic" category. Instead, I offer a group of five additional participants who express what I will call *conflicted skepticism*: while aspects of skepticism were present in their comments, these participants are still being influenced by hegemonic ideas about the importance of early detection. The remaining two participants are difficult to categorize because they knew almost nothing about mammography prior to the interview yet also did not seem to obviously express a broader default interventionist stance.

As I explored in chapter 1, early detection is a key structuring belief—a foundational filter and attentional anchor—organizing the disagreement between interventionists and skeptics in the medical field. Recall in addition that one prominent argument made by skeptic doctors and researchers was that patients are extremely—even overly—fearful of breast cancer because of both cultural messaging and the *screening paradox*—the growing cultural presence of women who have had a breast cancer diagnosis (many of whom were in reality likely overdiagnosed). They suggest that this fear drives patients to want mammograms even when they may not be beneficial. When interventionists discuss women's fear, in contrast, they primarily argue that women want the reassurance of screening. Given their salience to the disagreement, in what follows I use the topics of early detection and fear to focus my analysis as I illustrate the different attention types I identified among the patients I interviewed.

Default Interventionism

Interventionism-aligned patients, who make up 60 percent ($N = 18$ out of 30) of the patient sample, consistently express that early detection is essential and without negative consequences. These participants typically use phrases like "you need to catch it early" (Allison, age fifty, white, professor, has had two or three mammograms), "if it's preventive care, then the earlier, the better" (Rochelle, age fifty, Black, unemployed, never had a mammogram), and "what does it hurt to start it earlier?" (Catherine, age forty-four, Black, unemployed, never had a mammogram).

To some extent, then, the key idea of early detection structuring medical debates about mammography also organizes patients' beliefs. That being said, many patients are interventionism-aligned by default only and are totally unaware that there is any disagreement about early detection or mammography more generally. Even among those with general awareness of the debate, there is little specific knowledge; most have only the fuzziest notion of the particular points of disagreement or of important contested ideas such as overdiagnosis or the harms of mammography, which is why the majority of the participants fall into the category of *default interventionism.*

In addition to a default belief in early detection, fear is significant among the patients I interviewed. However, the roots and impact of their fear are more nuanced than the expert skeptic and interventionist characterizations suggest. What is notable among the patients I interviewed is that how their fear manifests is significantly dependent on their particular history with breast cancer and screening. To reflect this, I suggest that the impact of fear must be understood as the result of a process of *autobiographical attentional alignment* with the hegemonic narrative of early detection. That is, fear often nudges women from a default interventionism to become more aware and intentional about screening; however, this can mean pushing them toward being more attentive to either the risks or the benefits—in other words, toward either conscious skepticism or conscious interventionism. Which direction they lean depends on their autobiographical experiences, whether of friends and family with cancer, of their own medical treatment and testing, or otherwise.

This idea aligns with prior research demonstrating that most women with false-positive mammogram events experience an increase in fear, but that fear does not necessarily push them away from screening. For example, Schwartz et al. (2004, 75) found that 37 percent of their respondents described receiving the news that they needed further testing following a mammogram as "very scary" or the "scariest time" of their lives. Yet almost all of these patients were still glad they had the screening test. Indeed, women with prior false-positive mammograms are on the whole not found to be less likely to be screened (Brewer, Salz, and Lillie 2007; Hardesty, Lind, and Gutierrez 2016). It is possible, in fact, that in many cases the emotional intensity of such experiences could make them more conscious, vigilant interventionists. In other cases, however, as I will illustrate, false-positive screening experiences can drive patients toward conscious skepticism, or at least make them actively conflicted about screening. Regardless, prior screening experiences seem to serve as clarifying cognitive filters that make women more intentional about their views. One implication of my analysis is that, while skeptic doctors and scientists argue that dominant cultural discourses lead women to "misfear" breast cancer and thus want more screening (Rosenbaum 2014), and interventionists argue that women simply want the reassurance screening brings to them, what both of these narratives exclude is the group of women whose predominant fear is not of breast cancer but of screening and overdiagnosis, even if this is not the majority. They also do not acknowledge the important point that the screening paradox—although certainly a significant aspect of many women's personal experience with breast cancer and screening—is not the only autobiographical influence on patients' fear and attention.

Conscious Interventionism

Attesting to the power of the screening paradox, many of the women I spoke with describe a fear of breast cancer and connect that fear to the prominence of breast cancer in their autobiography. About half directly discuss a friend or relative with breast cancer who has impacted their views. For most, the effect of this experience was to increase their fear and motivate more active, intentional screening, essentially making them more conscious interventionists. For example, Tania, a fifty-year-old white contingent faculty member who has had six or more mammograms, discusses the way watching both her mother and a friend go through breast cancer treatment affected her, saying, "It was a really scary wake-up call." Frances, a forty-eight-year-old Black legal assistant who has had one prior mammogram, had two sisters die of cancer, and her reaction is to be more vigilant with her own screening. As she puts it, "It's better to know than to not know. And you die because of ignorance a lot of times or because you don't address medical problems." Nancy, mentioned already, discusses a friend diagnosed in her forties who she believes would not be alive if she had waited to get screened until she was fifty. Joanne, a fifty-year-old white technical writer and editor who has had six or more mammograms, similarly knew three women diagnosed prior to age fifty, and her reaction is to feel extremely reluctant to delay or space out screening unless there is overwhelming scientific evidence to convince her. Allison, the fifty-year-old white professor introduced previously, who has had two or three mammograms, and Jodi, who is forty-four years old, Hispanic/Latina, works as a teacher's aide, and has had one prior mammogram, both shared stories about friends who were diagnosed after missing just one mammogram or even in one case had an aggressive cancer appear between annual mammograms; in both cases, their friends' experiences added substantially to their anxiety.

The majority of the interview participants, then, had the experience of people in their immediate social world confronting a breast cancer diagnosis. Even if they personally never receive a diagnosis, breast cancer is part of their autobiography, with the cancer experiences of friends and family members providing templates of possible future trajectories for themselves, some of which are totally devastating. These imagined possible futures shape their feelings about mammography and screening behavior, typically making them more aware and active about screening. Many also perceive a collective fear of breast cancer within their social group. For example, as Tania, the white, fifty-year-old contingent faculty member quoted previously, describes, "I mean I have so many friends—I mean I am thinking of one close friend in particular who is just terrified that she's going to get breast cancer." This is in keeping with what the skeptical medical professionals I interviewed described earlier in this chapter—that is, patients are extremely fearful of breast cancer, and the broader cultural climate is one of collective fear and promotion of screening through the rhetoric of "early detection saves lives."

Some skeptics point out that patients can desire more screening than their doctors recommend, even when following the more aggressive guideline of annual screening starting at forty. This was best illustrated in the interviews with a subset of patients who represent the most extreme examples of conscious interventionism in the sample. This group is particularly terrified of breast cancer and very intentionally seek more intensive screening—and they perceive doctors and other gatekeepers as pulling back on mammography. For example, Megan, a forty-three-year-old white stay-at-home mother who has had six or more mammograms, describes her immediate social group as follows: "I think within the group I'd be referring to, they're mostly sort of high-achieving, aggressive sort of go-getter women, and they're like, 'Well, I want to be on top of this and know before—' I don't know. 'I'll kill you before you kill me.'" Megan also perceives doctors as pulling back on breast cancer screening and treatment of certain kinds of lesions:

> I guess my current understanding would be maybe that they're saying now less is better. Less exposure to, um, the radiation, less sort of intrusive, you know, taking a—a needle aspiration or whatever it's called, like that might be more harm than watching, you know, probing and poking might be worse than letting something rest. Um, I also feel like there is some sort of controversy around someone has stage 0 or stage 1 because I do have a friend the same age as we are who has just gone through radiation and chemotherapy. Um, I feel like at least from what I have read here in town, you know, some of the top breast people are saying, "Stage 0, don't even bother with it yet." Or I'm not really sure. I just get the sense they're feeling that the laypeople, me, myself, uh, are being too proactive or too alarmist. Um, I mean I think within the—the circle I have talked to about it, most women would say, "Oh, my God, definitely, cut my whole breast off and get it as far out of me as possible." But I am hearing them say, "No, don't go that far. Don't."

Nicole, a forty-six-year-old white hospice nurse who has also had six or more mammograms, is another example of someone who finds even the guideline of annual mammography beginning at age forty too conservative. She thinks there should be "liberal exceptions," particularly for patients with a family history of breast cancer, and also feels that patients should not have to do a lot of "arm twisting" to get mammograms before age forty.

Often when the participants knew someone diagnosed with breast cancer prior to age fifty, fear of cancer led them to become more directly aware and intentional about their own screening—to want more or better testing—and thus to become more conscious interventionists. For instance, Tamara, a forty-three-year-old white actuary who has had two or three mammograms, believes, "You can't take your chances because so many people have seen so many horrible things happen when breast cancer is concerned." For some of these patients, screening provides relief from fear, as exemplified by Vivian and Lauren. Vivian, a forty-year-old white school librarian who has not yet had a mammogram, tells me, "I get a little nervous, so sometimes I tend to go on the more screening side." She thinks of it as bringing "peace of mind." Lauren, quoted above about how her doctor had never mentioned the conflict, speaks similarly about screening providing "comfort" on an emotional level.

Many patients driven by fear to seek mammograms in a conscious, self-directed manner express significant discomfort with the idea of pushing back the starting point for mammography. Joanne, as mentioned already, has known three women diagnosed prior to age fifty; she says she would be reluctant to delay or space out screening. The evidence would have to be "overwhelming" to convince her to do so. "It almost has to be double." Often this uneasiness seems to be connected with the idea that "you never know" whether a problem is brewing unnoticed and "some women get cancer earlier" than fifty—perspectives fundamentally reflective of the social hegemony and taken-for-grantedness of the theory of early detection. "I don't feel comfortable with it, no. I don't. Because I feel like . . . you're basically playing Russian roulette with people's lives because some people might need it earlier. You never know. Every woman is different," said Catherine, age forty-four, who is Black, unemployed, and has never had a mammogram.

Underlying such comments that "you never know" are often concerns about aging and death, as in the case of Abby, a forty-four-year-old Black daycare provider who has had one mammogram. She feels that "after a certain age" you "just don't know what's going on with your body." Joanne, the fifty-year-old white technical writer and editor introduced previously, who has had six or more mammograms, similarly ties her resistance to delaying the initiation of screening until age fifty to unknowns in the aging process: "I mean the difference between 40 and 50 for a baseline is huge! You know, I don't know that it's so much of a difference every year versus every other year once you have had your baseline if you don't have any, you know, if you've never had a problem. That to me would be more—I don't know if 'reasonable' is the right word. I could see that guideline sort of being, you know, up for discussion. But the difference between forty and fifty to me is huge! I mean a lot happens in ten years!"

Explicitly linking discomfort with the idea of delaying mammography with fears about aging and death, Nancy (forty-six-year-old white counselor who has had four or five mammograms) says the experience of a friend who died of breast cancer in her forties, leaving behind two young children, made her fearful of delaying mammography: "I think 50 is too late and it—it does need to start sooner." Comments such as "early is better" or you should do it earlier because "you never know" illustrate that a default belief in the concept of early detection and associated ideas about the inevitability of cancer's progression over time forms the foundation for many patients' discomfort with delaying mammograms. Patients expressing this sentiment, as well as the related responses such as bringing up examples of friends and relatives who were diagnosed with cancer in their forties, or the idea that patients can only benefit—never be harmed—from knowing what is going on with their bodies, especially as they age, support the finding in prior literature that patients feel negatively about recommendations to delay mammograms until forty-five or fifty (Allen et al. 2012; Barker and Galardi 2011; Davidson, Liao, and Magee 2011; Friedman et al. 2013; Hersch et al. 2013; Kiviniemi and Hay 2012; Squiers et al. 2011). They also roughly reflect the mammography skeptic doctors' characterization of patients as led by fear to seek screening, sometimes sooner than it is medically beneficial. However, while fear was a nearly universal theme, there was variability among the patients between fear as motivation for more intensive screening (leading to conscious interventionism, as just described) and fear as increasing their skepticism of screening, which is the subject of the next section.

Conflicted Skepticism

For a smaller subset of patients, while fear drives them to get mammography screenings, it is reluctantly and with less comfort or relief. These conflicted skeptics are not fully convinced about mammography's necessity and often experienced the harms of screening or witnessed screening fail but nonetheless feel too fearful to stop getting mammograms. For fifty-year-old Tania, for example, who had had six or more mammograms by the time of our interview, "it is very frustrating that it feels like I am on this conveyor belt, you know, living in this age of great medical technology, then this is what it is. And I balk against that. Um, but I haven't totally, you know, stopped doing it because of the fear." Kelly, who at age forty-six has had two or three mammograms, simply states, "There's only so far skepticism can take you." These participants describe an internal conflict between their skepticism of mammography and their fear of breast cancer. For example, Kelly tells me at another point in the interview that the greater fear for her is not fear of cancer but "fear of overtreatment." Conflicted skeptics thus have an ambivalent perspective on screening, which can be understood as simultaneous attention to both the benefits and potential harms. Prior research emphasizes that ambivalence may lead one to delay or not get a mammogram (O'Neill et al. 2012, e192). What I am highlighting with the category of conflicted skeptics is a group of ambivalent women who are still getting mammograms, even if they do so reluctantly due to their more balanced awareness of the potential risks. Here it is also important to note that I understand ambivalence essentially as a form of elevated consciousness—a more balanced, nuanced distribution of attention in which multiple meanings are acknowledged simultaneously—as opposed to something negative or a synonym for unclear or confused.

I did not find significant evidence of the widespread avoidance in response to the conflict described by interventionist doctors and researchers among the patients I interviewed—not even among the conflicted skeptics, where it was arguably most likely to appear. Recall that one of the interventionists' arguments was that patients are always already looking for reasons to avoid mammograms, and that the controversy will therefore be used as an excuse not to get screened. They also suggested that patients are confused by the conflict, which further exacerbates this tendency to avoid screening. Some patients I spoke with did express that they are uncertain whether they should get a mammogram or which guideline to follow, as the following comments illustrate:

> I am highly educated. I am pretty empowered about, you know . . . there aren't very many barriers to me accessing things. I have excellent health care and I'm thinking like, "Yeah, like, I don't know. What am I supposed to do?" It's kind of confusing. Like so, what must it really be like for a lot of other people? (Maria, fifty-year-old white elementary school principal who has had four or five mammograms)
>
> I went for the first [mammogram] at thirty-seven. It seemed like shortly after that, you know, you're hearing, "Oh, women don't need those until they're forty." And I'm going, "Well, great, you know, I had one early that I didn't need." So I, um, I don't know. . . . So I thought, "Well, do I really need one at forty?" Like, you know, no, so it's been very confusing. (Nancy, forty-six-year-old white counselor who has had four or five mammograms)
>
> Well, it [the conflict over guidelines] makes it really confusing. That makes it really confusing for me to figure out. (Vivian, forty-two-year-old white school librarian who has never had a mammogram)
>
> I think for patients it [the conflict] is very confusing and for people who maybe don't have the benefit of either having the interest to follow their own health, and follow what's new, or don't know any better, it can really be a problem. (Joanne, fifty-year-old white technical writer/editor who has had six or more mammograms)

Nevertheless, since all participants were between forty and fifty years old, they are technically still compliant with the USPSTF guidelines. Further, most of the patients who expressed confusion had already had multiple mammograms prior to age fifty, suggesting that they are not necessarily avoiding screening. Although the confusion may give them pause about when to have their next mammogram, none expressed an intention to stop getting mammograms until age fifty. The only group that was "avoiding" screening in any meaningful way were the conscious skeptics, who I will discuss in the next section.

That being said, a small number of the patients I recruited from a low-SES urban medical practice offer characterizations of screening behavior more aligned with the idea of avoidance when discussing the attitudes and behaviors of others in their community—in particular Catherine, who is forty-four, Black, unemployed, and has never had a mammogram, and Frances, a forty-eight-year-old Black legal assistant who has had one prior mammogram. They expressed that the women they know tend to be too "nonchalant" with their health, and that the trend is not to treat medical problems adequately rather than to seek extra screening. Thus, for these participants, the cultural climate they observe in their poor urban community is more one of underutilization of health care and preventive screening rather than overuse.

While it is possible to interpret the behaviors observed and reported by Frances and Catherine as avoidance, a more nuanced analysis comes from considering how they reflect the paradox of the simultaneous overuse and underuse of health care, in which too much care for some is often coupled with too little for others (Hankin and Wright 2010; Rosich and Hankin 2010). It is striking how their descriptions contrast with the sentiments of some of the most anxious conscious interventionist patients described in the previous section, such as Megan and Nicole, who expressed that women in their peer groups want *more* screening than their doctors and even the more aggressive guidelines allow. This contrast is consistent with the literature on disparities in health and healthcare utilization (House 2002; Link and Phelan 1995; Phelan, Link, and Tehranifar 2010) and on the middle- and upper-middle-class roots of critiques of medicalization and overtreatment (Barker 1998; Bell 2009, 2010; Brubaker 2007).

Prior research has also documented race and class disparities in rates of mammography screening and breast cancer incidence and mortality (Bradley, Given, and Roberts 2002; Miller et al. 2019; Spadea et al. 2010; Yu 2009). Some of these works specifically point to the intersection of social class and health knowledge and beliefs; for example, Missinne, Colman, and Bracke (2013) draw on Shim's (2010) concept of *cultural health capital*, defined as the repertoire of cultural skills, beliefs, attitudes, and behaviors that optimize healthcare relationships, to argue that socioeconomic disparities in mammography uptake are traceable to class-based cultural knowledge and behavior about health and health care instantiated early in life, independent of adult earnings or education. Possibly reflecting such cultural health capital disparities, some of the participants in my study who were located in low-SES urban contexts spoke to me about inadequate attention to preventive care and underutilization of screening they observed in their communities. However, as discussed previously, I found that specific knowledge of mammography debates and guidelines was low among the majority of the women I interviewed regardless of class status, so I hesitate to draw that conclusion based on my limited data.

Conscious Skepticism

A small handful of patients among those I interviewed did actively avoid screening; however, their decision to do so was not a reaction to a state of confusion. In fact, looking across the entire sample of women age forty to fifty, these were among the most knowledgeable about the screening conflict. These *conscious skeptics* were not so much "avoiding" screening, then, as they were consciously "abstaining" from it, as all had well-developed reasons for their choices. Christina, for example, who is forty-three, white, unemployed, and has never had a mammogram, grew concerned about overdiagnosis and overtreatment after recently watching a friend and coworker suffer through treatment. She refers to the statistically small number of patients whose lives are saved by mammography in light of the much larger number who must be screened. In her opinion, many more women are overdiagnosed and overtreated due to mammography than are saved. As she puts it, "I don't want to go through years of suffering for those two cases in however many whose lives might be saved by it." Eva also chooses not to have mammograms, but again, like Christina, this is not because she is irrationally avoidant but because she has well-defined concerns about the harms of screening. Here she describes some of these concerns: "I have put out calls on local listservs and stuff asking for anybody that knows someone who follows what I understand to be the science, which is, 'We can't save your life with this mammogram and we are exposing you to, um, to radiation,' not to mention physical pain, not to mention I personally put a lot of stock in the problem of false positives because I have had bad experiences with that myself."

Eva's prior negative experience with screening increased her attention to potential risks within the cultural context of faith in screening, which made her more conscious and knowledgeable about the balance of screening's benefits and harms. This illustrates the finding by Rozbroj and his colleagues (2021, 9) that "participants who believed they had been overdiagnosed had a stronger conceptual understanding and more complex evaluations of overdiagnosis." The conscious skeptic patients in my study reflected this more complex understanding by fluently expressing the counterintuitive idea that early detection is not always totally beneficial or benign:

I don't think that early detection is necessarily better than not knowing if you had lived the same amount of time. And early detection is bad if it causes treatment that won't extend your life. So I am very skeptical of early detection, I guess. (Eva, forty-three-year-old white editor who has never had a mammogram)

I think there are a lot of people that are just looking at it as a positive net gain. Like, "What can it hurt? It might possibly save you from cancer. It might possibly save a whole bunch of people from cancer." And the people that are out there that are saying, "Hey, you know there were false positives," or "This early detection detected a cancer that was slow growing or not necessarily terribly malignant and didn't need to be treated so aggressively." Um, and now later now this woman now has another form of cancer and her treatment options are limited because of the aggressive treatment of the earlier cancer and now she is going to die anyway. And those people could go, "Well, do you really know that? All we really know is that we saved her from cancer ten years ago. Yay, us! And we're really sorry now." (Celeste, forty-one-year-old white editor who has never had a mammogram)

In summary, most of the patients I interviewed fell into one of four attentional types: default interventionism, conscious interventionism, conflicted skepticism, and conscious skepticism. The majority were default interventionists. This reflects their internalization of the broader culture of faith in screening and early detection. It also aligns with and reinforces prior research that has found that while laywomen's knowledge about mammography guidelines and the conflict that surrounds them is generally low, they tend to respond negatively to recommendations that reduce the frequency or push back the starting point for mammography. I also find support for the skeptic doctors' and physicians' characterization of patients as very fearful of breast cancer and for their arguments that it is that fear that drives many women to seek screening, contributing to the screening paradox. Reframed in the terms of the attentional types I am proposing, one effect of the screening paradox and the broader culture of fear is to make some default interventionists into more conscious, active interventionists. One nuance my analysis adds, however, is that fear can also make default interventionists into conflicted skeptics or even conscious skeptics, depending on their experiences with breast cancer and screening, in a process of attentional autobiographical alignment. An attentional shift to conflicted skepticism was illustrated in examples of patients who, despite feeling skeptical of screening and finding no comfort in it, continued to get screened.

Conscious skeptics in many cases actually feared screening more than breast cancer due to prior negative experiences with false-positive results.

Attentional Diversity: Attentional Exclusions, Doctor-Patient Interaction, and Attentional Deviance

One of the most significant benefits of attention as an analytical framework is that it can reveal the constitutive exclusions—or *patterns of inattention*—of any perspective or interpretation. One example of such an exclusion is the way that neither the interventionist nor the skeptic medical experts acknowledged the possibility of conscious skepticism and conflicted skepticism as relevant perspectives among patients. Several additional themes prominent in the patients' narratives were absent from the characterizations of the medical professionals and researchers I interviewed. The first is a prevailing lack of trust in the experts that was widely shared among the patients I spoke with.

Almost all of the patients I interviewed across all four attentional types expressed anger and frustration over the very existence of the disagreement about screening women in their forties. In reacting to my summary of the conflict, many raised the issue of what they perceive as conflicts of interest, pointing out that mammography is a for-profit service, which naturally leads to reluctance among radiologists to reduce screening:

> I do have enough of a cynical streak that I think that the people who make money off of the tests, particularly with our medical system that is so oriented towards making money, the people making money off of the tests make more money if women are given them earlier in their lives and more frequently. (Celeste, forty-one-year-old white editor who has never had a mammogram)
>
> They're looking at their bottom line. (Tamara, forty-three-year-old white actuary who has had two or three mammograms)
>
> I hate to say this, but I feel like it's true. I feel like sometimes I think a lot of it has to do with money. (Jennifer, forty-six-year-old Black mental healthcare worker who has had four or five mammograms)

A few patients mentioned financial conflicts of interest working in the reverse way, raising concerns that the growing cost of medical care is likely why governmental organizations are trying to pull back or withhold mammograms (Catherine, Jennifer, Rochelle). Other patients noted they are not particularly surprised by the lack of agreement among experts. For example, Christina (forty-three, white, unemployed, has never had a mammogram) feels that "people are just going to believe who they want to believe anyway," and Vivian (forty-two-year-old white school librarian) believes that "any of it is sort of a guess at this point, right? Because they're all giving different guidelines." Allison (fifty, white, professor, has had two or three mammograms) says she "expects no consistency," but then reflects on how that impacts patients: "I expect no consistency at that level almost. . . . At the same time, just as sort of the lived experience of it, I think you take all this competing information and go, 'Oh, f_ck that! Nobody knows what's right. I'm just going to do what's right for me.'"

Such cynical reactions were not limited to patients with either interventionist or skeptical leanings. For example, Allison is someone who emphasized early detection as essential. Christina, on the other hand, is more skeptical. At forty-three, she has not yet had a mammogram, and she plans to wait until age fifty. She was able to provide informed summaries of the concept of overdiagnosis, the harms of screening, and the minimal impact of screening on the breast cancer mortality rate. Similarly, accusations of conflicts of interest were issued in both directions—at radiologists who were seen as benefitting from the promotion of mammography beyond its demonstrated effectiveness, as well as at the organizations suggesting that less mammography is better, who were accused of using cost savings rather than patient outcomes as their primary goal. For example, on the one hand, some patients expressed frustration with what Kelly, the forty-six-year-old white journalist who has had two or three mammograms, calls the "mammogram industrial complex," by which she seemed to mean the many medical technologies, specialists, scientific research programs, lobbyists, awareness campaigns, and radiology facilities devoted to mammography and mammography promotion. Eva expresses frustration over her difficulty finding a practitioner who is honest and knowledgeable about the disagreement over age-based screening guidelines; instead, it seems most are content to simply push patients to be screened because that is what they have traditionally done: "I guess I am still frustrated that I can't find a doctor who goes, 'Okay, reasonable people disagree on this.' . . . Um, and I guess I am a little suspicious of the organizations that have the same sort of intractability. Um, the same sort of desire to stick with whatever they've done thus far."

At the same time, other patients express frustration that the medical establishment may be pulling back and withholding screening. Nicole provides one example of this reaction: "I don't think women should have to wait. . . . It's just like a lot of arm-twisting and, to couple that with the anxiety, it's just a lot of energy that I think that women shouldn't have to put forth."

One consistent thread within these expressions of frustration and lack of trust is that the lack of expert consensus felt unjust to many of the patients I spoke with in a specifically gendered way. The comments within this theme reference the social marginalization of women as reflected in medicine, and the exclusion of consideration of women's embodied experiences. Eva, for example, says that for her "there is like this sort of general question about how medicine treats women that all this triggers." Joanne makes a similar point: "Like my sarcastic side, I guess, wants to say, 'They can sure get a pill out for a man, you know, for—there's not a—nice way to say—but for a hard on.' They can sure agree and get that to market, you know, but no one can agree like on women's health." Further, participants with very different takes on mammography made similar references to gender. Nicole, for example, feels that the change in guidelines resembles healthcare rationing and that women should be allowed to start screening sooner, as reflected in the comment quoted previously that she does not think women "should have to wait" until they are fifty. She connects this with gender inequalities in health care when she states, "I don't know that it feels like it's women making these decisions for these guidelines necessarily." On the other hand, Eva is the participant who proclaimed herself "very skeptical of early detection." Yet both feel that the disagreement emanates in some significant way from gender inequality.

Several patients connect these feelings of gendered neglect or injustice to the embodied experience of getting a mammogram. One example is Nancy, who says she feels like her body is not fully considered during the screening process. She describes the technician as putting "some extra cranks on that machine." She also perceives the entire design of the technology as not taking into account women's actual bodies: "Like is there any way we could think of something that's cone shaped or conical rather than square flat things smooshing it?" This resonates with the other participants' comments above that medicine would have resolved debates about mammography already if men were the ones directly impacted and that it does not feel like women are the ones making decisions about mammography. In this vein, it is also interesting to note the total absence of talk about women's embodied experience of mammography as relevant in the interviews with doctors and medical researchers. Among the patients I interviewed, in contrast, over half raised the issue of how mammography physically feels. Some, like Nancy above, find the procedure very painful, and this contributes to their anxieties about getting screened. Samantha is another example. She tends to have low blood pressure and worries she might faint from the pain. Other participants pointed to the pain of the procedure as one reason they prefer the revised, less frequent guideline, suggesting that it is an important factor in their decisions about whether to get a mammogram:

> There are people who feel like the recommendation should stay at forty. Um, and those people would want me to get my breasts squished, so I'm not listening to those people. (Celeste)
>
> I would prefer doing it every two years because it hurts so much. (Jodi)
>
> I mean I just feel like two is good. That's just me. Because I feel it's a lot of pressure and discomfort on you. (Jennifer)

Not all of the patients I spoke with found mammograms as painful as these remarks suggest, however. In fact, four participants (Chyna, Abby, Frances, Joanne) told me the experience was less painful than they anticipated.

In short, patients on both sides of the screening debate expressed that they do not feel fully heard, accepted, or supported by their doctors or the medical establishment more generally. Among many of the patients I interviewed, then, there was a clear sentiment that their doctors' patterns of attention were out of sync with their wishes and concerns, even if they felt that way for different reasons. This was true regardless of whether they were seeking more mammograms or fewer, although patients concerned about overdiagnosis and the risks of mammography seemed to feel most acutely that their beliefs and perceptions were not in concordance with those of their doctors. This sense of *attentional dissonance* was also observed in the undercurrent of comments about how frustrating it was for patients that the profession lacks consensus about mammography and about the specifically gendered framework in which many participants situated the conflict, such as those patients who felt that this debate would have been long resolved if men's bodies and lives were at stake. Patients who were very fearful and wanted more aggressive testing also expressed that what the debates signified for them was that the medical establishment was trying to pull back on screening and may even view patients like them derisively. Those most likely to express that they experience *attentional conflict* with their doctors and feel more generally *attentionally marginalized* and socially ostracized for their views, however, were the participants who were the most skeptical of mammography. These patients often felt socially isolated, unable to share their feelings about mammography with friends and family. They also at times shared that they had difficulty locating a doctor who was open to their skepticism and followed the USPSTF guidelines.

These findings are consistent with prior literature identifying dissonance between doctors' and patients' patterns of relevance and attention as an important source of patient dissatisfaction, which I touched on in chapter 1 (Hesse-Biber 2014; Hunter 1991). Specifically in relation to screening, Silverman et al. (2001, 238) found that women's "mental model" of cancer differed from doctors': "Women and experts valued the potential harms of screening differently," they explain, such that doctors tend to be more skeptical of cancer screening than patients. Of course, this does not reflect the experiences of skeptic patients who are interacting with interventionist doctors. Further, recall that the vast majority of my participants reported that their doctors had never discussed the risks of screening with them. More closely reflecting this experience, Welch, Schwartz, and Woloshin (2011, 190) argue that doctors' default assumption is that most people want to be screened. This creates resistance for patients who prefer less testing because they have to question their doctors' default, taken-for-granted beliefs: "Disagreeing with a doctor who is suggesting more diagnosis can be challenging. Some people may feel too intimidated to say no when offered a test. They may be afraid of making their doctors mad, of being called (or feeling) irresponsible, and they may worry that they will come to regret the decision in the future" (188).

On a related note, Sulik (2009) argues that certain ways of engaging with medical technologies (including mammography) can help bridge such gaps of perspective between patients and providers. Patients' beliefs receive more legitimacy when they are cast in technoscientific terms that correspond with expert/medical knowledge (1069). On the other hand, patients' perspectives can be received as a threat to medical authority and dismissed when they do not conform with those of providers, even when they are exceptionally well informed. This phenomenon was illustrated in the experiences described by Christina and Eva, the conscious skeptics I discussed in the previous section.

Despite being two of the most well-informed participants about mammography guidelines and the varying recommendations, Christina and Eva both describe feeling that their doctors were dismissive when they raised questions about them. They also understand themselves as what I call *attentional deviants* when it comes to mammography—people who are isolated and out of step from the broader culture in ways that lead to tension and conflict with others and to feelings of discomfort discussing their beliefs and decisions. Christina, for example, says her mother disagrees with her so strongly that they cannot even discuss mammography; in fact, she says she doesn't know "anyone else who feels this way about it." Other women she knows "just see it as something you do." Eva similarly describes feeling detached from her peer group on this issue. She says that she tries to be understanding and accepting of her friends "who feel they should get mammograms, which is most of them" but also describes worrying about whether she will have to have an uncomfortable conversation with a friend who was recently diagnosed with breast cancer about why she does not have mammograms. An additional example is Celeste, who, like Christina, reports that her views on mammography are a source of conflict with her mother: "She has wrung her hands, and gone, 'Why would you do that [not get a mammogram]?'" Like the other skeptical participants, she describes feeling socially isolated in her views.

Perhaps because they do not feel that their views are widely shared or well accepted socially, such participants tend individualize their attentionally deviant perspective by calling it "quirky," or saying "it's just me, but . . ." For example, Kelly refers to the "quirks of how I feel about doctors," Celeste says it is "based on my own personal belief system," and Eva clarifies that "this is just a thing about me. . . . And I can't make that judgment for other people." This tendency to individualize their beliefs as "just a thing about me" rather than a reasonable, well-informed response to the current conflict over guidelines (despite the fact, as mentioned previously, that these participants are probably the most well informed on the scientific disagreements) emanates directly from their feeling of being out of step with their peers and the broader cultural climate, which they perceive as pro-mammography. This not only detracts from the validity and strength of their position but also demonstrates the resistance to change created by hegemonic collective sentiments such as early detection and the sense of isolation experienced by individuals with socially deviant attentional patterns.

The aim of this chapter was twofold: first, to center the voices of the women age forty to fifty, about whom most of the debate among experts in the mammography conflict is purported to be concerned; and second, to examine whether patients' narratives of mammography track with the two primary attention types organizing the conflict in the medical field, interventionism and skepticism, or whether patients' patterns of relevance and focus offer an attentional counterpoint to the patterns of focus structuring the scientific conflict. Most patients I spoke with were default interventionists. They were not really aware of the conflict over mammography, although some had a vague notion of overdiagnosis, and many were clearly influenced by broader cultural discourses of health and prevention, specifically early detection. In this sense, their patterns of attention overlapped with those organizing the debates among experts only in a very general way. There is significant support present in the patients' narratives, however, for the claims of skeptical doctors and scientists about widespread fear of cancer and the screening paradox driving women to seek screening and to respond negatively to any suggestion that early detection is not imperative. I offer the following refinements of this argument through my analysis of attention and autobiographical alignment: While most patients started out as default interventionists, in many cases the autobiographical experience of the screening paradox—the increasing presence of breast cancer in their lives—created cognitive and attentional shifts that heightened their interventionism, making them more active in seeking screening and thus moving them from a default interventionist pattern to a conscious interventionist pattern.

For a smaller subset of women, however, prior negative experiences with screening introduced skepticism into their attentional pattern rather than crystallizing interventionism. Conflicted skepticism emerged when default interventionism was not fully abandoned, whereas conscious skepticism was observed when the challenge to early detection paradigms was more thorough and transformative. Importantly, neither the distinction between conflicted and conscious skepticism nor that between default and conscious interventionism is fully captured by the binary opposition between interventionism and skepticism among experts. This relates to an additional prominent idea expressed by the patients I interviewed that was not reflected in the medical debates: feeling cynical and mistrustful of doctors. Some of this emanated specifically from a feeling of gendered injustice—that women are not being considered appropriately in the debates—but more generally, many patients expressed feeling attentionally out of sync with their doctors, and this was the case regardless of their beliefs about mammography guidelines.

In this chapter I have explored how the patterns of attention and concern among the patients I interviewed compare with those organizing debates among experts, illustrating attentional diversity and mapping out the attentional roots of not just the conflict among experts but also of tensions between doctors and patients. Having done that, in the chapters that follow I return to foregrounding an analysis of how the attentional norms of interventionism and skepticism function to animate and sustain the mammography conflict among experts. Where relevant, I weave patients' narratives throughout the book to provide support or illustrate an attentional alternative or connection. First, in chapter 3, I recast disagreements over mammography as an attentional battle, highlighting heightened emotion, rhetorical maneuvering, and accusations of conflicts of interest. Through this focus I demonstrate that by analyzing how each group pays attention we can more deeply understand the cognitive mechanisms by which the emotion of the conflict is intensified, and through which the two groups differentiate themselves and discredit the validity of the other side's norms of attention and relevance. In chapter 4 I discuss how each attentional type differentially weighs key concerns in the debate, such as the most relevant expertise for evaluating mammography (clinical versus population data), the importance of treatment versus early detection, or the avoidance of death versus the quality of life, and I illustrate how these value weightings are deployed as an attentional strategy to discredit the other. In chapter 5, my focus shifts to the different conceptions of temporality created by skeptical versus interventionist patterns of attention, manifesting, for example, in notions of early versus late detection and debates about age cut points, which I frame as an additional battle strategy in the attentional conflict over mammography.

Chapter 3

Attentional Battles over Mammography

In this chapter I reframe disagreements over mammography as an "attentional battle" (Zerubavel 2015, 57), or a conflict over how both popular and scientific attention should be focused. Because relevance is socially defined, such seemingly basic questions as whether a detail, concept, or piece of evidence should be considered relevant and attended are often sources of significant conflict. In an effort to support the validity of one attentional pattern, such disputes often involve *attentional differentiation*, or efforts to polarize positions through emphasizing differences in attentional focus. The salience of attention to differentiation is illustrated in the social problems literature in the concept of *claimsmaking*, which involves emphasizing some aspects of a potential social problem but not others and promoting some causes and solutions while excluding others (Best 2017, 9). Along with differentiation, attentional battles typically also involve *attentional discrediting* through claims of "correct" and "incorrect" focus as well as the establishment of "attentional taboos" (Zerubavel 2015, 60) and forms of "attentional deviance" (Zerubavel 2018, 59). *Attentional battle* as an analytical focus thus draws out instances where relevance is contested, with differences in attention called upon to polarize a disagreement, or where one group attempts to marginalize or discredit another's attentional norms.

The concept of attentional battle offers a number of distinctive analytical benefits for analyzing cultural conflicts. First, as just alluded to, attentional battles are by definition multiperspectival, or there would be no basis for dispute. Analyses of attentional conflicts are thus intrinsically comparative, taking into account a diversity of possible interpretations. As such, approaching something as an attentional battle also facilitates diffractive analysis (i.e., analysis focused on juxtaposing differences) of each side's constitutive exclusions, or patterns of inattention. As I have emphasized throughout, the sociology of attention takes as a starting point that all attention presupposes inattention, and further that what is not attended in any interpretation is both empirically larger and arguably more socially significant than what is selected for focus. This is both because we are typically unaware of our patterns of attentional exclusion, and because, as Barad (2007, 214) argues, exclusions represent interpretive openness and "foreclose the possibility of determinism." A sincere engagement with exclusions across differences of perspective thus aims to cultivate a humbler awareness of and accountability for one's own patterns of inattention.

Further, rather than treating any one perspective in isolation, the concept of attentional battle directs focus to the rhetorical and cognitive organization of a conflict as a whole, allowing for recognition of, among other things, the *attentional relationships* among polarized patterns of attention; this can include, for example, identifying instances where formally similar attention patterns and norms are used by each side, but with totally different content and objectives. A focus on attentional relationships can also reveal attentional hierarchies and contingencies in which some ideas serve as foundational filters or attentional anchors that fundamentally structure the attention patterns of the conflict as a whole. In the case of the attentional battle over mammography, as I suggested in chapter 1, early detection functions as such a foundational filter, defining the patterns of attention on other topics (e.g., how one understands the USPSTF change of recommendation). Such a focus on the attentional relationships comprising the attentional map of a conflict as a whole thus also reveals *layers of anchored attention*. For example, although skeptics' and traditionalists' interpretations of the USPSTF guidelines are contingent upon their view of early detection, these interpretations in turn anchor other patterns of attention (e.g., how they perceive the number of organizations supporting each guideline, or how the quality of the evidence is understood), as I will illustrate in this chapter.

Finally, a focus on attentional battles allows for a clearer delineation of two conceptually distinct dimensions of cultural conflicts—*battles over attention* and *battles for attention*. Battles *over* attention are disputes over *how* to pay attention, as exemplified by the idea of attentional discrediting. At the same time, attentional battles are also struggles *for* attentional dominance, or competitions for public exposure and acceptance of one's viewpoint. Battles for attention are similar in many ways to *framing contests* as previously studied in the context of social movement scholarship. The concept of "framing" was primarily popularized by Goffman (1974, 21), who defined frames as cognitive structures that serve as "schemata of interpretation." Beginning in the 1980s, frame analysis was used to advance a constructionist approach to social movements that emphasized the cognitive interpretations used by participants (Benford and Snow 2000; Ruiz-Junco 2013; Snow et al. 2014; Snow and Benford 1988). The development of this approach has generated a rich conceptual vocabulary related to framing processes (for a review of these concepts, see Benford and Snow 2000), of which the most relevant to the present discussion is *framing contests*. Opposing camps in a "framing contest" (Ryan 1991) frame and reframe reality through developing and promoting "counterframes" (Benford 1987), or rival discourses on reality. These framing contests are processes of "meaning work," which Benford and Snow (2000, 613) describe as "the struggle over the production of mobilizing and counter mobilizing ideas and meanings." In this way, the conceptual vocabulary of framing contests acts as a reminder that social movements are as much about publicly promoting a particular set of meanings as they are about motivating action, and over the past several decades, social movement scholars have accordingly devoted greater focus to meaning making in social movements.

This work has effectively highlighted metamessages that social movement actors use to define an issue as deserving or undeserving of attention, but it has generally stopped short of analyzing the organization of attention *within* a particular social movement frame. This lack of focus on patterns of attention within a frame may emanate in part from the conceptual structure of the frame metaphor itself. For instance, as I have argued previously, although frame offers a clear metaphorical representation of "in" (attention) and "out" (inattention), it also suggests that the attended and inattended are separated by a metaphorical border or boundary (the frame), as opposed to interwoven within a given interpretive space (Friedman 2013, 27). This representation conceptually isolates the attended from the inattended, as opposed to understanding them as interconnected, which is a primary reason I argue for filter analysis as opposed to frame analysis. Murray Davis (1983, 285) makes a similar argument when he explains why he chose to use "filter" as opposed to "frame" in his typology of sexual worldviews: "The term 'frame' directs the reader's attention to the different organizations of experience within and without a boundary. I prefer the term 'filter,' which directs attention to the modifications experience undergoes as it passes through a contextual scheme."

In addition to encapsulating the analytical benefits of the filter metaphor over frame, Davis's comment also helps to illustrate a key reason it is beneficial to distinguish between battles for attention and battles over attention. While battles for attention emphasize legitimation contests between filters, focusing on their outward-facing attempts to gain attention and discredit one another, battles *over* attention highlight the organization of attention *within* a particular worldview or movement frame, clarifying the underlying internal nuances of attentional filtration; this can illuminate why a particular frame may have been applied in the first place, as well as the attentional relationships among otherwise seemingly opposed perspectives, among other insights.

In addition to more clearly differentiating conceptually between battles for attention and battles over attention, the concept of attentional battle also provides a new approach to understanding the emotional intensity of cultural conflicts. Battles over attention and battles for attention are both fundamentally about what is selected for focus, and what is deemed "irrelevant" and ignored or dismissed; attentional battles thus frequently involve a sense that attention is being offered and withdrawn, won and lost, which can heighten emotional tensions: "Whichever criteria are applied, selection will always entail a wide range of possibilities not realized, actions not carried out, issues left unaddressed, and people not getting their turn. The sheer impossibility of simultaneously paying attention to all existing events, things, and people makes attention a rare commodity, and, by consequence, also accounts for the fact that from attention, competition ensues—competition in which there are winners and losers, for a gain in attention for A is a loss of attention for B" (Schroer 2019, 4). Thus, one further benefit of analysis in terms of attentional battle is that it can help identify the attentional roots of some of the heightened emotion of cultural conflicts.

This chapter examines how the interventionist and skeptic doctors and scientists I interviewed engaged in attentional battle—differentiating themselves through references to attention and relevance, and discrediting or marginalizing the other side's attentional norms. I also look at how each side characterized media representations of mammography, tracking their discussions of the struggles for attention faced by interventionism and skepticism. Given that the media is often viewed as "setting the attentional agenda" for the broader public (Zerubavel 2018, 70), competitions for attention frequently focus on media representation and involve claims about which attentional patterns are selected for media focus and which are left out. Using a content analysis of news reporting on mammography in four high-circulation publications, I then contextualize the participants' claims about how the media has portrayed mammography by examining whether media attention has in fact been more favorable to one side or the other. First, however, I begin with the topic of emotion, because part of what makes something an attentional *battle*, as I just alluded to, is that disagreement is impassioned. Indeed, anger and frustration are palpable in disagreements over mammography. What I hope to accomplish through examining this emotion through the lens of attention is to reveal some of what fuels the high emotions of the debate, offering an opportunity for deeper mutual understanding and more effective communication—and perhaps ultimately even a path toward resolution to the conflict.

Attention and Emotion in the Mammography Wars

The twenty-nine physicians and medical researchers I interviewed consistently described debates over breast screening guidelines as both emotionally charged and highly polarized. In fact, Dr. Malcolm, a surgeon and epidemiologist, believes mammography screening is "the most polarized and emotional issue in contemporary oncology and perhaps even contemporary medicine," and to Dr. Light, a radiologist and professor, the conflict is "as widely polarizing as any topic in medicine that I am aware of. It is extremely emotional, personal, and I think, unfortunately, societally divisive." Some interventionist participants even directly state that they feel personally attacked by the screening recommendations coming out of the USPSTF, which they perceive as sending the message that "what I do is not only worthless but harmful" (Dr. Cashman, radiologist). Emotion runs particularly high in such feelings of insult and dismissal by the Task Force's revised recommendations and in the frequent interventionist descriptions of working "in the trenches" with breast cancer patients, "saving lives."

For some, the intensity of the conflict over mammography has led to fatigue and even disengagement from dialogue. For example, Dr. Franklin, a primary care physician and researcher, admits: "Quite frankly, I get tired of breast cancer. It's a very sort of dangerous place to be, if you will, as a researcher." Dr. Light, the radiologist and professor quoted previously on how divisive this debate has been, describes a "rampant fatigue" around the issue of mammography due to the lengthy and contentious debates that never seem to advance:

> We don't want to hear about it. We don't want to have another presentation on this stuff.... This rampant fatigue—a combination of words that I think somewhat antithetical: rampant fatigue—about this topic. Because it's tiring.... We're tired of this debate, and we're tired of the counterpoints, and we don't even want to hear about it anymore. That's how emotional this has become. So I think there's a—almost a sense of this fatigue factor suppressing, interfering, obstructing further dialogue because it doesn't seem to be an avenue to get minds to meet on this.

Dr. Light portrays the conflict over mammography as having become uncomfortably stagnant—a deadlock of perspectives that seems unable to be resolved—in part due to the divisiveness and emotionality one faces when trying to engage.

A number of participants, including Dr. Malcolm and Dr. Kraft, made the additional point that one reason the conflict is so heated and the dividing lines so immovable is that the debates are about something other than the data:

> There is complete polarization.... I can only deduce from this polarization that we're dealing with ideology and not data. (Dr. Malcolm, epidemiologist and former breast surgeon)
>
> I was struck by how polarized they were because... there was a vast... quantity of evidence, and the idea, you know, you can imagine lots of arguments when there is not much evidence. But when there is a huge amount of evidence, it seems surprising that there would be so much argument. You'd think the evidence would kill the argument. But absolutely not. That was what was surprising: how polarized the debate was, given how extensive the evidence was.... So it was actually a very interesting example of how you would like to think that the data would settle the argument, and it didn't. The prior positions were too entrenched. (Dr. Kraft, epidemiologist)

One of the contributions the sociology of attention can potentially offer to the mammography debates is to help clarify what underlies this highly emotional polarization of perspectives if not disagreements about the scientific data. By bringing to light the different organizing beliefs and patterns of attention behind the conflict, it may also begin to unlock the entrenched positions, despite the high emotion involved.

I divide the discussion that follows into two sections: conflicts *over* attention, and competitions *for* attention. When discussing conflicts over attention, I draw out the contrasting norms of attention each side uses to differentiate themselves and polarize the debates, as well as how attention is used to discredit and marginalize through claims that the other side is using the "wrong" framework for attention. In discussion of competition for attention, the focus shifts to the recognition and attention skeptics and interventionists feel each perspective receives in the media and other outlets for the public dissemination of ideas. As part of this discussion, I also present the results of a content analysis of news reporting on mammography to provide context for their claims.

Conflicts *over* Attention

Attention requires differentiation, as it is not possible to notice or select something that cannot be separated out from other attentional options (Zerubavel

2015, 26). Thus, contrasts and discontinuity necessarily underlie attention, and efforts to emphasize and increase such contrasts—through *attentional polarization*—are central to the work of an attentional battle. In what follows, I use the example of how skeptics and interventionists describe the USPSTF and the 2009 change to the Task Force's mammography guidelines to illustrate this attentional work of differentiation and polarization. As I have already suggested, while interpretations of the USPSTF are contingent on how skeptics and interventionists view the foundational idea of early detection, how one makes meaning of the USPSTF is in turn an attentional anchor for other key distinctions in the attentional battle over mammography.

Attentional Polarization: Characterizations of the USPSTF

The 2009 USPSTF guideline change is a primary focus of debates over mammography. Participants' view of this change informs the organization of their attention, and the patterns of relevance and focus they promote. Interventionists typically seek to discredit the USPSTF guideline, often through references to expertise—that is, *expert organizations* all recommend earlier screening—or else by pointing out the smaller number of organizations supporting the USPSTF change (i.e., the USPSTF is the *only one* who differs; *everyone else* recommends retaining the earlier recommendation). Dr. Jones, a radiologist, draws together the themes of expertise and number when she explains her position in the screening-age debate:

> I will say what my professional opinion is first, which is supported by the American College of Radiology, American Cancer Society, American College of Surgeons, Society of Breast Imaging, and so on I could go. But basically starting at age forty and yearly after that. . . . And that is based on Level 1 scientific evidence, and it's, you know, what I have been taught and practiced for the past twenty years. . . . But those of us in breast imaging know that younger women tend to get more aggressive cancers, so it doesn't make sense to screen them less often. We're hoping to catch them earlier.

Echoing Dr. Jones' refrain of "and on I could go," Dr. Andrews, an ob-gyn and breast health specialist, states that the question of age "is probably the biggest area of controversy between the guidelines of ACOG and American College of Surgeons and American College of Radiology and American Cancer Society [Dr. Andrews laughs here, seemingly in response to the long list]—and the U.S. Preventive Services Task Force."

Many interventionists focus their criticisms of the USPSTF on the point that there were no specialists in breast cancer on the panel charged with debating the merits of mammography, with the result that their recommendation was based "only" on computer modeling and "the subjective opinion of the panel members, none of whom had any expertise in caring for women with cancer" (Dr. Adams, radiologist). Dr. Cashman, also a radiologist, similarly argues that the panel did not include any "experts in the field":

> There is a lot of things wrong with their, um, analysis and their conclusions. The first thing that is wrong is that there are sixteen members of this Task Force: about twelve physicians and the rest were, uh, nurses, or nurse practitioners or other researchers. And of the twelve physicians, seven of them were either internal medicine doctors or family practice doctors. None were radiologists that do what I do, that screen and diagnose breast cancer. None were surgeons and do breast surgery, and none were oncologists or other specialists that take care of breast cancer patients. And so they had no experts in the field on this panel.

In terms of attention, interventionists thus stress that in evaluating which guideline to follow, what is relevant to attend is how many organizations support the guideline, and whether those organizations represent the opinions of specialists in breast cancer.

Rather than the number of organizations, skeptics emphasize the quality of scientific evidence supporting each recommendation. They also argue for attending to international comparisons to assess the USPSTF recommendation. For example, skeptics point out that the USPSTF issues guidelines only after a careful scientific process of evaluating the state of the research, whereas other organizations (even if more numerous) are not held to as stringent a scientific standard. As Dr. Price, a clinical oncologist with additional training in public health, puts it: "The Task Force uses a different process, you know, a more formal process of systematic evidence review." Dr. Jackson, a family medicine doctor and academic researcher in public health, similarly contrasts the "evidence-based" process of the USPSTF with what he disparagingly refers to as a "consensus-based" process used by some other organizations: "a lot of organizations out there including medical organizations that do not do evidence-based guidelines and they basically just do, you know, what's called consensus-based guidelines, so basically just a bunch of guys sitting around a table saying what they personally think." In addition to using a more strictly scientific process of evidence review, skeptics pointed to the differing standards or criteria by which various organizations judge mammography to be successful, emphasizing that from a scientific standpoint, just finding a cancer (detection rates) is not adequate. It is necessary to demonstrate a positive impact on mortality rates: "Different organizations use different standards making their recommendations. For the American Cancer Society and particularly those who advise them, the mere fact that you find an early cancer is sufficient to say, 'This is adequate for screen.' But organizations like the U.S. Preventive Services Task Force recognize that that's not the way you evaluate whether screening is effective, but whether or not you can demonstrate that screening results in reduction in deaths from breast cancer. They use more strict criteria and are more careful in assessing the evidence" (Dr. Michaels, academic researcher specializing in cancer).

In addition to arguing that the USPSTF uses more scientific standards of evidence than other organizations, skeptics also compared the United States to other countries, pointing out that far more mammograms are performed in the United States than in other comparable nations, and thus that the USPSTF change brings the country into closer alignment with international consensus (although even the revised guideline is more aggressive than most, it turns out). Dr. Light, who is a radiologist, stresses that the age forty guideline "is the world's most aggressive by a margin. We do more mammograms per person than anywhere in the world by a huge difference. Even those who promote mammography the most, like Sweden, do a third to half of what—well, a half to two thirds what we do." Dr. Price, the clinical oncologist and public health expert quoted previously on the USPSTF's stringent process of evidence review, similarly uses international comparisons to support the soundness of the USPSTF's guideline change and to argue that those who wish to retain the more aggressive standard are out of step with international consensus:

> The U.S. tends to have quite different guidelines than the rest of the developed world and Western countries. In contrast with most countries, many of our organizations in the United States, save one—well, not save one, save more than one. But many of our organizations recommend regular screening in women from age forty on. The U.S. Preventive Services Task Force, however, currently ... doesn't recommend screening for women in their forties, but does recommend routine screening beginning at age fifty. That's a little bit more in concert with other Western nations, which tend to start screening at age fifty.... The Task Force is currently much more aligned with the majority of recommendations around the world.

The intention of such comments about international consensus, as with their arguments above about focusing on more stringent forms of scientific evidence, is to emphasize and polarize the different norms of attention used by skeptics and interventionists.

However, when engaged in this process of attentional differentiation, as can already be seen in this series of examples, interventionists and skeptics are not only showing that they use *different* norms of attention and relevance. They are also arguing that the other is focusing attention on the *wrong* things, deploying narratives of "incorrect" attention to invalidate one another. In the next section, I examine more directly these efforts to discredit and marginalize through references to attention by digging more deeply into disagreements over expertise, touched on already, as well as introducing examples of accusations of bias and conflicts of interest.

Attentional Discrediting and Marginalization: Competing Definitions of Expertise and Bias

Underlying the interventionist and skeptical positions are contrasting beliefs about the forms of expertise relevant to making recommendations about mammography screening. I have already noted that interventionists criticize the USPSTF for not including any experts in the field of radiology or the clinical treatment of breast cancer. The problem with this omission, they argue, is that it limited the panel's interpretation of the issues in a number of important ways. For example, Dr. Kramer, a family medicine doctor and director of a major cancer center, explains the necessity of a clinical perspective to really evaluate the meaning of a false-positive screening experience for a patient, as opposed to "just looking at the numbers":

> So that's where I'm coming from as a clinician is my own personal experience that I don't think they [USPSTF] have. If that false-positive was so bad, then most of the women wouldn't be coming back next year, because "I don't want to go through that again." That's my own interpretation of why I have a different value weighting and why I think a lot of clinicians have a different value weighting than does this group, which—it's just some people feel it's the best way to approach these recommendations is to have people more looking at the numbers. But I think that there's a lot of problems with just looking at the numbers because then you have taken the value weightings out of it.

The clinical "value weightings" Dr. Kramer emphasizes in her remarks are based on firsthand observations and experiences working with patients with breast cancer. This knowledge is often more about emotion and individual patients' lives than numbers and science. For example, taking into account the devastation of breast cancer in young women and weighing that adequately, regardless of what the statistics say, are the central concerns of the following comments by Dr. Andrews, an ob-gyn and breast health specialist:

> The data shows that mammograms have reduced mortality in forty-year-olds. That's very clear. So what we have to say is, you know, can we compare this and say, you know, it's of equal value to save the life of a sixty-year-old and a forty-year-old? And that's very difficult for me as an actual practitioner and probably it kind of summarizes why a lot of people like me who have taken care of a lot of breast cancer patients come down on the side that they do about this. . . . And so I think that's why we're all looking at the same data; it's just like, you know, what's the value of that life?

The emotional experience of working with cancer patients, with the feeling of life or death on the line, deeply shapes the perspectives of cancer specialist clinicians such as Dr. Kramer and Dr. Andrews, leading them to at times discount or dismiss (i.e., attentionally invalidate) statistical rationales for ones that better reflect the emotional stakes of their work of trying to save patients' lives. Dr. Shoumer, an oncologist, further illustrates this perspective: "Where many of the people in the controversy I think failed to really understand the problem is that when you save a life, that cannot possibly be compared to the anxiety of being recalled or the inconvenience of having an additional view. So I think much is being made out of comparing apples to oranges in this controversy, and of course the controversy comes largely from people who are statisticians and therefore do not see patients."

Within these discussions of the necessity of direct clinical experiences was also a clear derision toward academic scientists who "sit at a desk all day" working with numbers, as Dr. Shoumer illustrates when he remarks that there is a big difference between those working "in the trenches" with patients, "and people who sit at a desk thinking about 'What would be the level of evidence needed in order to prove without a shadow of a doubt that a hypothesis is correct or not?' . . . I think there's a serious cultural difference between those in the trenches and those, you know, thinking about perfection in clinical trials." With regard to attention, the argument being made by Dr. Shoumer and others is that population data inappropriately dominate the attention of academic researchers.

It is instructive to further distinguish ethical values from epistemological values as distinct points of differentiation and discrediting in the attentional battle over mammography. Parker, Rychetnik, and Carter (2015) specifically identify two types of values Australian experts applied in their interpretations of mammography screening programs: ethical values (e.g., ideas about benefit and harm or fairness) and epistemological values (values about the validity of different forms of evidence and analysis). As just described, the clinical value weightings applied by interventionists encompassed considerations that were both ethical (e.g., saving a life cannot be weighed equally with anxiety or inconvenience) and epistemological (e.g., you can't just look at the numbers) in nature. When articulating these different values, interventionists are performing both *attentional polarization* and *attentional discrediting*. This was also true of the skeptical participants, although the salience of epistemological values was more pronounced in their narratives.

Skeptics argued that scientific objectivity and expertise in population data analysis—not clinical work with cancer patients—are most relevant to setting screening guidelines. While clinicians may have expertise in the treatment of breast cancer, they are not experts in the interpretation of statistical data, which is, skeptics point out, the key task set before the USPSTF. It is therefore entirely appropriate that the Task Force be composed primarily of people with "expertise in evidence," and even that the debate focus "only" on the data and numbers. Dr. Jackson, a family medicine doctor and academic researcher in epidemiology, exemplifies this view: "These are almost always issues of population-based science, which really has essentially nothing to do with clinical medicine. . . . As a matter of fact, being a radiologist I think would bring you the opposite. It would actually—it would make it more difficult for you because not only do you not understand a key science that you need to understand, but you already have a bias because you're a radiologist and you know, hey, if you're a carpenter and everything looks like a hammer and a nail." Here Dr. Jackson claims that not only do radiologists not have the needed training for the task of setting medical guidelines based on population data, but their training may bias them in ways that make it uniquely difficult for them to attend to the most relevant information.

Dr. Markman, a professor of medicine and epidemiology, makes a similar argument that the form of expertise needed for the USPSTF is "critically appraising studies and synthesizing evidence" rather than "expertise in reading x-rays" or "knowing how to give chemotherapy." Not only is this not the form of evidence needed, but clinical breast cancer experts have emotional investments in the disease and their role in treatment that can make them particularly resistant to focusing on what is most relevant to the question of population screening guidelines. Many skeptical participants considered this an important form of bias (or restricted attention). Dr. Obermeyer, a family medicine doctor, shares the following anecdote to illustrate his view that the emotions of clinical practice can limit one's view of the evidence:

> And you need to be very careful. I mean I have even heard some of my colleagues here say, you know, "I know the guidelines say this, but guess what? I had a twenty-five-year-old woman who just had a mastectomy because she had pretty advanced breast cancer." Um, you know, to base a population-based screening on that one person, um, I mean, I understand where the emotions come in there. Um, from an evidence standpoint, that's just not practical and that sort of comes out with your Numbers Needed to Treat as well as Numbers Needed to Harm. Um, and looking at those specific numbers, you know, just it's not weighted towards that young woman, which is a very unfortunate, sad situation. I feel for her. But I think, "Well, where do you stop? Do you say, okay now, you know, every woman that's in their twenties that I see, I need to make sure that I am, you know, ordering mammograms on them." I mean, where do you stop?

Dr. Blakely, a primary care physician, explains that she feels the tension between population-based recommendations and clinical experience in her own practice. As she characterizes it, her clinical work with patients can sometimes "push" her "away from the data": "I am trying to form a really informed opinion of my own by really looking at the data, and you know, my clinical experience sometimes like starts to creep in and push me away from the data, and I keep coming back and trying to interpret the data to fit my population." What Dr. Blakely is describing is the tension between two very different notions of what is relevant, only one of which ("the data") she thinks is scientifically creditable and ought to be attended.

When advocating restricting attention to scientific research, skeptics repeatedly made the argument that the scientific evidence supports their view. Anyone who follows "the data," they often suggested, would be a skeptic. As Dr. Samuels, a primary care physician, puts it: "If you paid attention to the evidence" you would be a skeptic. Dr. Kraft, an epidemiologist, similarly states: "I don't know of any data that would justify saying do it [mammograms], even every two years, let alone yearly." Several participants made this same point by emphasizing that they were previously supportive of earlier screening but were ultimately "forced" by the evidence to change their view. Dr. Malcolm, an epidemiologist and breast surgeon, is one such example: "I myself was a strong proponent of mammography for a very long time. . . . And then I sort of held that view until evidence, uh, forced me to change my mind."

Skeptical and interventionist participants thus *attentionally polarized* their positions on mammography screening in part around two competing sets of epistemological values, best represented by their different conceptions of expertise—"clinical" expertise and expertise in "data science." I will have more to say about these competing foci of attention in chapter 4, when I discuss mental weighing. Here the essential point is that, when each side claims that the other *lacks the necessary expertise*, or *applies the wrong values*, to properly attend and interpret mammography, they are engaging in a process of *attentional discrediting* as part of an attentional battle.

Attentional discrediting also occurs when both skeptics and interventionists accuse the other of having problematic conflicts of interest. For instance, both attributed financial motivations to the other, with skeptics arguing that many interventionists are financially self-serving in advocating for more frequent screening, and interventionists arguing that the USPSTF (and its supporters) are motivated by a desire to cut healthcare costs in recommending reducing the frequency of screening. Dr. Jackson, a family medicine doctor, and Dr. Light, a radiologist, are illustrative of the skeptical perspective. Both argue that many of those who recommend earlier and more frequent screening stand to benefit financially from doing so:

> You have the basically the radiology groups who obviously benefit from more mammograms, the surgical groups that benefit from more women getting diagnosed because they do more surgery, and the oncology groups who obviously benefit because, you know, more women get diagnosed and they do more treatment. Um, no one really said, "Wait a minute. You know, do these people have a conflict of interest?" (Dr. Jackson)
>
> I really think there is a business no one wants to admit . . . that there is an underlying financial motive to keep doing what we're used to doing. . . . So I do think there's a suppressed or not-to-be-acknowledged factor that drives them to continue to profit financially from the business. So there's that underlying motivation. I'm sorry that it exists as far as I'm concerned. (Dr. Light)

Skeptics also emphasized that neither they nor the USPSTF benefit in the same way from being skeptics. They do not profit financially from screening or not screening. Dr. Jackson continues: "The U.S. Preventive Services Task Force has, you know, absolutely no bias coming in whatsoever. They're not an interested party. They don't benefit from doing mammograms, they don't benefit from not doing mammograms. They just completely look at the evidence and say, you know, 'Where is the weight of the evidence?'" As Dr. Markman, a professor of medicine and epidemiology, explains, the Task Force is governed by a strict conflict of interest policy that explicitly excludes anyone who could be biased by financial interests: "The Task Force has a very strong conflict of interest policy. At the very beginning of every single session, they go through every single person on the Task Force with every single topic they're going to talk about at that meeting and they say, 'Do you have any not just financial, but do you have any intellectual conflict of interest here?'"

In a related vein, Dr. France, a breast surgeon, believes that—far from benefiting him—being a mammography skeptic has in fact been professionally damaging at times: "You have to consider which side has the biggest conflict of interest. Being a screening skeptic does me no favors. I haven't made money. . . . It has been against my best interest to take this position. So there is no conflict of interest on my side. I am just a clinical scientist who goes where the data leads." Dr. Samuels, the primary care physician quoted above about the scientific support for the skeptical view, shares the following anecdote about how she counsels her patients to think about the conflicts of interest at play, which similarly emphasizes that skeptics do not benefit financially from the perspective they promote:

> When my patients say, "Well I got a letter from the radiologist saying it's time for my mammogram." And I say: "Well, the recommendation is every two years." And they say, "Well I just had one last year, but my radiologist says I need another one." And I say, "Well, the radiologist makes money every time you have a mammogram. I do not, and neither does the government. So we don't lose money and we don't gain money. We just—it just is. So try to weigh that when you're trying to decide."

Although a less prominent theme in the interventionist narratives, some participants suggest that skeptics are also biased by financial motivations, although not typically for direct personal gain; these interventionists argue that the USPSTF was interested in saving on healthcare spending and thus that they overattended to cost cutting—as opposed to patient outcomes—in their decision to change their recommendation. For example, Dr. Smith, a family medicine doctor, and Dr. Jones, a radiologist, both feel the Task Force had a goal of reducing healthcare costs:

> They're [USPSTF] looking at the cost and the overall cost and they're saying we're doing too many mammograms. I'm looking at it and saying, "I'd rather do too many mammograms and catch a breast cancer." (Dr. Smith)
>
> My hunch is that healthcare dollars are shrinking and everybody's looking for ways to cut costs. And mammography seems to be under

constant attack, and its, that's my gut feeling—I can't substantiate this any other way—but is that it's financially driven, the attacks on mammography. (Dr. Jones)

It should be noted in this context that several skeptical participants were vehement in pointing out that the USPSTF is explicitly precluded from considering cost during their analysis process. Dr. Obermeyer, another family medicine doctor, for example, raises and dismisses this critique: "I mean there's a lot of people that say, 'Well, when you factor in cost efficiency of a test, maybe you're being less sensitive to patient care issues.' Um, you know, interestingly enough, despite the USPSTF not doing that, I think a lot of people make that accusation."

Beyond such financial conflicts of interest, both sides also accused the other of having other kinds of attentional blockages and biases—intellectual biases, cognitive biases, outside influences—that limit their ability to clearly and accurately perceive certain aspects of screening or pieces of relevant evidence. For example, Dr. Jones, the radiologist and interventionist quoted previously, feels that, even if not directly benefiting financially, skeptics are motivated to pursue counterintuitive ideas about mammography as a means to advance their academic careers through publishing: "I think part of the motivation is people who are in the scholarly fields trying to advance themselves, advance their CVs, move up in professorship levels, and find a niche. . . . Because it seems like it gets published in fairly reputable journals, and it certainly gets a lot of media attention. . . . That's my gut feeling is that the motivation has to do with, uh, money and ego." Dr. Adams, another radiologist with interventionist views, feels that the members of the USPSTF were influenced by several "leaders in trying to reduce access to screening" who were not on the panel but were powerful in shaping their conclusions. "It is pretty clear that most of the USPSTF actually did not understand the data and were guided in their conclusions."

In the other direction, skeptics were very consistent in pointing out that interventionists are not only financially motivated in a direct way, but that their deep investment in the idea that mammography is good for patients has cognitively biased their attention, creating problematic blockages and exclusions. Skeptics argue that this fundamental belief in the positive contributions of mammography, which is supported by other related beliefs (e.g., in the importance of early detection), makes it deeply counterintuitive for interventionists to accept ideas about the harms of mammography—especially overdiagnosis. Dr. Freeman, a breast surgeon, exemplifies this point with a story about giving a talk about mammography to a group of radiologists and being struck by their cognitive resistance to even the most basic points he was making because he was an identified skeptic:

> I was asked to be part of this seminar and to give a talk. And I started just by saying—stating really how I—how mammography screening is thought to work. . . . And I said . . . if we don't have treatment for . . . breast cancer, there probably wouldn't be any reason to screen because it—then you would detect it earlier, but we couldn't do—you couldn't alter the state of the cancer. And right there I was stopped by a radiologist . . . an older woman. She raised her hand up and said, "I don't believe you." And I was a little bit surprised by that. And I said, "Well you don't have to believe me, but this is just the way it works. And there's no disagreement on this. This is just the way it works. We don't have—we cannot—we cannot prevent cancer by mammography screening. . . ." I think because I am skeptical to mammography screening, she didn't want to hear anything of what I said. She was blocking whatever I said, and I thought that was very, very interesting to see. And I thought, "She's probably scared that I'm going to stop her from doing her work." I mean that's all, that's what she's been trained to do. I mean, she's been doing that for the last I mean twenty years maybe, and she doesn't have anything else to fall back on.

Dr. Markman, a professor of medicine and epidemiology, also discusses interventionists' cognitive resistance to the harms of screening due to their financial interests and other beliefs:

> People have—there are certain, um, I don't know whether "conflicts of interest" is the right word, but certain ways of seeing things that are encouraged by where they sit. The American Cancer Society actually gets a fair amount of their money from people who have had breast cancer in the past or who have relatives who have had breast cancer and they—their work as to fighting breast cancer is I think one of the ways in which they continue to survive. That is, uh, part of their lifeline for funding. So they're encouraged to think in terms of every single death from breast cancer is a tragedy, and it is in a way, but what they are not as good at thinking about is the issue of diminishing return. So as you screen more and more intensively, that is screen starting at a younger age or going to an older age or screen more frequently, for example, or screen with MRIs or tomosynthesis as opposed to film screen mammography, that all those ways of screening more intensively may get you a little bit, but increasingly they start costing you more in terms not only of money, but in terms of harm caused.

At another point, Dr. Markman calls this "decision-based evidence" (as opposed to "evidence-based decisions"), which he describes as follows: "[Interventionists] do what psychologists tell us all humans do, which is they end up with a decision that they really believe in and then they pick and choose evidence that confirms what they already believe." Returning to the concept of battles over attention, the significance of such arguments about conflicts of interest and cognitive exclusions is that they are intended to invalidate the other side's attentional norms and commitments by establishing that their attention is biased by financial motivations and deeper psychological and emotional investments that lead them to apply "incorrect" standards of relevance and attention to the evaluation of mammography.

Competitions *for* Attention: Media Representations of Mammography

The focus of the preceding discussion was attempts by both skeptics and interventionists to marginalize or discredit the other as having the "wrong" focus or giving "insufficient" attention to the "truly relevant" ideas. This sometimes took the form of accusations of bias or conflicts of interest that preclude attending to the issues accurately or scientifically. Each group also extended analogous criticisms to the broader culture through discussions of media bias. For example, interventionists argue that there is an "anti-screening bias" that leads to the "wrong" focus of attention in media coverage of mammography. Such criticisms highlight another aspect of attentional battles, which is the quest for greater public and scientific recognition of one's perspective. When, for example, interventionists complain that the messages of skeptics get more media coverage, then, this is also part of the attentional battle over mammography—competition *for* attention.

It is undeniable that media play a significant role in shaping our attention, telling us what to think about and directing the public's collective focus through what is reported: "By figuratively *spotlighting* certain issues and events while downplaying or even completely ignoring others, they [media] in effect shape our collective sense of relevance, thereby basically determining what we collectively attend and inattend to. Thus, by choosing which issues and events make newspaper headlines and become the lead stories on radio and television newscasts, for example, editors and news directors actually effect what we come to consider the most important issues and events" (Zerubavel 2015, 70). This is true not only of mass media but also of academic publishing, which can be conceptualized as another attentional battleground in which the information that becomes available for scientific discussion and focus is decided.

In the interviews, skeptics and interventionists presented totally polarized accounts of the distribution of media attention and broader social recognition of debates about mammography. In brief, skeptics argued that pro-mammography messages—for example, "early detection saves lives"—have been heavily promoted for so long that as a result the skeptical viewpoint, which is a corrective to this one-sided narrative that only emphasizes the benefits of screening, is totally counterintuitive and therefore very difficult for the public to understand and accept. The cultural and media forces supporting mammography, in this view, are much stronger than the forces raising the question of the possible harms.

Dr. Freeman and Dr. Price exemplify this skeptical position, providing vivid descriptions of what they see as strong and consistent pro-mammography cultural messages:

> It has been a massive campaign sort of influencing women to undergo mammography screening, and I'm sure you're aware of the campaign back in the '70s where if you haven't had a mammogram, you should have, um, something other than your breast examined or something like that. Indicating that if you don't undergo mammography screening, you are not taking care of yourself or you might even—you might even be stupid.... And I think that the forces behind pushing women or nudging women to undergo mammography screening are much stronger than the forces who are saying, "Well, hang on a little bit. Are you sure this is something you want to do? Have you really understood the benefits and the harms?" And there are no campaigns against mammography screening, saying that women with breast cancer have their diagnosis because of mammography. (Dr. Freeman, breast surgeon)

> Until recently, most news stories have focused simply on the benefits of screening. Um, and as a matter of fact, even as the knowledge about harms accumulated, still most stories were devoted to the benefits or even anecdotes. That is, someone who is diagnosed with breast cancer and did well.... And I think that may have changed recently as messages about overdiagnosis became a little more widely known to the press. Uh, but for decades, the message has been, "The most important tool is mammography," "Mammography saves lives," and so it's been sort of over simplified, or at least rested on a narrow spectrum of information regarding the benefits and harms.... But the messages have been, I think, distilled down to sound bites and, uh, ads, that leave no room for uncertainty about the benefits and don't even mention the harms. So I think it's been

oversimplified and the medical profession has in essence gotten across messages that are quite strong. (Dr. Price, oncologist)

Both of these participants feel strongly that cultural discourse has historically been narrowly focused on the benefits of mammography and has failed to acknowledge what they believe are important and increasingly well-documented harms of screening.

Dr. Thomas, a primary care physician, similarly emphasizes that cultural discourse has strongly favored mammography—in his view in ways that exceed the scientific evidence:

> The other issue we need to explore is how we communicate about screening. So it was sold, it was oversold in the beginning, and that has gotten us in trouble as a result. . . . There were groups who were advocating for annual mammography for all people before we had evidence that it worked. And when the evidence came out and it was ambiguous, then it became—there was something wrong with mammography. Well, in fact, there was nothing wrong with mammography. What was wrong was people who were advocating with good intention ahead of the evidence. So I think that we still have to undo that damage. . . . So I think we are still suffering the consequences of what was said to be an important, clear, simple message, which was in fact an oversimplification and got us into trouble.

Fundamentally, the skeptical view is that the weight of cultural emphasis has been strongly in favor of screening for a very long time. This has involved asymmetrical attention to the benefits of mammography without acknowledging the harms.

As a result, in the battle for attention over mammography, skeptics face the not insignificant challenge of overcoming the counterintuitiveness of overdiagnosis. As alluded to several times already, overdiagnosis and the harms of screening more broadly are counterintuitive in large part because of the longstanding cultural narratives about the benefits of screening and the importance of early detection just discussed. In addition to being untenable within the dominant cultural logic, overdiagnosis is also counterfactual because basically everyone diagnosed with cancer is treated, so we do not have specific overdiagnosed individuals to point to as examples (Hofmann 2014; Rogers 2019; Rogers, Entwistle, and Carter 2019). Without confirmatory personal anecdotes, the only evidence available to support the existence of overdiagnosis lies in abstract estimates using population data. Stories of women whose "lives were saved" by screening and early treatment are incredibly powerful in focusing our attention on screening's benefits, while the narratives available to skeptics to demonstrate the harms of screening are not nearly as compelling. Of course, such personal anecdotes, which rarely capture the nuances of early detection, are also easily taken up in the media (Welch, Schwartz, and Woloshin 2011, 160).

While skeptics perceive prevailing cultural beliefs about mammography to be too simplistically focused on the benefits of mammography, uncritically promoting the logic of early detection, interventionists offered a very different narrative for how mammography is portrayed in the media and perceived in the broader culture. One of the most dominant themes in the interventionist narratives is that, as Dr. Jones, a radiologist, puts it, "mammography seems to be under constant attack." Interventionists perceive the current cultural climate as "anti-mammography" and argue that publications critical of mammography have recently dominated both the popular and medical literatures. Some further argue that many of these publications have significant methodological problems; others just feel that more "anti-screening" papers are accepted by academic journals than "pro-screening papers," and that these papers also receive disproportionate media attention. The result, they argue, is that misinformation about mammography circulates to the public, creating confusion and leaving a negative impression of mammography.

Dr. Jones, the radiologist who said mammography is under "constant attack," elaborates by arguing that mammography receives more criticism than any other screening test: "There has never been a test—a screening test that has been scrutinized the way mammography has. Certainly not colonoscopy, pap smears, even screening for—for any disease in such large, randomized control trials and multiple trials." Dr. Jones finds that mammography is held to a higher and unfair standard in the scientific community and news media, one that is more stringent than other medical tests and procedures. She feels that this creates a misperception that mammography is less trustworthy or effective than other tests, which can have undesirable consequences when relayed to consumers:

> I don't think we see any other medical test that is consistently in the news and attacked the way mammography is, whether it's lung cancer screening, colon cancer screening, hypertension, diabetes, you know, everybody just takes it for granted, or even going for a physical exam every year. No, I am not aware of any study that ever looked at, you know, took a large population of patients and had them get physical exams every year by a

primary care physician and those who didn't and see who had a lower mortality rate. It's just not, you know, it's not there. And no other—there is not another cancer screening test that's ever been done that's looked at that. Um, for colonoscopy, or pap smears, or skin cancer screening, I mean it makes inherent sense, but I rarely see anybody attacking those fields. So, it's disappointing and it's disheartening, and it's I think very, very damaging, especially to the—to the women who are on the fence about getting a mammogram, or fearful of getting a mammogram.

Unlike skeptics, who describe a decades-long and unrelenting cultural promotion of mammography, then, most interventionists seemed to think that a small group of "anti-screening" researchers are reshaping the cultural narrative with attacks on mammography that receive unwarranted media attention. Dr. Cashman, another radiologist, describes the cultural climate as follows: "There's an underlying anti-screening sort of movement with the medical literature, and then that has been picked up by the public, uh, media [which] has magnified it beyond its merit." This "anti-screening movement," he explains, is really based on the work of a small group of researchers whose work received a lot of media attention: "a couple of very vociferous and very dedicated anti-screening researchers who have gotten publications published and have gotten mainstream media to pay attention to these publications because they're sort of contrarian for one thing." He goes on to specifically single out reporter Gina Kolata of *The New York Times*, whom he views as responsible for a significant amount of the media coverage of the "anti-screening" research.[1]

Dr. Adams, a radiologist, further elaborates on each of these points. Remarking on the quality of the academic publications critical of screening, he states that they are "simply not scientific" and yet "given undeserved credibility":

> Those whose goal is to reduce or eliminate access to screening have managed to get papers published in the medical literature that should never have passed peer review. Their methods are not supportable and their conclusions are simply false. They have claimed that screening is leading to massive "overdiagnosis"—cancers that would regress or disappear had they not been detected. It turns out that these papers are simply not scientific.

The problem is not only that the research in these papers is methodologically flawed, he argues, but also that academic journals have refused to publish critical reactions to them:

> Women and physicians are confused because misinformation has been disseminated while explanations as to the fallacy of the arguments have been prevented from being published so that the misinformation is taken as facts. It is outrageous that scientifically unsupportable papers have been published. The public is unaware that they are being misled. Some journals have been complicit. For example a Letter to the Editor of the *New England Journal of Medicine* signed by more than forty experts in breast cancer as well as several societies. . . . was refused publication.

Thus, Dr. Adams feels that biased publication practices have led to public confusion. He specifically mentions the concept of "overdiagnosis" as one that is scientifically unsupportable yet has been steeped into the cultural narrative surrounding mammography due to the media attention it received.

Dr. Cashman makes a similar point about the confusion generated by the public circulation of certain "negative" concepts about screening. He specifically points to the term "false positive" as distorting for the public: "Some of it is, you know, the criticisms of mammography, from maybe a scientific standpoint we use terms like 'false positive' or 'unnecessary.' And then when the public hears this, they think that's a bad thing. They think, 'Well, then it must be flawed and it must not be worth doing because I'm hearing these negative descriptions of mammography.' You know, something that's false sounds bad, something that's unnecessary sounds bad." In short, whereas skeptics perceive a decades-long, one-sided cultural narrative that early detection and mammography save lives, interventionists perceive mammography as under significant and unwarranted critical scrutiny, with both academic and trade publishing outlets favoring perspectives that challenge orthodoxies.

Notably, when I asked Dr. Price, an oncologist and mammography skeptic, about the interventionists' claim that recent media has been biased toward the skeptical viewpoint, he answered, "Well, what they may be reacting to is the change. And they may be perceiving the same change that I am perceiving, except that I am saying that I think it's a good thing. You know, because it's more balanced. . . . I mean I know very high-level radiologists, chairs of departments and such, who will say . . . 'Mammography is under more scrutiny and more fire than I have ever seen in my twenty or thirty years of practice.' And, you know, they're right. They are. It is, I think, justifiably. But it's not—I still think that there's a heck of a lot of positive mammography media out there." In suggesting that skeptics and interventionists are perceiving the same discourse two different ways, Dr. Price is highlighting the power of their preexisting cognitive filters in defining how they attend to what is presented in the media.

Mammography in the Media—A Content Analysis

Given these very different depictions of the tone and focus of media discourse on mammography, the remainder of this chapter sets out to directly assess the state of media coverage of mammography from the first USPSTF guideline announcement in 2002 until the American Cancer Society guideline change in 2015. Is it true, as interventionists suggest, that the media has an anti-screening bias? Has there been an increasing focus on the harms of screening over time, or is the weight of cultural emphasis still primarily on early detection and the benefits of mammography? To answer these questions, I conducted a content analysis of the entire body of reporting on mammography from 2002 through 2015 in the four U.S. newspapers with the highest circulation: *The New York Times*, *The Los Angeles Times*, *The Wall Street Journal*, and *USA Today*.

During this period, 589 total articles mentioned mammography. About half of these (294) appeared in *The New York Times*, and the rest of the sample was split more or less evenly between the remaining three publications, with each contributing approximately one hundred articles (17 percent) to the sample. In terms of article type, about 10 percent (sixty-two) were editorials, whereas 37 percent (215) were reported news stories, features, or news analyses. The remaining articles took a variety of other forms, such as profiles or letters to the editor. The reporting on mammography was not evenly distributed throughout the period under analysis, with by far the highest concentration of articles (107, or 18 percent) appearing in 2002. The year with the next highest number of articles published was 2009, with seventy-eight articles (13 percent). To a significant extent, the distribution of the articles roughly reflects the timing of major announcements about mammography guidelines. The original USPSTF guideline announcement recommending annual mammograms at age forty occurred in 2002. The revised age and frequency guidelines (fifty-plus, biennial) was announced in 2009, and the re-review and confirmation of that guideline took place in 2015. The ACS guideline change to age forty-five was also announced in 2015. While there were corresponding peaks in the number of articles published during 2002 and 2009, levels of coverage in 2015 were roughly consistent with the five preceding years (2010–2014). (See figure 3.1.)

Upon deeper analysis, despite mentioning mammography, not all 589 articles provided enough material for substantive thematic analysis, and therefore some were excluded from the full content analysis (248 were excluded of the

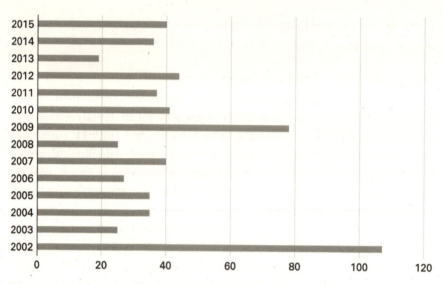

Figure 3.1. Number of publications on mammography, by year (2002–2015) (*N* = 589)

589 total articles). Examples of excluded articles included roundups of breast cancer product promotions, articles about celebrities (e.g., Melissa Etheridge) diagnosed with breast cancer, reporting on the Affordable Care Act that mentioned insurance coverage for preventive screenings such as mammography, and other articles that discussed health care more generally, using mammography only as an example. After eliminating these types of articles, the sample was reduced to 341 total news pieces.

Of these 341 articles substantively focused on mammography, 179 (52 percent) mentioned the guidelines for frequency and timing of mammography screening, and 147 (43 percent) mentioned that there is disagreement about these recommendations. Not all of the 179 articles discussing breast screening guidelines included enough information to be categorized as favorable or unfavorable to the USPSTF revision, and some focused on other guidelines, such as the ACS's 2015 revision. After removing those articles, of the remaining 119 that could be categorized, slightly more were favorable to the USPSTF revision (*N* = 44, or 37 percent) or were evenhanded in their discussion (*N* = 43, or 36 percent) than were explicitly supportive of the earlier guideline (*N* = 32, or 27 percent). (See figure 3.2.)

However, when looking at the entire sample of articles, not just the subset that included specific discussions of age and frequency guidelines, 68 out of 341 articles included criticisms of the USPSTF, and a slightly larger proportion mentioned the benefits of mammography (226, or 66 percent) than the harms of

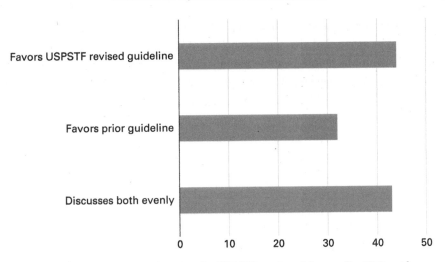

Figure 3.2. Number of articles favoring the USPSTF 2009 revision vs. the 2002 guideline (*N* = 119)

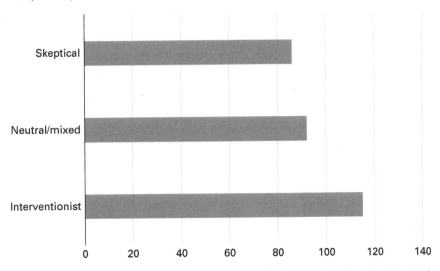

Figure 3.3. Overall tenor of discussion of mammography by number of articles (*N* = 293)

screening (216, 63 percent). Note that in some cases articles mentioned both the benefits and harms of mammography, which is why these results total more than 100 percent. Of the 341 total articles, 293 could be classified in terms of their overall *perspective on mammography* (not limited to the disagreement about age/interval of screening). Of these, 115 (39 percent) reflected the interventionist position, 86 (30 percent) reflected the skeptical viewpoint, and a similar proportion (*N* = 92, 31 percent) presented a neutral or mixed discussion. (See figure 3.3.)

Articles were categorized as skeptical or interventionist because they promoted one or more of the defining beliefs of each perspective. Skeptical articles, for example, pointed out the limitations of early detection frameworks that only focus on the benefits of mammography without acknowledging the potential harms of early and frequent screening. They were also likely to point out the culture of fear surrounding breast cancer, and many mentioned overdiagnosis. Articles categorized as interventionist, on the other hand, often pointed out that the USPSTF included no breast cancer specialists and that the most important harm to be avoided in mammography screening is the harm of dying from breast cancer. This was sometimes expressed through the narrative that women are strong enough to endure the harms of false positives and recalls for additional screening—and in fact prefer this to the risk of "missing" a tumor. Some interventionist articles also emphasized that in certain cases tumors are very aggressive, and therefore even spacing out screenings by an additional year could risk a woman's life.

In general, the interventionist claim that the media unfairly favors critical perspectives on mammography is not supported by the results of this content analysis. In terms of overall tone, many articles were evenhanded in reporting both positions, but between skepticism and interventionism, more reflected an interventionist viewpoint. The balance of emphasis in the articles varied slightly by article type, with editorials (perhaps not surprisingly) the least likely to present a mixed or neutral perspective at 13 percent ($N = 8$) of the sixty-one total editorials. Interventionism and skepticism were equally represented in editorials at just over 40 percent each (twenty-six and twenty-seven articles, respectively). In contrast, a neutral or mixed emphasis was the most common categorization in informational news stories (38 percent, $N = 38$ out of 100), news analyses (43 percent, $N = 25$ out of 58), and features (52 percent, $N = 11$ out of 21). Thus, while no particular article type consistently favored skeptical views, neither did any favor interventionism.

As highlighted in chapter 1, early detection is a central point of attentional differentiation between interventionists and skeptics. When examining the portrayal of early detection in the news, one sees again a somewhat higher representation of favorable or interventionist perspectives compared with skeptical views. Recall that many skeptics are critical of the idea of early detection because they feel that it has been overemphasized and that it oversimplifies how cancer progresses, ignoring the evidence and significance of overdiagnosis. Interventionists, on the other hand, tend to argue that early detection remains the most important factor in cancer mortality. For example, when discussing the role of improvements in treatment, they tended to bring the focus back to early

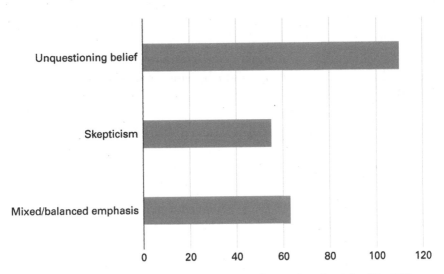

Figure 3.4. Perspective presented on early detection by number of articles ($N = 228$)

detection, arguing that better treatment only works when tumors are detected early. In the news data, when early detection was mentioned ($N = 228$), twice as many articles uncritically emphasized early detection's importance in line with interventionists' views than expressed any form of skepticism about early detection (110 vs. 55 articles, respectively). In addition, slightly more articles presented a mixed or balanced discussion of early detection ($N = 63$) than were directly supportive of the skeptical viewpoint. (See figure 3.4.)

On the whole, then, while the data are multivalent in places, interventionist ideas were more consistently prominent than skeptical ideas in newspaper coverage of mammography. Although slightly more of the articles specifically discussing the age and frequency guidelines under debate either favored the revised USPSTF guideline over the prior, more aggressive approach or were balanced in their discussion of the different recommendations, when analyzing the broader media discourse on mammography, interventionist perspectives dominated. This may reflect the cognitive resistance discussed by skeptics to concepts like overdiagnosis and the harms of screening that fundamentally challenge the received wisdom about breast cancer. The coverage of early detection may be shaped by this resistance as well, since criticisms of the theory of early detection were relatively absent from the news reporting relative to the coverage of the guideline changes that are their logical extension. That is, it may be that shifting mammography's initiation to later and advising less frequent mammograms, while controversial, is more accessible and easier to accept than the more radically challenging skeptical ideas that motivate those changes, for example, overdiagnosis, the harms of screening, and the complexities of early detection.

Another claim that was raised in the interviews was that coverage of the skeptical perspective and references to the harms of screening have increased over time. This was present, for example, in the skeptics' suggestion that, while still less emphasized than the interventionist view, there has been increasing recognition of the skeptical perspective and the harms of mammography over time; skeptics view this both as a sign of progress and as what interventionists are likely reacting to when they claim that the media is biased against mammography. In a prior literature review of forty-two articles specifically addressing overdiagnosis, Pathirana, Clark, and Moynihan (2017) did find increasing references to overdiagnosis over time. Although they found very few mentions of this concept prior to 2013, references increased each year from 2013 through 2017. To look at this question, I compared the number of articles in my sample reflecting an interventionist versus a skeptical viewpoint and those mentioning the harms of mammography over time to assess whether there was an overall upward trend in references to critical perspectives on mammography. The crosstabulation of these questions does not reveal a clear pattern of increasing criticism of mammography. Articles expressing skepticism about mammography seem to follow a pattern of peaking with each official guideline change and then dropping down again. Thus, the years with the highest number of skeptical articles are 2002 ($N = 22$ out of 66, or 33 percent) and 2009 ($N = 22$ out of 55, or 40 percent), with a smaller peak in 2015 ($N = 10$ out of 26, or 38 percent). In the intervening periods, the numbers were generally lower, ranging from zero to two skeptical articles annually between 2003 and 2008, and from three to eight articles in the period just following the 2009 USPSTF guideline change, 2010 to 2014. (See figure 3.5.)

However, the percentage of articles in the sample from each year mentioning the harms of mammography did increase over time. It was the highest in 2014 at 86 percent ($N = 19$ out of 22 total articles in the sample from 2014), whereas in 2009 it was 73 percent ($N = 45$ out of 62 total articles that year), and in 2002 it was 59 percent ($N = 47$ out of 79 total articles). For comparison, in 2002, 73 percent of the articles mentioned the benefits of mammography ($N = 58$ out of 79 articles published), in 2009 it was 60 percent ($N = 37$ out of 62 total articles), and in 2014 it was 82 percent ($N = 18$ out of 22 articles). (See figure 3.6.)

Another prominent theme regarding media coverage discussed in the interviews, as mentioned already, was either criticism or support of *The New York Times* reporter Gina Kolata's coverage of the issues. Skeptics tended to characterize Kolata's work as fair and informed, whereas some interventionists found her

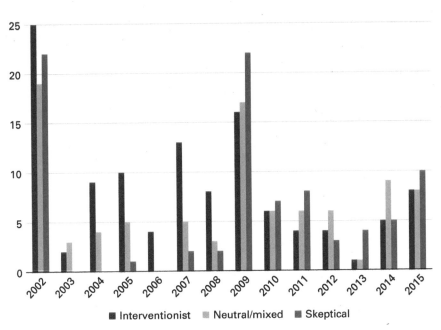

Figure 3.5. Number of interventionist, neutral, and skeptical articles by year ($N = 293$)

to be biased against mammography and unwilling to devote equal attention to the benefits of mammography in addition to the harms. This raises a broader question about whether the four publications analyzed differed in their emphasis, with some—perhaps *The New York Times*, given the singling out of Kolata's work—more likely to emphasize the harms and limitations of mammography. To evaluate this claim, I compared the proportion of articles from each source using three data points: (1) Was the overall valence of the article skeptical, interventionist, or mixed/neutral?; (2) Were the harms of mammography mentioned?; and (3) Were the benefits of mammography mentioned? The results of this analysis do not support the claim that *The New York Times* is predisposed to the skeptical viewpoint or the harms of mammography. In fact, *The New York Times* had a higher proportion of articles categorized as interventionist, whereas *The Los Angeles Times* had the greater proportion of skeptical articles. In terms of the likelihood of mentioning the harms versus the benefits of mammography, across all four publications, more articles mentioned the harms of mammography than did not. However, all four publications were also more likely to mention the benefits of mammography than not. For instance, in *The New York Times*, 124 articles mentioned the

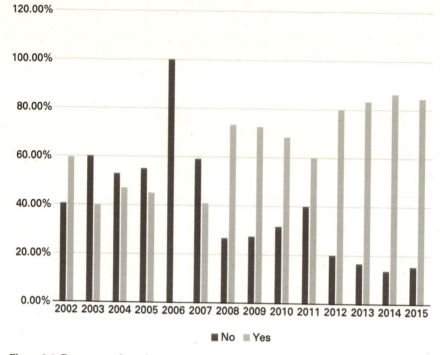

Figure 3.6. Percentage of articles mentioning the harms of mammography by year ($N = 340$)

benefits of mammography, while 115 mentioned the harms. Similarly, there were thirty-two mentions of the harms and thirty-five mentions of the benefits in *The Wall Street Journal*. *The Los Angeles Times* was the only publication where mentions of the harms were more frequent than mentions of the benefits, with forty-three articles mentioning the harms and only thirty-seven the benefits. Of course, these are not mutually exclusive measures: Many articles mentioned both the benefits and harms. Overall, though, if anything, the emphasis in the analyzed coverage of mammography once again slightly favors the interventionist perspective and the benefits of mammography. (See figures 3.7 through 3.9.)

In this chapter I foregrounded the antagonistic, combative aspects of cultural disagreements over mammography by analyzing them as an attentional battle. Through this lens I examined how interventionist and skeptic doctors and scientists differentiated themselves and polarized their positions through discussions of their differences in attention and relevance. To illustrate this, I focused on how each group described the salient facts to note about the USPSTF and the most important evidence and expertise for evaluating mammography. I then examined how each group rhetorically invalidated the other through claims that their attentional norms are incorrect, distorted, biased, or self-serving. I subsequently

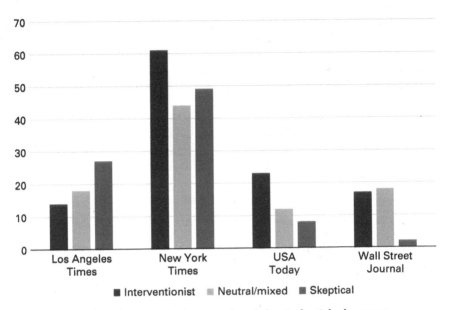

Figure 3.7. Number of interventionist, neutral, and skeptical articles by source

turned to the other aspect of attentional battles—competitions for attention—for a discussion of how interventionists and skeptics portrayed the broader cultural presence of their frameworks of relevance and attention, with particular emphasis on their perceptions of publishing and media coverage. Finally, I presented the results of a content analysis of U.S.-based news coverage of mammography from 2002 to 2015 to provide context for these claims about how much attention each perspective has received. On the whole, this analysis provides validation for skeptics' claims that cultural discourse is supportive of mammography and early detection. It also demonstrates how powerfully our attentional commitments shape how we perceive and portray reality, since the two groups experience cultural narratives and media coverage of mammography totally differently depending on what they select for focus. Some of this selection is likely a conscious strategy of the attentional battle they are waging with one another, while some is very likely unconscious bias deriving from their investment in either supporting or critiquing mammography.

The emotion of the conflict was also apparent in both the interviews and the news coverage. A focus on mammography as an attentional battle allows this deep contentiousness defining conflicts over mammography to clearly surface. Perhaps even more importantly, though, it provides an understanding of how disputes over how we should pay attention and what ideas receive more public attention in debates about mammography serve to sustain and fuel the

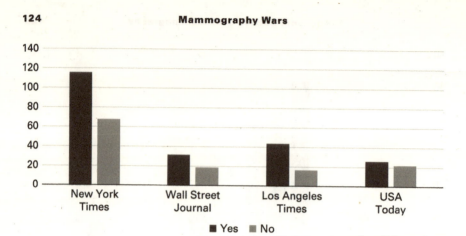

Figure 3.8. Number of articles mentioning harms of mammography by source

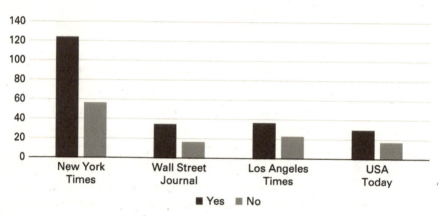

Figure 3.9. Number of articles mentioning benefits of mammography by source

divisiveness and high emotion that have surrounded mammography from its earliest beginnings. Additionally, this focus provides a window into how scientific data is being perceived and used in the context of this battle over and for attention. Given the heightened emotion, references to research and data often seemed more about differentiating and discrediting the other side than directly evaluating the scientific "facts." In the next chapter, I further extend this line of argument through a discussion of mental weighing, which similarly demonstrates that the treatment of data and evidence—for example, about the risks and benefits of mammography—is not based strictly on empirical or scientific risk; rather, it depends on interventionists' and skeptics' attentional battle strategies, including how they differentially mentally weigh concepts like overdiagnosis and early detection.

Chapter 4

Attentional Weight

Relevance, Risk, and Expertise in Mammography

Dr. Kramer, a general internal medicine doctor by training who currently leads a cancer center, uses the metaphor of a balance to illustrate how her interventionist beliefs and clinical experiences working with breast cancer patients provide what she calls "value weightings" that she applies when evaluating mammography: "If you had a see saw and on one side was a 100-pound block of concrete and that's the benefit. I feel that the harms are equivalent to a feather and that's what I'm piling on the other side. And I could put a whole lot of feathers on there and still the benefits outweigh [them]." Such "value weightings" shape how she perceives the evidence and lead her to different conclusions about mammography than others with different values. Specifically, based on her application of weight, the benefits of mammography are much more significant and "weighty" than the harms. At another point in our interview, she remarks that the composition of the USPSTF panel during the deliberations about mammography did not reflect her "value weightings," which again are specifically based on her experiences treating breast cancer patients, since no breast cancer experts were included:

> There was not a breast cancer expert on the U.S. Preventive Services Task Force panel. In fact, the lead was a pediatrician, but with a lot of knowledge of interpreting data. Okay. But how many—how many women has she told they have breast cancer and seen their lives just become devastated and, you know, walked that walk through with them as they're undergoing treatment and dealing with family members and young children and stuff like that? And so, you know, I see the devastation that

causes and I see that women get upset with a false positive—that, you know, (exhales) "Oh, but I'm so glad that it—it's negative." And then they come back the next year. So it didn't affect them enough to turn them off of it. So that's where I'm coming from as a clinician is my own personal experience that I don't think they have.... That's why... *I think a lot of clinicians have a different value weighting* than does this group, which—which it's some people feel it's the best way to approach the recommendation is to have people more looking at the numbers. But I think there's a lot of problems with just looking at the numbers because you have taken the value weightings out of it. (emphasis added)

In remarks resonant with Dr. Kramer's description of the clinical "weight" that she uses to measure the harms against the benefits of mammography, but reflecting a skeptical perspective, Dr. Franklin, a primary care physician and academic researcher, tells me what he believes is the reason for the starkly different interpretations in the mammography conflict:

It's a close call and *people probably weight the data in different ways.* The strongest proponent, you know, will focus on the data that are most favorable and the opponents or the skeptics will say... "First, most of these data don't speak to anything that's happening now. Uh, women are well aware of the need to present when they have an early breast lump. So in the early trials, you know, come on, it's a totally different world. And second, our treatments are so much better. And whenever treatments get better, the benefit of early detection will become less important." (emphasis added)

Dr. Jackson, a family medicine doctor and academic researcher in epidemiology, similarly evokes the role of *mental weighing* in the conflict when he describes the way that preexisting mental investments lead to certain evidence getting "more priority" in decision-making. Here, he highlights the way that taken-for-granted ideas like early detection can lead to a pattern of heavily emphasizing the benefits of mammography: "These organizations, they often kind of start with a bit of a bias that, you know, 'More screening is good and more testing is good and more treatment is good.' And then tend to kind of look at the evidence that supports that, and then the evidence that doesn't necessarily support that kind of *gets less priority* in their decision-making" (emphasis added).

Finally, Dr. Brown, a breast surgeon, uses the terms "interpretation" and "messaging" of data to explain that the same data can take on totally different significance, depending on the application of mental weight: "I mean one person might say, 'Oh, 3 percent, that's huge!' But then you can get somebody to say, you know, 'Oh, 3 percent, that's nothing.' So I think it depends on interpretation of data and how they want to message it and how they want to present it." Building on these and similar descriptions, in this chapter I focus on how interventionism and skepticism as frameworks of attention shape the way adherents apply *attentional weight* and use mental weighing to discredit one another in the attentional conflict over mammography.

The "value weightings" Dr. Kramer and others describe in the above passages remind us that values direct attention and mental weight—even when it comes to science. In other words, what we accord higher value is defined as "relevant" and thus more likely to be given attention. Conversely, when something is not valued, our attention is diminished. When considering a screening program specifically, as Harris et al. (2011, 30) put it, "it is not possible to weigh the benefits and harms of a screening program without using judgment about the weight of various health benefits and harms." Stated differently, "scientific evidence can only help us describe the continuum of benefit versus harm"; any cut point or point of intervention in this spectrum is a value judgment (Quanstrum and Hayward 2010, 1077). Values are often implicit, however, and alternative meanings of the values being applied are not easily recognized (Parker, Rychetnik, and Carter 2015, 6). What the sociology of attention contributes to this conversation about values and interpretation in medicine is to link values to attention and to propose comparative analysis of patterns of attentional weight as an analytic approach to revealing these implicit values. Accordingly, the analysis I present in this chapter is situated at the nexus of values and attention, identifying how the competing structures of attention in disagreements over mammography are connected to different values and applications of weight. Importantly, the concept of attentional weight as a manifestation of values does not imply a binary understanding of relevance—yes/no—but asks, How much attention? Relative to what? Attentional weight is not a question of total inclusion or exclusion, in other words, but of what is considered more or less worthy of how much attention. A map of attentional weight is therefore similar to a heat map, depicting gradations of intensity of relevance and focus.

As a concept, attentional weight emphasizes the connection between attentional norms of relevance and the broader concept of *mental weighing*. In general terms, mental weighing can be understood as the assignment of social emphasis and deemphasis that colors how we give meaning to and experience the world (Mullaney 1999, 271). As Mullaney (1999) argues, the mental weights we assign are largely determined by the "lens through which we view the world"

(278), or our frameworks of attention. These sociocognitive lenses or filters lead us to perceive some things as more "weighty," or as "counting" or signifying more than others.

The assignment of attentional weight is illustrated powerfully in the cultural semiotics of marking, which was inspired by work in linguistics by Roman Jakobson and Nikolai Trubetzkoy and then later taken up and developed further by Jakobson's student Linda Waugh (Jakobson and Waugh 1979; Trubetzkoy 1969). Built around the distinction between the marked and the unmarked, or the remarkable and the unremarkable, the focus of a cultural semiotics of marking is the social aspects of what "stands out" to us (the marked) and what does not (the unmarked) (Zerubavel 2018, 1). The unmarked is what is ordinary, uneventful, expected, and taken for granted—and thus not noticed or given any special linguistic mark. The marked, in contrast, is what is unusual, special, or deviant—which is typically marked linguistically as a "special case" or "exception." This connection between linguistic marking and deviance or anomaly is illustrated, for example, in terms such as "male nurse" and "ethnic food."

The relationship between marking and attention is that the marked is by definition attended to, while the unmarked represents the expected background of our phenomenal world, which is typically not attended. There are thus "pronouncedly asymmetrical amounts of cultural attention respectively paid to the marked and unmarked" (Zerubavel 2018, 6), wherein the unmarked is characterized by its cultural invisibility. This asymmetrical cultural attention is also connected to social weight. Not only is what is marked attended to more than the unmarked, but the marked also carries much greater "weight," or significance (Zerubavel 2018, 11), despite the greater privilege that often inheres in unmarked default categories, such as "white" and "male." Mullaney (1999), for example, demonstrates how we assign semiotic weight to culturally marked and unmarked behavior by documenting the way that culturally "marked" acts "count" more than unmarked acts in defining our social identities. Cultural marking and mental weight are thus interrelated with attention in multiple ways. Not only does cultural marking determine what we pay attention to, with our attention asymmetrically trained on the marked, but conventions of relevance and attention also dictate what is marked or unmarked in the first place, and "marking battles" (Zerubavel 2018, 28) can result from conflicting notions of what should be given mental weight—illustrating the connection between mental weighing and the attentional battles discussed in chapter 3.

As alluded to already, such decidedly conventional notions of how much attention to give to a particular facet, detail, or concept are not just about *whether* to pay attention but also about how *much* attention and emphasis to give something. Stated another way, "attentional weight" is an "analog," as opposed to "digital," concept. Zerubavel (1991, 34) describes the distinction between digital and analog thinking as follows: "'Digital thinking' has a staccato character somewhat evocative of the on/off nature of the conventional light switch . . . in marked contradistinction to the smooth, legato style of the dimmer or the traditional analog clock." For instance, arguably the most central issue with respect to mental weighing and mammography is how skeptic and interventionist doctors and scientists weigh the risks and benefits of mammography. Yet this is not simply a question of whether they are entirely inattentive to either the risks or benefits, but rather of how much and what kind of attentional weight they allot to each, which is patterned by their broad attentional type and linked to the other ideas and data points they select as "relevant" to attend. The evidence and facts thus take on totally different significance depending on how one applies attentional weight. However, this weight is not a yes/no, either/or choice, but a question of degrees of attention and emphasis.

As exemplified by the semiotic distinction between the marked and the unmarked, patterns of attentional weight are often evident in what is linguistically and epistemologically emphasized and deemphasized. For example, the application of mental weight was linguistically illustrated in the interviews with doctors and scientists when they used marking terminology that suggested abnormality or deviation from a default position, such as "over," "under," "early," or "late" (see Zerubavel 2015, 7). Thus, terms such as "early detection," "overdiagnosis," "overbelief," and "overtreatment," or the idea that mammography has been "oversold," are all indicators of heightened attention and mental weighing and of underlying default beliefs or unmarked norms that differ for interventionists and skeptics.

Tracking the theme of mental weight through the interviews, in this chapter I focus on how skeptics and interventionists weigh the forms of expertise and evidence that are most valid for the evaluation of mammography, as well as the risks and benefits of mammography. It is of course not only doctors and scientists who apply attentional weight to the evaluation of mammography—or to scientific evidence generally. For this reason I also present an analysis of the most prevalent patterns of mental weight found in patients' evaluations of the risks and benefits of mammography and their own personal risk of breast cancer. Prior research has found that patients do not perceive risk in terms of statistics or scientific data, whether regarding breast cancer or otherwise (Bloor 1995). There is therefore a disjuncture between evidence-based medical knowledge and patient perceptions, even when doctors provide statistical information (Hesse-Biber 2014, 124). This is the reason, for example, that Rosenbaum (2014) writes about "misfearing" breast cancer. What we do not understand well enough, however, is how these risk perceptions are organized and patterned cognitively, which an analysis of the organization of attention and weight can help clarify.

Sharp disagreement about the harms of screening is at the center of debates about early detection and mammography. The concept of "harm" in the context of breast cancer screening is generally understood to encompass false-positive results, unnecessary biopsies, overdiagnosis, and overtreatment (Carter, Castro, and Morcos 2018), although some argue that it is important to expand this definition to include anxiety and other psychological considerations as relevant harms of screening (Harris et al. 2011, 28; Welch, Woloshin, and Schwartz 2008). Hicks (2015, 168) even suggests the definition of harm could be broadened to include wasted time and financial harms. Parker, Rychetnik, and Carter (2015, 5) find three distinct patterns of how experts defined harm, some of which, they argue, correspond with particular professional roles: researchers working with population data tended to define harm as overdiagnosis, whereas clinicians working with identifiable patients defined harm as receiving false-positive results and getting overtreated. A third view focused on women's experience of the screening process, emphasizing physical discomfort and inconvenience without considering overdiagnosis or false positives as forms of harm. For many involved in debates about mammography, the fact that there are such divergent beliefs about the existence, nature, and magnitude of screening's harms is the very reason to reconsider how early and often we screen.

Prior research on the harms of mammography has primarily appeared in medical journals and has largely focused on demonstrating, estimating, or debating the existence of overdiagnosis and the harms and benefits of screening more generally (Bleyer 2015; Bleyer and Welch 2012; Carter, Castro, and Morcos 2018; Hendrick and Helvie 2011; Independent UK Panel on Breast Screening 2012; Iwase et al. 2017; Kopans 2010; Myers et al. 2015; Raftery and Chorozoglou 2011; Wilt, Harris, and Qaseem 2015). A smaller body of research approaches the topic of mammography's harms by looking at the effect of some of the most widely recognized harms—specifically false-positive mammograms and unnecessary biopsies—on patients' attitudes toward mammography, quality of life measures, and subsequent screening behavior (Davidson, Liao, and Magee 2011; Hardesty, Lind, and Gutierrez 2016; Lewin et al. 2018; Tosteson et al. 2014). These studies generally find that experiencing the harm of a false-positive mammogram does not negatively impact later adherence to screening guidelines (Davidson, Liao, and Magee 2011; Hardesty, Lind, and Gutierrez 2016; Lewin et al. 2018; Tosteson et al. 2014). In one study, in fact, a prior false-positive mammogram made patients less likely to be open to even doctor-recommended delays in mammography (Davidson, Liao, and Magee 2011). Lewin et al. (2018) summarize these findings as indicating that the harms of false-positive mammograms and biopsies may be exaggerated. Others, however, argue that anxiety is a significant harm of screening—particularly when the results fall into the "grey zone" of ductal carcinoma in situ (DCIS), the most common breast-cancer-related diagnosis (Welch, Woloshin, and Schwartz 2008).

With the possible exceptions already noted (e.g., Parker, Rychetnik, and Carter 2015, who identify different patterns of focus in definitions of harm), the existing research has left unaddressed the cognitive frameworks and applications of mental weight underlying different definitions of harm that are my focus here. In addition, methodologically, prior work primarily approaches the issue of the harms of mammography using quantitative data analysis techniques—for example, large-scale literature reviews or meta-analyses (Bleyer 2015; Myers et al. 2015; Raftery and Chorozoglou 2011; Independent UK Panel on Breast Screening 2012; Wilt, Harris, and Qaseem 2015), computer modeling (Carter, Castro, and Morcos 2018; Hendrick and Helvie 2011), chart review (Hardesty, Lind, and Gutierrez 2016; Iwase et al. 2017; Lewin et al. 2018), or survey research (Davidson, Liao, and Magee 2011; Tosteson et al. 2014). By analyzing in-depth interview data through the lens of attention and mental weighing, here I take a more fine-grained approach, tracing the nuances of how both doctors and scientists, and patients themselves, make sense of the idea of screening's harms.

The Harms of Screening: Feather or Block of Concrete?

The mammography skeptic doctors and scientists I interviewed insist that there are significant and often unacknowledged harms associated with screening, primarily overdiagnosis and overtreatment. They also consistently emphasize the psychological effects of being recalled for multiple screenings and biopsies. These harms are, in their view, documented and real, even the rule rather than the exception, and yet the cultural "overbelief" in early detection makes it difficult to conceive that screening could any cause harm at all. Dr. Jackson, a family medicine doctor and epidemiologist explains: "The concept of, 'Well, there could be more harm than benefit' is sort of a hard concept for people to understand. . . . 'What do you mean? How can there be harm from getting a mammogram? How can that be harmful?' . . . It's definitely potentially harmful, but that's a difficult concept for people to understand." On the other hand, interventionists reject or minimize (i.e., give "negative" mental weight to, or make less or light of) arguments about the harms of screening. "The harms are a feather," is how Dr. Kramer, the interventionist quoted in the opening of the chapter, puts it. Interventionists also characterize overdiagnosis as an "abstract" or "purely theoretical" idea without clear application to clinical practice, and dismiss other harms, such as anxiety, as insignificant when compared to what they consider the "real" harm to be concerned with—dying of breast cancer. One can see the application of mental weight by interventionists manifest in descriptors such as the "real" harm, "minimal" harm, and "purely theoretical." Skeptics' mental weight, in contrast, is evident in terms such as "*over*diagnosis," "*over*treatment," and an "*over*belief" in early detection. I illustrate each of these points in greater detail in the sections that follow, beginning with the skeptics' characterizations of overdiagnosis.

Overdiagnosis: The Most Important Harm (That's Hard to Understand)

Like many skeptical participants, Dr. Raff, an academic medical researcher, feels that overdiagnosis is the "most important harm of breast screening": "It's a topic of all the top journals now . . . All of them publish articles on overdiagnosis. It's no longer a debate about whether there is overdiagnosis. . . . There is a consensus at least in the scientific community that this is a problem, and it's something that we need to deal with." Dr. Price, an oncologist, similarly describes overdiagnosis as a "serious harm": "I would say that overdiagnosis occurs in breast cancer screening. I don't have any doubt about that. It is a serious harm when it occurs . . . and the evidence that has emerged over the last decade suggests that there was more overdiagnosis than we thought. And so that's been part of the reason that some groups have said the balance of benefits and harms is different than we thought 20 years ago and 25 years ago." Using terms like "serious" and "important," then, skeptics such as Dr. Price and Dr. Raff give significant weight to the harm of overdiagnosis in their mental evaluations of the "balance of benefits and harms."

At the same time, despite emphasizing its significance, and although it is documented at the population level and acknowledged by most major journals, skeptical participants consistently referred to overdiagnosis as "counterintuitive." Dr. Price, for example, goes on to say: "So we have grown up to learn or to think that all cancer is bad and a cancer is a cancer and all cancers progress. And so it's highly counterintuitive even to most physicians that there could be overdiagnosis." Dr. Franklin, a primary care physician, similarly describes overdiagnosis as "hard for people to understand," emphasizing that this is because it cannot be demonstrated at the level of the individual patient: "And then there's the harm that's, you know, hard for people to understand, but in fact exists, that is finding something that's labeled breast cancer. Um, maybe it's ductal carcinoma in situ, but maybe it's an invasive breast cancer that in fact never goes on to grow. And this is a new idea, but it's no longer debated about whether it happens; the debate is now how often does it happen, and it's very hard to know ... because we tend to treat everybody." In addition to its counterintuitiveness, here Dr. Franklin is also pointing out overdiagnosis's counterfactuality: there is no way to definitively prove overdiagnosis at an individual level, despite it being "obvious" at the population level, because all cancers are treated as if they will progress, relying on a paradigm of early detection and treatment. Thus, conceptualizing overdiagnosis is always based on the counterfactual condition: "If we did not treat all tumors, some of them would not go on to cause harm." Further, as a counterfactual, no real patients know they have experienced overdiagnosis.

Thus, even though overdiagnosis is perhaps the most important concern skeptical participants have about screening, all of this combines to make it incredibly difficult to conceptualize and accept as a tangible harm. Another way to say this, using the metaphor of mental filters, is that early detection as a mental filter or paradigm of thought creates an attentional blockage when it comes to overdiagnosis. Interestingly, interventionists and skeptics largely agree that overdiagnosis is both counterintuitive and counterfactual. However, while from the skeptic perspective overdiagnosis is weighed as important and thus the point is that this creates a distorting node of inattention, from the interventionist perspective overdiagnosis is at best "a feather" in terms of mental weight, and therefore "irrelevant" and appropriately excluded from attention. In terms of attentional weight, while the skeptical framework gives significant emphasis to overdiagnosis, interventionists again view it as "a feather" or even apply *negative attentional weight* by invalidating the concept and thus restricting what "counts" as a harm. In this way, we see that the *inclusiveness* of the definition of the harms of screening can make the harms carry more or less significance. These expansions and contractions of what "counts" as a harm is the focus of the next section.

A "Cascade" of Harm

It was most common for skeptical participants to take an expansive view of the harms of screening in the interviews, both temporally and in terms of what is included as a harm. They emphasized that the harms of screening can unfold over time rather than occur only at the time of the initial screening, and that harm should not be defined as exclusively physical but should include psychological risks as well as those that are only able to be documented at the population level. Dr. Blakely, a primary care physician, exemplifies this expansive understanding of the harms of screening when she lists a series of harms that can be initiated by intensive mammography screening:

> How many unnecessary biopsies are being done? How much unnecessary surgery is being done? And those things are, you know, cause extreme morbidity. It's not just cost. And of course it's cost, you know, of course money is involved in that. But it causes mental anxiety, you know, a terrible amount of anxiety and angst and misery. It also causes physical morbidity: infections, bleeding, I think rare death. But, you know, that could be a consequence of unnecessary biopsies as well. Um, so you really have to, you know, you're looking at risk and benefits, but people don't want to hear about unnecessary biopsies. They're willing to go through an unnecessary biopsy if it means that they're going to, you know, rule out that it's cancer.

As reflected in Dr. Blakely's reference to "anxiety and angst and misery," her understanding of what screening's harms encompass includes both physical and emotional effects.

This expansive view of screening typical of the skeptical participants was most thoroughly described by Dr. Markman, a professor of epidemiology, who refers to the temporal expansion of screening's harms as the "screening cascade," or the "cascade of harm," a concept used in the medical literature to encourage a very broad definition of screening's harms: "When one is assessing the value of screening, it is important to count the benefits versus the harms and costs from the *entire cascade*" (Harris, Wilt, and Qaseem 2015, 713, emphasis added). Dr. Markman explains the concept of the screening cascade as emphasizing that "screening is not simply a single task, but a series of tasks, a series of events, really, that can end either in harm or benefit." He goes on to describe in great detail the series of harms patients potentially face at each stage, beginning with the nervous anticipation and anxiety patients may initially feel when waiting for the test and then the results, which he considers the first harm of the cascade for those who experience it: "Well, you can see that the anticipation. Again, for some women, and I'm not saying this is universal, but for some women that anxiety increases. So there we have some harm; people are waking up at night having disruptive thoughts." In addition, he points out, anxiety further increases if a call back is required for additional testing due to an abnormal or indeterminate mammogram. All of this anxiety is prior to even being diagnosed with cancer. Subsequent to a diagnosis, he emphasizes the harms of overdiagnosis, and treatment side effects:

> Then let's say that you have—you're told that you do have cancer. Well, the cancer could be something called ductal carcinoma in situ, which is not really an invasive cancer, but most people think of it as—as an

invasive cancer. Or it could be invasive cancer, and invasive cancer is heterogeneous also in that there are certain types of invasive cancers that will never kill you that are slow growing. There are other kinds of . . . invasive cancers that are very fast growing, and they're going to kill you because we don't have good treatment for those. Uh, so but we can't tell all of that at the very beginning. . . . So everybody gets treated. . . . Well, I've just said that a bunch of those women—and our best estimate now is that somewhere around a quarter of the women who were detected by mammography with breast cancer are probably overdiagnosed. So now a quarter of the women going to treatment, surgery, radiation, chemotherapy, Tamoxifen, um, hormonal therapy, those women are being treated for nothing. They don't—they're getting in the end, no benefit. They don't know that. And we don't know that, physicians. But in fact, they are.

Finally, beyond the physical harms of overdiagnosis and overtreatment, which, while certainly rarer than the anxiety and stress surrounding the initial mammogram and follow-up testing, is estimated by Dr. Markman to apply to a quarter of women diagnosed with breast cancer, there is the additional psychological effects of labeling. Again giving weight to less-recognized psychological harms, Dr. Markman describes the experience of labeling as follows:

By the way, telling you you've got breast cancer, that's an effect that we call labeling. So we've just now taken out a mark and put it on your forehead and said "breast cancer." And you—you feel differently about yourself suddenly. . . . So those women have been labeled. Their lives are basic—are really changed. Now some of those women do fine with that change and, um, you know, there are lots of women who can take that threat and actually make it into a positive. But it's not every woman and certainly I think for almost every woman, there is clearly a change in their lives and the way they think about themselves. And I am not—I think that that's a negative. And so that has to be considered.

I quote Dr. Markman's comments at length because they effectively capture the way that expanding and contracting the aperture of our attention influences mental weight. By thinking expansively about what counts as a harm, and giving significance to all aspects of the "screening cascade," skeptics use *attentional expansion* to make the harms of mammography more "weighty." However, one challenge faced by those promoting a broadened definition of screening's harms is that only a small subset of these harms are actually measured in the existing research, leading to a lack of available supporting evidence. As Carter (2021, 32–33) describes, "the range of possible harms is wide," yet "these harms are arguably insufficiently recognised and measured." Interventionists, on the other hand, consistently *removed* weight from the harms of screening, in part through *contracting attention* and restricting what counts as a harm, usually by pointing out that overdiagnosis is just an "academic" or "theoretical" issue, and that it misses the "real" harm of breast cancer, which is the possibility that a patient could die. Recall also in this context that because overdiagnosis is counterfactual, it is nearly impossible for skeptics to tell a specific story about an individual who was harmed by overdiagnosis, whereas interventionists can use the powerful rhetorical tool of personal anecdotes to give additional weight to the benefits of screening.

The "Real" Harm—Death, Not Overdiagnosis

On the topic of overdiagnosis, interventionists' primary argument is that doctors do not have the ability to apply overdiagnosis clinically to individual patients since they do not know with certainty which specific tumors will grow quickly or slowly. Therefore, the concept is "just theoretical" and ought not be given much weight in cancer detection and treatment. Dr. Andrews, an ob-gyn and breast health specialist, for example, refers to overdiagnosis as "somewhat academic" and therefore "slightly irrelevant." Dr. Cashman, a radiologist, similarly attempts to lessen the gravity of overdiagnosis as a harm by arguing that it has been "wildly overestimated" and does not provide information that can be applied to a specific patient:

> So and then I guess the final thing, which has thrown sort of a wrench in all of this, is the concept of overdiagnosis. And that has been wildly overestimated by a lot of these again anti-screening researchers that have claimed that, you know, 30 or 50 percent of all breast cancers that are diagnosed are unnecessary—unnecessarily diagnosed and that they would have never killed the patient in the long run and that's sort of their—their big argument. "You're finding all of these cancers that wouldn't have otherwise hurt the woman and you're putting them through surgery and radiation and chemo, which could hurt the woman and you should have just left them alone." Well, better studies have shown that the rate of overdiagnosis is in the low single digits. Uh, so probably 5 percent or less. Um, and the problem with the whole concept of overdiagnosis is that we have no way of knowing which cancer that we diagnose will or will not kill the patient.

As a general rule, interventionists are dismissive of overdiagnosis, mostly because it is not clear how to apply it clinically. Interventionists also reframe discussions of the harms of screening using an emotionally powerful rhetorical and attentional substitution of the harms of *breast cancer* for the harms of *screening*.

The harm that interventionists argue is most significant, and to which skeptics do not give adequate weight in their view, is the harm of dying from cancer. As Dr. Cashman went on to say, "You know, the one thing—the one thing the Task Force, for all their emphasis on the harms of screening mammography, the one thing—the one harm they did not talk about at all and that harm was the harm of dying of breast cancer." Dr. Kramer provides an additional illustration: "I am maybe putting a greater value on the benefits, too. So it goes both ways. Um, they're going, 'Yeah, you can get, you know, this amount of benefit by doing it annually. But you get 81 percent of it, so almost that amount, if you do it every other year.' And I'm like, 'Whoa, whoa, whoa! That—that's women dying!' And so, you know, I think it's different weight on both the benefits and the harms."

Rhetorically, these statements shift attention from the harms of *screening* to the harms of *breast cancer*. That is to say, the comparison alters the equation to weigh the harms of screening against the harms of breast cancer, rather than weighing the harms of screening against the benefits of screening. When interventionists make this argument, they are creating a false equivalence, since interventionists and skeptics are expressing the benefits and harms in two entirely different units, women with cancer vs. the entire population. Using "two different metrics," as Harris et al. (2015, 29) point out, "makes it difficult to decide whether the magnitude of benefits is greater than the magnitude of harms." However, this attentional shift is rhetorically effective in adding fear and emotional weight to the debate about the harms of screening in a way that both minimizes the "weight" of the expanded set of harms emphasized by skeptics and reinforces the logic of early detection. Dr. Adams, a radiologist, provides another example of this false analogy between the harms of screening and the harms of breast cancer when he further attributes this comparison to patients: "Most women and supporters of screening agree that these [skeptics' concerns] are certainly not equivalent to dying from breast cancer." The use of the language of equivalence in Dr. Adams' comment directly invokes mental weighing to minimize the significance of the harms that skeptics describe as so important by adding weight to the harm of "dying" and to patients' perspectives.

As I touched on already, language can play a significant role in directing attention and shifting mental weight. Calling something "cancer," as interventionists are doing in these examples, as opposed to using the term "abnormality" or other noncancer terminology, changes how patients and physicians respond. Using the term "cancer" adds weight to a diagnosis, making patients more likely to seek treatment, which is why some suggest removing it from biologically less risky abnormalities such as DCIS (Allegra et al. 2009; McCaffery et al. 2016). In a similar vein, Welch, Schwartz, and Woloshin (2011) argue more broadly for a clearer distinction between "disease"—which "implies something that makes, or will make, a person ill" (54)—and mere "abnormalities" to avoid adding undue mental weight to benign findings (xvi), a shift also recommended by Moynihan, Doust, and Henry (2012). Linguistically signaling the removal of mental weight even more explicitly in an effort to lower the intensity of subsequent interventions and protect patients from overdiagnosis, Welch and his colleagues (2011) use the terminology of "*pseudo*disease" and "*incidental*omas" for such less-harmful abnormalities (54, 99–100). In contrast, when interventionists use the term "cancer" to rhetorically shift away from the harms of screening and toward the harms of dying from the disease, they are directing attention in a way that increases the mental weight applied to the benefits of mammography.

I have already referenced the differences in the scope of what skeptics and interventionists find constitutes a harm, with skeptics typically advocating for a broader definition that includes psychological and emotional as well as physical harms. This is intended to acknowledge the many, many patients who experience significant stress associated with mammography, especially those who have to endure repeated ambiguous or false-positive results and follow-up testing. For example, among the patients I interviewed, twenty-three had had at least one mammogram prior to being interviewed, and of those twenty-three, sixteen (70 percent) had been recalled at least once for additional screening or testing. For some patients, rescreening occurs every time they have a mammogram, a process that can take months to resolve. Despite this, interventionists tend to dismiss all but the most physically dangerous harms (recall, for example, the participants who said the harms were like a "feather," or that the only real harm to be concerned with was "dying," not stress, unnecessary testing, or overdiagnosis). In the interventionists' narratives, this dismissal of the emotional aspects of screening as not requiring significant attention somewhat ironically often came coupled with language advocating for the patient's perspective, arguing that patients would rather face the "minimal" potential harms of screening than risk the "greater" harms of breast cancer. As mentioned already, this requires a rhetorical substitution of *breast cancer* for *screening* and assumes that all cancers are lethal. In light of this, when advocating for the patient's perspective, interventionists seem to be thinking only about the patient who is ultimately diagnosed with cancer as opposed to the much larger number who are not—for whom the risk of death from breast cancer is not applicable, but who do in many cases experience the cascade of harms, particularly emotional ones, related to screening. Thus, the patients each group has in mind when characterizing the harms of screening also appear to differ, with interventionists focusing on patients with breast cancer (weighing their experiences more heavily), and skeptics focusing on the larger population of women being screened, most of whom do not have cancer, and therefore can only be harmed, not helped, by screening.

These differences in the imagined victim, and in what even constitutes a harm, are directly aligned with the prior cognitive investments of each mental filter. For interventionists, this is a belief in cancer's inevitable progression if left untreated, and in the necessity of early detection. For skeptics, the salient beliefs are overdiagnosis and the importance of taking a broad population rather than individual perspective when evaluating the effects of screening. I explore skeptics' and interventionists' differing emphases on population- versus individual-level data in the final section of this chapter. First, however, I examine how the patterns of mental weight applied to mammography's risks and benefits by doctors and scientists I have just described relate to the attentional weight patients themselves use in evaluating mammography.

Autobiographical Alignment and Mental Weight: Patients Weighing Mammography's Risks and Benefits

Patients also have to weigh the risks and benefits of mammography. I have previously cited prior research indicating that understandings of risk are never strictly scientific but instead are significantly colored by prior experience and broader social and cultural influences (Bloor 1995; Hesse-Biber 2014). This was certainly true of the patients I interviewed for this project, most of whom shared stories about friends and family members with breast cancer, as well as their own prior screening experiences, that they believe influenced their feelings about the relative risks and benefits of mammography. In many cases, these experiences affected their thoughts on the issue far more profoundly than any scientific debates or even the recommendations of their doctors. In chapter 2 I introduced the categories of *default interventionism*, *conscious interventionism*, *conflicted skepticism*, and *conscious skepticism* as the salient patterns of attention the patients I interviewed used to make sense of mammography. I further argued that, depending on their specific autobiographical experiences with breast cancer and screening more generally, patients might either become more conscious, aware interventionists or might become more skeptical of the default cultural logic of early detection. In this section, I return to these four attentional types to specifically examine how the process of autobiographical alignment leads patients to differentially weigh the benefits and harms of mammography.

Many of the patients I spoke with dismiss the very idea that screening could have any risks, reflecting a taken-for-granted belief in the benefit of early detection. These default interventionist patients thus evaluate screening based on the assumed validity of early detection paradigms without any specific, conscious evaluation of the benefits or harms. For example, Catherine, who is Black, forty-four years old, and has never had a mammogram, states simply, "You're saving somebody's life. You know, what does it hurt to start it earlier?" Rochelle (forty-five, Black, currently unemployed, never had a mammogram) similarly cannot imagine "how you would justify waiting," and Tania (fifty, white, contingent faculty, six or more mammograms) wonders, "Why would you wait?" In terms of mental weight, such statements can be understood as applying zero weight to the harms of screening, or possibly even applying a negative mental weight, but again, in the case of default interventionists, this tipped scale in favor of mammography's benefits is assumed, rather than consciously stacked. The distinction between broad and narrow definitions of risk I described among the skeptic and interventionist doctors and scientists is also helpful here as an initial way of parsing the patients' narratives. In keeping with a tacit overweighing of the benefits of mammography just described, in general, default interventionists also assumed a narrow concept of risk in which the only consideration was the physical risk of the test. This is similar to the finding in prior research that the vast majority of women are not aware of other risks of screening, such as overtreatment or overdiagnosis, and thus may not be weighing the benefits of mammography against a full consideration of the harms (Silverman et al. 2001).

Conscious interventionists also expressed an asymmetrical pattern of mental weighing in favor of mammography's benefits, but with a heightened ability to articulate how they are weighing the risks and benefits and why the benefits clearly outweigh the risks for them. For example, Joanne, a fifty-year-old technical writer/editor who has had six or more mammograms, explains that for her, the evidence of the harms of screening "almost has to be double" to shift the balance away from the benefits, suggesting that she is aware that her mental "scale" is weighted in favor of the benefits by default: "For me personally, the evidence would have to be overwhelming that a) it's harmful to me personally to actually have the tests done and b) overwhelming that there is data and evidence that proves that it doesn't have to be done the way it's currently being done." Joanne is able to clearly articulate that her mental stance automatically assigns the benefits a higher level of additional significance and considers the harms "a feather" in comparison (as Dr. Kramer described earlier)—or even assigns them what appears to be a negative mental weight, explicitly stating that the harms would have to be "double" or "overwhelming" to bring them into balanced consideration with the benefits. Joanne also seems to have a narrow, strictly physical definition of risk in mind when she explains that her mental calculus was to weigh the risk of the screening "causing a problem" versus the possibility of "missing" a tumor: "I guess everything is a risk these days. And so which are you more afraid of: the screening possibly causing a problem or not having it and missing something?"

Vivian (forty-two, white, school librarian, has never had a mammogram), another conscious interventionist, similarly seems to consider the only risks to be physical when she refers to the treatment her mother-in-law had for her breast cancer and concludes that screening seems worth the trouble to her "if the worst case of early detection is you go through that stuff." There is also evidence among the conscious interventionist patients of the rhetorical and attentional slippage between the harms of screening and the harms of breast cancer observed among the interventionist doctors and scientists. As Vivian goes on to clarify, she is not weighing the risks against the benefits of *mammography* in her thinking, but the risks of mammography against the risks of *breast cancer*: "I mean like you could die instead."

As I described in chapter 2, attesting to the power of the screening paradox, many of the patients I spoke with discussed friends or relatives with breast cancer whose experiences have affected their views. Most of these patients described the prominence of breast cancer in their autobiography as increasing their fear. However, I also observed that how fear affects patients' thinking is significantly dependent on their particular history with breast cancer and screening in a process of *autobiographical alignment* with the hegemonic narrative of early detection. The typical pattern observed among interventionist patients with significant autobiographical experience with breast cancer among friends and family is that their fear makes them more conscious of the benefits of screening and elevates their own personal sense of risk. Megan, a forty-three-year-old white stay-at-home mother who has had six or more mammograms, is someone whose fear has significantly elevated her perception of her own risk of breast cancer and pushed her toward conscious interventionism. She feels "like it's like a time bomb (laughs). I don't know why. It's something that always makes me nervous." She later acknowledges that her feeling of being at elevated risk is probably not based in science but in her social experiences within her family and in her broader reference groups and communities: "Probably on a non-scientific level, maybe because they're very large, the Jewish thing, and my mom has incredibly lumpy breasts. She has had trouble with mammograms for a long time, but also never had any cancer scares. Um, what else? You know, maybe being in the Bay Area and knowing a lot of women getting diagnosed." Many others expressed a similar feeling of "social risk," in which experiencing increasing numbers of friends and family members diagnosed and treated for breast cancer has made them feel that they, too, are more likely to be at risk, regardless of whether those affected have any impact on their actual hereditary risk. This once again highlights the need to evaluate risk as a social perception (Bloor 1995; Hesse-Biber 2014), in this case reflecting autobiographical experiences and the prevailing sentiments of one's social networks.

Among those participants who do have a significant hereditary risk of breast cancer, such as mothers, sisters, or maternal aunts or grandmothers with the disease, many described a sense of fatalism about their own likelihood of getting the disease. Some even expressed that they believed they would definitely see a breast cancer diagnosis in their lifetime, essentially a belief in 100 percent likelihood that reflects social and emotional, rather than scientific, significance.[1] Nicole is forty-six, white, works as a hospice nurse, and has had six or more mammograms. Three aunts and her mother have all had breast cancer diagnoses, which feels like "a big, black cloud." She says that she has made her peace with the idea that she, too, will have breast cancer. "I don't really need to know statistics. It's probably going to happen to me."

Motherhood and family obligations more generally was another autobiographical factor that influenced how the patients I interviewed weighed the benefits of screening, usually with the same attentional pattern as knowing friends and family with breast cancer—that is, by increasing fear and focusing attention more directly on the benefits of screening. The theme of motherhood surfaced in the narratives in several different ways. Most prominently, there was a sense of wanting to be healthy for one's children, or being particularly fearful about leaving children behind if one were to become ill or die. For Rose, a forty-five-year-old white admissions director who has a child with significant special needs, the sense that she must stay as healthy as possible for as long as possible was particularly acute:

> It's indelibly linked. Uh, yes. For every—for many mothers, I am certain that it is not only the case for me and my particular kid. But for my particular kid, [my husband] and I are, you know, the primary care providers for a kid who is always going to need a very intensive level of support. And while we are always working on ensuring that that support is there

beyond us, uh, or in addition to us, we're really it in ways that I do think about, "What, you know, what are the choices I can make to keep myself in as good a shape or as sane (laughs) as possible?"

Samantha, a forty-seven-year-old white professor who has had four or five mammograms, similarly connects her fears about breast cancer to motherhood and to worries about what would happen to her child if she were to die: "I have more fears now that I am a mother about it. Um, when I can also like be really mindful, I can get really big and think—or get really high above and see the like bird's-eye view of like, 'Okay, you know, my daughter has wonderful sisters of mine who will take care of her.' You know, and like again, not to be cavalier, but knowing that, um, that people will survive without me. But there is definitely a lot of, yeah, a lot of it is connected to being a mother."

In a variation of this theme, some participants suggested that not having children might change their calculation about risk and benefit. Vivian, for example, reflecting on her aunt's choice not to treat her breast cancer, finds it more comprehensible because her aunt is single and does not have any children: "I guess for her, given her, given her life, right, that she doesn't have children or a spouse, so there is not like anybody she is beholden to decide to do something different—not that any of us are, but you know what I'm saying. Like there's no kids."

While for most participants their autobiographical experiences with breast cancer and screening served to add fear and emotional weight not just to their own sense of personal risk but also to their belief in the benefits of screening and early detection, for a few, such experiences instead served to fuel their skepticism and attention to the harms of screening. These participants tended to emphasize examples of overtreatment, or of cases in which even with early detection and treatment, the person still died. In other words, such skeptical patients emphasize the risks of overdiagnosis and overtreatment, as well as the *outcomes* of diagnosis, rather than just the benefit of "catching a cancer early." One example is Kelly (forty-six, white, journalist, has had two or three mammograms), who discusses a cousin who had a DCIS diagnosis that Kelly felt was overtreated: "And, you know, she had like a double mastectomy and like she is in her sixties now and it never came back. So, you know, my take on it is probably she never needed to be treated. I don't know if she would have that take. But like, so yeah, I mean but I mean I guess I feel—I feel that I am a stubborn enough person that if—if I was diagnosed and it was stage 0 . . . I would not even get radiation because I don't believe that, you know, that it's actually life threatening." Rather than emphasizing the point that her cousin survived, which might add significance to the importance of early detection, here Kelly instead stresses the harm of overtreatment.

Christina (forty-three, white, unemployed, has never had a mammogram) is another example. In the following she describes a friend who died despite having a mastectomy and chemotherapy. Instead of encouraging her to weigh early diagnosis more heavily, this experience made her skeptical of treatment: "And who knows what the, you know, chemotherapy that she had right after her daughter was born, and the radiation, and all that. Who knows how long that prolonged her life? But it didn't save it. She died at forty-two, which is the age I am now. And, you know, I—I don't want to go through that." These skeptical takes on the risks and benefits of early detection again exemplify the way that, rather than being strictly scientific or numerical, the meanings assigned to risk are infused with autobiographical experiences, specifically as these discourses align (or not) with dominant cultural discourses and scientific definitions.

Further, in contrast to interventionist patients who seemed only to weigh the most serious and rare physical risks of screening such as misdiagnosis, unnecessary treatment, or complications from biopsies, skeptic patients expressed a more expansive conception of risk similar to the one advocated by the skeptic doctors and physicians. These patients, for example, have concerns about less well-known physical risks such as radiation exposure:

> It raises my risk cancer from—although I think it's probably pretty minor—but, um, exposing me to radiation without a good reason is negligent. (Eva, forty-three-year-old white editor, never had a mammogram)
>
> I am worried about [radiation from] mammograms and—and potential risk of cancer and so . . . if there's not a really good reason for me to have a mammogram, then I definitely wouldn't want one. (Jocelyn, forty-seven-year-old white medical school instructor/researcher, three mammograms)

They also emphasized the importance of emotional considerations. This was particularly prominent among participants who had previously experienced a false-positive screening. While certainly concerned about the potential physical risks, these participants were very clear that emotional factors weigh quite heavily in how they understand the risks of screening and in their personal decision-making about whether and how often to be screened. For example, Jocelyn had two previous experiences with false positives: one with her own mammogram and another with her mother's false breast cancer diagnosis and subsequent unnecessary treatment. Avoiding such emotionally painful experiences in the future is a major factor in her thinking about mammography:

Well, I mean it's definitely something that I have personally lived through. When I got my first call back about my very first mammogram, I think it was something like the 22nd of December. It was right before Christmas. They didn't tell me anything other than I appeared to have a mass in, you know, in my breast tissue. Um, and, "Yeah, everybody is closing for the holidays. (Laughing) So you can come back in a few weeks." So I basically spent, you know, a couple weeks over the week of Christmas, you know, going, "I'm fine. This is, you know, I'm forty. Things are terrible viewing in mammograms at forty" and, um, from, you know, "They have seen a mass, I am sick, I am dying, and now I'm going to wait for a couple of weeks." So for me, avoiding that experience, and that's, you know, and my outcome was really good. I didn't end up having a bad experience. And my mom actually was falsely diagnosed with breast cancer when I was in maybe eighth or ninth grade. We were told that she didn't have a lot of time left. And it was a complete misdiagnosis. She didn't have cancer at all. She did have I think at the time they called it fibrocystic disease so she had, um, fibrous tumors in her breast, but they weren't cancer. So for me, you know, having gone through that with my mom, and then gone through it with myself, I mean I—I take that very seriously. . . . My mom ended up having surgery and radiation and, you know, all these treatments for something that really should have been left alone. So, I know in my case, all I did was get some follow-up imaging and then I was released. So I do know that it can end up in much more involved processes with surgeries, and treatments, and so forth.

Given her own experience being called back for further evaluation of a mass that turned out to be nothing, but even more so her terrifying experience with her mother's misdiagnosis and unnecessary treatment, Jocelyn is highly concerned about and seeks to avoid at all costs the anxiety she associates with breast screening.

Similarly, Eva, quoted previously about her concerns over radiation risk, had two prior frightening false-positive experiences, one with a pap smear and another with a prenatal screening with her son, that also weigh very heavily in her evaluation of the risks and benefits of mammography:

It has to do with weighing . . . I personally put a lot of stock in the problem of false positives because I have had bad experiences with that myself. Not with—not with boobs but with an ultrasound during my second pregnancy and with a pap smear. . . . I have sort of just recently come around to this idea that like, I have these two settings and I really freak out about negative tests that turn out to be nothing. The precancerous cells on the pap smear, which turned out to be nothing, was one. But even more so, I had an ultrasound with my son, where they found what's called an echogenic bowel. His bowel looked white like bone, and I got acquainted with all of the things that could be a sign of, including Down syndrome, but also worse things. And it was just, not only an extremely stressful 24 hours before we figured out that he did not have the condition that would make him blind when he was born and live to the age of two, but it was—there was this question for the rest of my pregnancy, "Is there something wrong?"

Although not everyone had experiences as intensely stressful as those described by Jocelyn and Eva, many participants who had been recalled for additional screening following a mammogram described it as quite anxiety provoking and sometimes drawn out over many months. Such experiences are quite common: although the exact numbers are debated, at least 10 percent of women, and likely a much higher number (possibly up to 50 percent), particularly of those getting their first mammogram, will be recalled for a second screening.[2] As mentioned previously, among the women I interviewed who had had a mammogram, 70 percent had to return for further evaluation at least once, and for some this occurs every time they get screened.

One additional experience that prominently colored how the patients I interviewed mentally weigh the risks and benefits of mammography had to do with billing and insurance coverage. Insurance coverage was an important consideration for many patients, even those with traditional health insurance plans but particularly so for those with high deductible plans or who are under- or uninsured. Many participants shared stories about unexpected charges for follow-up screenings, which are billed as diagnostic rather than preventive care and are therefore not covered fully by many insurance providers. They described being taken by surprise by these fees, and many said that they now opt to get screened less frequently, knowing they are likely to have to pay for the follow-up screenings. Kelly, for example, who was forty-six at the time of the interview, has decided to stop screening until she is fifty after receiving an unexpected bill and learning about the USPSTF change of recommendation.

I have a high deductible insurance plan and I had, you know, then ObamaCare now made mammograms free. But what they don't tell you is that if they do anything past one pass with the mammogram, none of the rest of it is free because they code it as diagnostic. Even though they hadn't actually found anything. I was not in there because there had been a lump detected. So the fact that like they couldn't correctly read the film after the first time they did it, I was charged for the second go around on the mammogram and then I was charged several hundred dollars for the ultrasound. And then like after that, I started reading articles where they said that . . . the United States Preventive Task Force said you don't even need to start until you're fifty. And then like another group was like, "Well, you can start at forty-five and do it every other year." So after that, after I got charged all that money for the stuff, I was like, "Screw this! I'm not going to even start until I'm fifty!"

Tamara similarly received an unexpected bill for one of her follow-up screenings and now weighs cost heavily when deciding how often to get screened:

So it was actually a very complicated and expensive process, and I ended up kind of irritated. I went to my ob-gyn and she felt it, and she said, "I don't think that's cancerous. But you'd better go get a mammogram." . . . They did the mammogram and they said, "Well, we don't think that's cancerous, but we think we should schedule you for an ultrasound." And so then we did an ultrasound and they said, "Well, we still don't think that's cancerous, but we should go on ahead and do a biopsy." So they—they were very careful and they checked very thoroughly for this thing that turned out to be a very common, uh, nobody anywhere along the way thought it was cancerous. And in the end, my bill was $2,000. . . . And so I have to look at it and go, "Okay, every time I go in for a mammogram, it's going to cost me $2,000 and it's going to be out of pocket." So I just have to—I can't go every year. That's crazy (laughs).

Tania, who had a similar experience to Tamara and Kelly of being surprised by her bill for follow-up screening, describes her mental calculation as trying to balance the stress of waiting against the cost of the screening:

It was two summers ago. Um, was that I ended up paying about $900 for—out of pocket for, um, gosh it was the follow-up ultrasound, and then I think it was a second mammogram and ultrasound that I paid for. So that was—that seemed extreme to me and that's where I feel like, "Okay." And it was—and it was fine, which is great. I am grateful. But it's that balance of, you know, the fear, the knowledge that I have crappy insurance or no (laughs)—I mean I do have coverage but, um, and will have to pay a lot out of pocket, is it worth the stress of waiting, you know? Yeah, it's balancing those things.

Popular media has featured similar stories about women being surprised by charges for follow-up screenings after their mammograms (Lewis 2020; Werner 2019). Surprise medical billing more broadly was also the focus of significant political attention in recent years, leading to the passage of the No Surprises Act in 2021 ("Surprise Medical Bills" 2021), although the focus of that Act is out-of-network charges and emergency care rather than the distinction between screening and diagnostic testing. However, also in 2021, U.S. Senators Jeanne Shaheen and Roy Blunt reintroduced the bipartisan *Access to Breast Cancer Diagnosis Act*, which explicitly focuses on eliminating copays and other out-of-pocket expenses for diagnostic tests following screening mammograms ("Shaheen & Blunt Introduce Bill" 2021). Given the existence of these Acts within the current cultural narrative of breast cancer in the United States, and given the prominence of this theme among the patients I interviewed, it is notable that billing concerns were totally absent from the doctors' and scientists' narratives about what influences women's mammography behaviors. Along with prior experiences with breast cancer among friends and family, prior screening experiences, and feelings about motherhood and other family obligations, the women I interviewed frequently described negative experiences with surprise billing as weighing heavily in their thinking about whether to get screened.

In summary, analyzing the risks and benefits of mammography in terms of different applications of mental weight brings more nuance and clarity to how patients conceptualize and weigh the benefits and risks of mammography. Generally speaking, the allotment of attentional emphasis in patients' evaluations of mammography's risks and benefits shared the characteristic patterns of the skeptic versus interventionist medical professionals, although the patients' orientation to either interventionism or skepticism was driven significantly by their prior autobiographical experiences—most profoundly, their experiences with breast cancer among friends and family, prior negative screening experiences, motherhood, and medical billing and insurance issues. The distinction between broad and narrow definitions of harm, for example—where the pivotal question is whether and how much weight should be allotted to emotional stress—distinguished the patients' narratives in similar ways as it did those of the doctors and specialists. Additionally, both the patients and the medical experts varied in whether they placed more weight on the harms of screening or the harms of breast cancer. In this way, the attentional norms of interventionism and skepticism also provide some insight into the organization and balancing of patients' concern with respect to the risks and benefits of mammography—although without understanding the relationship between these attentional norms and their prior autobiographical experiences, it is only a partial picture of the patterns of their attentional and emotional weight.

It is not only a more detailed understanding of such divergent reckonings of risk and benefit that is revealed by a focus on mental weighing, however. Another key area of dispute regarding mammography, as we have seen, is the appropriate source of medical authority and data (whether clinical or statistical) to use to evaluate mammography. Here, too, using attentional weighing as an analytic lens can reveal the underlying cognitive structure of these disagreements, as I explore in the next section.

Identified and Statistical Victims: Clinical Authority versus Population Science

When deciding whether to recommend mammography for a patient in her forties, clinicians must navigate two frequently contradictory sources of information: population-based statistical data may suggest one course of action (e.g., to delay initiating screening until age fifty), while face-to-face interactions with individual patients may motivate physicians to suggest more aggressive care. Aronowitz's (2007) historical analysis shows that conflicts about how to weigh statistical data against what he calls "the clinical gaze" have been present since early debates about mammography, with statisticians and other critics pointing out the methodological limitations of an individual-level perspective while others argued that aggregate data were equally "illusory." Consider in this light the following comments from a 1940s surgeon quoted by Aronowitz: "'There are those who on a purely *statistical* basis,' surgeon Robert Janes disdainfully noted in 1944, 'tell us that we have not in any way influenced the mortality rate from carcinoma of the breast in all these years.' For Janes and other defenders of the . . . 'do not delay' campaign, it was the aggregate statistical impression, rather than the clinical gaze, that was illusory" (167). Since the insertion of statistical ideas into debates about mammography, then, cancer expert clinicians have been railing against limiting cancer treatment (i.e., giving too much weight) to what is demonstrated to be effective on a *purely statistical* basis, while those who work with population statistics dismiss (i.e., take weight away from) such critiques as making decisions on a *purely individual* basis.

This tension is not unique to mammography; the application of abstract statistical data to an "identified" victim frequently provokes resistance from clinicians and patients in health care more generally, where it is criticized for giving inadequate attention to the individual. In such a view, population medicine is framed as the opposite of "personalized medicine," with health care being determined outside of the clinical encounter—and thus outside of patients' and their doctors' control, and without consideration of their unique situation. This tension between population-based data and clinical practice was an important theme in the doctors' and scientists' narratives. In chapter 3 I discussed the conflict between clinical expertise and population science as an example of attentional discrediting, a form of rhetorical maneuvering in attentional battles. There I introduced Parker et al.'s (2015) distinction between ethical and epistemological values to distinguish examples of attentional polarization and discrediting based on claims of fairness and benefit/harm from those about validity and evidence. In this chapter, digging more deeply into the cognitive organization of these polarized epistemological and ethical values, the focus is tracing the differing standards and patterns of attentional weight that underlie arguments for and against each form of expert knowledge.

Perhaps the most prominent claim in the interviews relating to expertise came from interventionists, who place significant weight on the clinical relationship and therefore take issue with the fact that doctors and scientists who are not directly involved in screening or treating patients for breast cancer have been given the authority to determine screening guidelines by serving on the USPSTF. Interventionists also raised the related argument that most criticisms of mammography come from people who do not routinely treat cancer patients. Dr. Adams, a radiologist, exemplifies this latter point: "The opposition to screening is coming, primarily, from doctors who do not actually care for patients with breast cancer. They either do not practice medicine, or are primary care doctors who see very few cases of breast cancer each year in their practice so for them it is not a big problem."

At times, these criticisms take a quite derisive tone, as when Dr. Shoumer, an oncologist, expresses the interventionist emphasis on clinical expertise as follows: "Those of us who deal with patients day in and day out have a different view of the world than people who sit at a desk and work on computer models." Dr. Cashman, also a radiologist, is similarly dismissive when he refers to someone on the Task Force as "basically an office physician." Such comments reflect a strongly held belief that doctors with direct experience diagnosing and treating breast cancer patients have expertise essential to determining mammography guidelines—expertise that research scientists who do not practice clinical medicine clearly lack, as do other clinicians such as primary care doctors. Interventionists accordingly place significant value on clinical specialists' knowledge and experience and support clinicians doing what they feel is best for a patient even when it does not fit into what Dr. Brown, a breast surgeon, refers to as "the box of guidelines and standardized medicine and the numbers." Dr. Raymond, a radiologist, similarly stresses that "the emotional state of the patient has to be taken into account all the time, and many people don't do that. They just sort of strictly go by the science—and we just can't."

Those participants critical of allowing generalist clinicians or research scientists to define mammography guidelines further argued that, unlike cancer specialists working directly with patients, general practitioners and research scientists do not have to confront the application of screening guidelines to actual patients with breast cancer. Such upsetting experiences humanize the debates for clinical cancer experts, adding emotion—and thereby putting them more in touch with what is actually being discussed during a clinical encounter, for example, a real forty-year-old woman who might not have a tumor found for ten years if screening is pushed back to age fifty. Dr. Andrews, an ob-gyn and breast health specialist who treats many breast cancer patients, describes the impact of such emotional clinical experiences on how she weighs the value of mammography: "It's a little easier for a primary care doctor . . . Versus someone who is like a cancer doctor who has, you know, seen some poor lady that was like 43 with metastatic breast cancer. And when you see that, you're just like, 'Oh, my God, you know, if we could have done anything to stop this outcome, it would have been worth it.'"

Not only do these participants feel that working directly with breast cancer patients gives them an important perspective on the real-life impact of screening policies (and thus the ability to properly weigh the evidence), but for some, it feels insulting that their expertise was not included in the USPSTF deliberations. In fact, at least for some radiologists, the debate feels like outsiders are underweighing their contributions and suggesting that what they do is not valuable. Dr. Cashman is a radiologist who expresses feeling unjustly dismissed in this way: "And I just do breast imaging as a radiologist and I don't even do any other type of body imaging other than just breast and breast cancer imaging. . . . Um, and it has been sort of—I mean for lack of a better term, insulting to me to see all of these other people, who don't do what I do, that aren't in my field, and that don't have the understanding even of the basic research behind what I do, say that what I do is not only worthless but harmful."

Embedded in such discussions of the importance of the perspective and knowledge gained from directly diagnosing or treating patients with breast cancer is an additional reason the perspective of the clinical breast cancer expert is viewed by interventionists as essential to debates about mammography: The numbers cannot tell the whole story, and thus should not be overweighed when evaluating mammography. Participants who argue for the importance of the breast cancer specialist's perspective emphasize that such work forces one to confront the real human beings that statistics represent in a highly abstracted way. This leads to an awareness of the ways that guidelines and population-based estimates can feel rigid, cold, and overly restrictive when dealing with real people's suffering, and to placing less weight on "just the numbers" as a result of that awareness. For example, Dr. Brown, a breast surgeon, explains that population-based percentages are not that relevant, and it becomes difficult to always follow standardized medical guidelines when clinicians are asked to, as she describes it, "put a human face against a population."

> Because it—it's just kind of like, you know, a woman has a 10 percent—a 12 percent chance of getting breast cancer, but when she has breast cancer, it's a 100 percent chance that she has it, if that makes sense. We do frequently say that. So, um, yeah, it's trying to put the human face against a population. It's one of the difficulties in just health-care providers accepting guidelines. At the end of the day you're a clinician; you have to do what you think is best for the patient, and that doesn't always necessarily fit into the box of guidelines and standardized medicine and the numbers you have been provided with.

Part of the reason guidelines and numbers can feel limiting to these participants is that patients not only have a "human face," as Dr. Brown put it, but they have agency, they have emotions, and they ask questions. In the clinical encounter, you have to convince them of the best course of action. For example, Dr. Mack and Dr. Blakely both describe patients feeling resistant to the idea of "watchful waiting" once a tumor is discovered, which nonetheless might be the proper response in some cases given what is known about overdiagnosis:

> It's a terribly hard sell. If someone's got a cancer, they want it out. That's it. It's got to go. (Dr. Blakely, internist and head of a cancer center)
>
> I've never had anyone walk out of my office, very few patients that were in their right mind, and walk out of my office and say, "I absolutely want to ignore this." (Dr. Mack, breast surgeon)

As alluded to in these comments, one of the challenges in accepting new guidelines and changing established clinical practices, especially when they involve less aggressive treatment as in the case of mammography guidelines, is that it can feel like withholding care, which is emotionally uncomfortable for both physicians and patients. Dr. Neff, an academic medical researcher and mammography skeptic, explains this discomfort:

This is a lot to take in. It's a lot to explain. It's a lot to believe, to trust. Um, it's a lot—it is a lot. And it's easier—and when you talk with clinicians about anything, it's easier to keep doing the thing you have been doing. It's harder to change. And it's easier to make a change that involves doing something than a change that involves doing less.

The emotional dynamics of the clinical encounter are not just about patients' resistance, then; the physicians' emotions are also at play.

Doing nothing, or doing less than what might have been done in the past, when confronted with a person suffering with cancer—or even a woman who just *potentially* has breast cancer—is difficult cognitively and emotionally, even when statistics indicate that it is, on balance, the most rational course of action. At the same time as emotions push doctors and patients away from "doing less"—making more conservative treatments and guidelines less likely to be accepted—emotions also pull physicians toward active treatment and the possibility of "helping" or "saving" the patient. Dr. Mack, the breast surgeon quoted above who said that no patient in her right mind wants to "ignore" a tumor, shares the following anecdote that illustrates her emotional response to successfully treating a cancer patient:

> I just had a case of a forty-four-year-old woman who had some mammographic findings, and she had a needle biopsy and it was DCIS. And we took it out and her margins were positive. And I re-excised her again and none of this is showing in mammography, and she had more disease. . . . So one has to be careful and in generalizing. I certainly would not like to see someone say, "Oh, everyone who has got a needle biopsy of DCIS stop, don't have any further treatment." Because I think for her, the fact that she only had 3 millimeters of invasion, that we were able to cure her with a mastectomy and she's not going to have to take any additional treatment. I think she's going to do very well. And *I have probably cured her.* But I imagine if I had waited for her to get an invasive—present with a bigger invasive breast cancer, she would have in all likelihood needed to receive chemotherapy and would have to have hormone therapy for another five or ten years. (emphasis added)

Dr. Cashman similarly emphasizes the feeling that he is saving lives: "I know that I save lives, which very few other physicians of any specialty could probably say." Many interventionists feel such experiences are important sources of their specialized expert knowledge and their willingness to do whatever it takes, statistics aside, to cure a patient—points that they feel are "underweighed" by skeptics. At the same time, skeptics point to precisely this experience—working with cancer patients in an emotional context—as potentially distorting breast cancer expert clinicians' ability to correctly weigh and apply the relevant science.

As opposed to the interventionist perspective that being a clinical expert brings important insight and appropriately tempers population guidelines with the realities of clinical medicine, skeptics view emotional encounters with cancer patients as clouding one's thinking, making it hard to objectively weigh the scientific evidence and guidelines. Such experiences bias the clinical expert toward more, rather than less, testing and treatment. They also make certain kinds of data more salient to them than others, particularly data that can be applied in a clinical context and data that suggest they, the clinicians themselves, can save a patient's life. Other data—data that are not applicable on an individual level, or that suggest that any treatments they can offer may not benefit a patient because of overdiagnosis—are considered less relevant and can even be difficult for interventionists to perceive and accept and are therefore "underweighed" in their thinking. Dr. Raff, an academic medical researcher, describes the limitations of these clinical norms of relevance:

> If you as a clinician see individuals every day with this particular disease, and you see young people dying from breast cancer and leaving their children and husband behind . . . it's terrible! And if you see this every day, it—I'm quite sure it changes your perspective. It changes the way you weigh the benefits against the harms. . . . The mortality reductions become very, very important to these people. So, and they have a hard time seeing these overdiagnosed patients because, you know, it's just you cannot identify an individual who's been overdiagnosed, just like you can't identify an individual patient who has been saved by breast screening. So, but when you see someone who has had a screen-detected breast cancer, it's much easier to think that "we made a difference to this woman" than to say "well, you know, maybe we gave her a diagnosis that she didn't need."

Dr. Samuels, a primary care physician, provides a similar critique of the clinical expert's mindset, arguing that they see things through a "different lens" and have "an emotional disciplinary mentality" due to working with patients with cancer all the time, which changes their perception of the risks and benefits of screening:

> I think it goes way deeper than, you know, sort of the financial motive, even for radiologists. I think there's this—there's this, um, belief maybe

tied to their working with patients with cancer all the time that in early detection and in that—that stuff that, that makes them—it—it impossible for them to weigh the same evidence, you know, in the same way. So, you know, even if they're looking at the same data, they're looking at it through a different, you know, through a different lens. And so I think it's a kind of an emotional disciplinary, um, mentality or world view that's shaping how they're seeing, you know, the risks and benefits.

Dr. Samuels specifically points to overdiagnosis as one of the attentional oversights of the clinical expert. By not granting appropriate weight to overdiagnosis, he explains, interventionists can misperceive whether treatment is working, since many patients appear to do better with treatment and do not die: "What they don't see is what would have happened if the patient hadn't been treated. And hadn't been screened."

Dr. Franklin, a primary care physician, also stresses the point that patients may appear to do better because of overdiagnosis rather than successful treatment of a dangerous tumor. He describes it as a "numerator-denominator problem," referring to the mortality rate from breast cancer, which is defined by the number of patients who die from breast cancer (the numerator) divided by the population of patients diagnosed with breast cancer (the denominator). What skeptics such as Dr. Franklin point out is that when we diagnose more breast cancer, it makes the mortality rate *appear* smaller, regardless of whether many of those cases are overdiagnosed: "When you're focused on the individual patients with cancer, of course whenever you start diagnosing more cancer, the typical cancer patient appears to do a lot better. . . . It's the numerator-denominator problem. You start inflating the denominator and of course everything starts to look better." This is also sometimes discussed as part of the screening paradox introduced in chapter 2; in fact, Dr. Freeman, a breast surgeon, uses that term to describe the inflation of the denominator through screening and diagnosing more cancer—and further notes that it is not only inflating the denominator that creates distortions in the mortality rate. When patients are overdiagnosed, he explains, they simultaneously increase the denominator and artificially decrease the numerator (because they would not have died regardless, since they were overdiagnosed): "The more you screen, the more you overdiagnose, and the more of these patients will survive, so it's called a screening paradox."

In addition to pointing out the ways that interventionists' notions of relevance and applications of mental weight are distorting, skeptics also advocate positively for placing much greater weight on population data than interventionists. For example, Dr. Markman, an epidemiologist and professor of medicine, argues that the expertise most needed on the Task Force is expertise at assessing scientific evidence, rather than expertise in diagnosing and treating breast cancer:

> I can just tell you that what is needed in making recommendations is expertise in evidence. It's not expertise in reading x-rays. Expertise in reading x-rays, expertise in knowing how to give chemotherapy, that's a different kind of expertise. You don't want people on there who are not experts at reading evidence. The people on the Task Force have been trained in, are knowledgeable about, are very good at critically appraising studies and synthesizing evidence so that you put it all together. That's a complicated thing to do. It's not a simple thing; it's a complicated thing to do and you have to, you know, have some statistical expertise and epidemiologic expertise and critical appraisal expertise, and you have to be able to put all that—so those are the people you want on the Task Force.

Dr. Jackson, a family medicine doctor, also emphasizes that the truly meaningful questions in the mammography conflict are not about the practice of clinical medicine, but about population science. In part, Dr. Jackson reflects critically on his own clinical training when making the point that clinical experiences should not be given weight when deciding the age at which a population screening program should start:

> These issues are almost always issues of population-based science, which really has essentially nothing to do with clinical medicine or, you know, I mean you might have to have a very rudimentary understanding of the clinical medicine, but so I'm a physician myself and so I'm sure I could probably be accused of this as well. But physicians often think that, you know, "Oh, well, we understand." "You know, we're radiologists and we understand pros and cons of breast cancer." Well, actually, no, you have actually learned nothing about it in your—I mean I went to medical school, and we learned nothing about clinical epidemiology. I didn't learn it until my master's in public health.

Dr. Blakely, who is a primary care physician, similarly finds her experiences working with patients tempting to rely on, but she keeps "coming back and trying to interpret the data" because she understands the analysis of population data as the proper source of guidance when counseling patients about mammography. Still, clinical experiences—for example, stories of particular patients who had a tumor identified through a mammogram prior to age fifty and went on to have successful treatment—are emotionally powerful and play a prominent role in the interventionists' accounts.

Interventionists use these emotional stories about saving the lives of identified victims to add weight to clinical expertise and the benefits of early detection. Such dramatic clinical stories often function as "trump cards" in the debate, automatically outweighing all other forms of evidence because they are about "saving a life" (Timmermans and Oh 2010, s97). Population-level evidence never takes the form of a trump card story, however. The statistical victim is always unidentifiable due to overdiagnosis' counterfactuality and the lack of adequate data on the other harms of screening. Without their own trump card stories, skeptics face a challenge balancing the weight of attention to fairly account for the harms of screening.

In the face of this challenge, skeptics tend to argue that individual cases are not actually scientifically relevant and should not be given much weight (i.e., they are overattended by interventionists). As Dr. Michaels, an academic researcher, puts it, "I think we've got to recognize you can't assess the efficacy of screening on the basis of an individual." For skeptics, then, emotional stories about individual patients with cancer are not relevant to the question of population screening guidelines, which requires one to abstract from these "identified" victims to the less emotionally charged "statistical victims" who are not seen at the level of clinical care but who are, in their view, the real victims of more aggressive screening programs.

The cognitive tendency to disproportionately focus one's attention and resources on specific, identifiable victims relative to statistical victims was originally noted by economist Thomas Schelling (1968). This bias favoring the identified victim was subsequently supported and clarified by a wealth of research, although the reasons for and implications of this cognitive bias are still debated. Some of this research points to the role of emotion (i.e., it is more difficult to "feel" for statistics than for a known, identifiable person), often using dual process theory as a framework. Taking this perspective, the identified victim effect is an artifact of different styles of cognitive processing that are related but not reducible to emotional investment (i.e., the intuitive System 1 vs. the calculative System 2) (Railton 2015; Small 2015). Much of this work seeks ways to elevate concern for statistical lives, such as the overdiagnosed, since the identifiable victim effect can distort sensible allocation of resources (Small 2015), as the skeptical perspective suggests. The emphasis is thus that we should work to *overcome* the identified victim effect, which irrationally diminishes our concern for those who are most statistically at risk or in need. Interestingly, other research has begun to counter such criticisms of the identified victim effect by highlighting the *value* of emotional reactions and the limits of purely statistical reasoning. Rather than dismissing as irrational the System 1, emotional, intuitive thinking that drives our preference for the identified victim, this work highlights the rational calculation that is actually present in intuitive preferences. Such affective responses, this work argues, *are* responsive to evidence, and reflect important "social competencies" (Railton 2015).

Debates over the role of emotion in screening decisions also intersect in interesting ways with the sociological literature on values, objectivity, and feminist research methods, specifically criticisms by some feminists of quantitative positivist methods as impersonal, abstracted from, and devaluing of individual experience. Qualitative approaches, these feminist critics of positivism argue, are better at capturing dimensions of the social world that have been traditionally and normatively central to women's experiences: the private sphere, emotion, relationships. Grounded in everyday life, qualitative methods also value the evidence of experience, feelings, and beliefs, whereas positivism emphasizes rationality, objectivity, and detached observation. In trying to eliminate bias, quantitative positivist approaches reject emotion and personal experience as legitimate evidence, whereas feminist critics question whether statistical significance always aligns with social or personal significance and whether rationality is the only or even the proper way to judge whether something is valid or important (Epstein 1988; Grant, Ward, and Rong 1987; Hill Collins 2009; Stacey 1988).

Applied to skeptics' and interventionists' arguments about how to weigh clinical expertise versus population statistics in the case of mammography, such arguments encourage us to consider the alternative forms of insight and validity available in clinical encounters with "identified victims" as opposed to the strictly rational conclusions drawn on the basis of statistics, basically reflecting the interventionist valorization of clinical and individual experience. This critique is also present in the broader literature on standardization and population-data-based quality improvement programs, where analysts point out that the translation of statistical probabilities into meaningful, individualized information is always problematic and may even exacerbate health disparities, particularly given that researchers rarely provide adequate guidance on how to apply population findings to particular groups (Beckfield, Olafsdottir, and Sosnaud 2013, 135; Fosket 2004, 295; Hankin and Wright 2010, s12; Moynihan, Henry, and Moons 2014). Such a view of course stands in contrast to the standard methodological critique of qualitative research with small samples of participants as lacking generalizability, that is, that such approaches may not be ideal to identify explanations either not observable on an individual level or obscured by the particularities of one's sample. Such critiques of qualitative methods also typically point to biases resulting from the human encounter of interviewing and ethnography—such as emotion and subjectivity—limitations which are seen as less present when working with population statistics on a computer. In the analogy with the mammography conflict, then, interventionist clinicians are aligned with qualitative researchers and feminist critics of positivism, whereas skeptics, who emphasize the biasing emotions of the clinical encounter and argue that we cannot assess the validity of screening on an individual level, are aligned with positivist critics of qualitative methods.

A few participants, however, dismiss such disputes over which type of victim and what form of expertise are more important on the basis that they rely on a false set of distinctions. For example, Dr. France, who is a skeptic but also a clinical breast cancer specialist and surgeon, reframes the purported conflict between clinical and population perspectives, arguing that, rather than viewing the population science as a threat to the individual, we should focus on the ways the individual patient benefits from population statistics: "I've worked with large data sets all my life and I have worked with patients all of my life. . . . And it's sheer nonsense to say that if you [worked with patients with cancer] you'd think about it differently. The individual patient benefits from someone who can interpret the data. So they're not mutually exclusive." However, note the way that Dr. France's argument that clinical care is always enhanced by the application of population data is actually in line with skeptics' arguments for giving more attentional weight to the data. At the same time, he sidesteps the more challenging point being raised in arguments about revaluing the identified victim as well as those raised in feminist research methods, which is that unresolvable epistemological differences may underlie statistical analysis versus the clinical encounter. The emergent research on the identified victim effect, for instance, encourages the consideration of the alternative forms of insight and validity available in clinical encounters with "identified victims" as opposed to the strictly rational conclusions drawn on the basis of statistics. Like the interventionists in the interviews, this research bucks the trend of seeking ways to increase the weight given to the statistical victim over the identified victim and suggests that individual-level, emotional, intuitive thinking has an important role to play in medicine, one that should not be supplanted by purely rational, data-driven processes.

While debates about breast cancer and mammography clearly reflect this broader unresolved tension in health care between identified and statistical victims, mammography skeptics' and interventionists' disagreements about expertise and attentional weight also seem uniquely emotionally charged. Perhaps this is because of the high-profile, broadly applicable nature of mammography guidelines—the way the questions being debated about mammography affect all women, and affect them in early midlife, when family and career obligations are often at their peak—which makes these debates feel especially "weighty." There is also clearly an aspect of ego involved, especially for those radiologists who feel that the validity of their entire professional role is being questioned, as exemplified by Dr. Cashman, who I quoted earlier as saying it is "insulting" that people who do not work in the field are saying that his work is "not only worthless but harmful." More generally, though, the work of treating cancer patients is frequently emotional, whether due to confronting patients' pain and fear of death, or the emotional highs and lows of feeling like one is either saving—or failing to save—someone's life. Several participants shared stories about their experiences treating patients diagnosed with breast cancer prior to age fifty that went on to do well. The highly emotional nature of being a cancer doctor also seemed to fuel the dismissiveness expressed toward those who approach the question of mammography from the perspective of either a clinical generalist or a research scientist. For example, as mentioned previously, Dr. Blakely (internist and director of a cancer center) disparaged the perspective of "people who sit at a desk all day and look at computer models," and Dr. Adams (radiologist) similarly made disdainful reference to "doctors who do not actually care for women with breast cancer . . . so for them it's not a big problem." The implication in such comments is that the emotion and individual patient focus that defines the work of clinical cancer specialists is *valuable* rather than distorting, adding motivation, urgency, even contextually appropriate desperation and thus keeping what they perceive as life-or-death questions in their proper perspective. Skeptics, in this view, are underattentive to such clinical realities and overattentive to statistical ideas like overdiagnosis that cannot be applied to the individual patient in front of them.

One further challenge posed by the application of statistical conclusions to clinical care, especially when it involves limiting testing or further interventions, is that it can be perceived by both the patient and the provider as though care is being "withheld" or the patient is being "abandoned" (Aronowitz 2007, 177). In the face of uncertain outcomes, it is more comfortable for both patients and doctors to *do something*, which allows one to feel as though one is asserting some control, rather than doing nothing. Further, even in cases where medical professionals and patients may wish to do less rather than more, the system within which care is delivered can also make this challenging (Armstrong 2021). As I mentioned in the introduction, population guidelines and other quality improvement measures often indirectly encourage more, rather than just more medically necessary, testing and treatment (Armstrong 2021; Hicks 2015). Moreover, in a system in which clinicians already feel like their professional autonomy is being eroded, doing nothing exacerbates that uncomfortable feeling for both patients and providers.

My analysis aims to add to this conversation a consideration of how the cognitive and attentional structure of the concept of early detection also contributes to resistance to doing nothing. This is in part through the ways an early diagnosis paradigm makes the harms of intervening in the asymptomatic population through screening, particularly overdiagnosis, essentially inconceivable. More generally, though, doing nothing is a fundamental challenge to the very premise of early detection. As Aronowitz (2021, 56–57) put it, "Why diagnose cancer if not to do something?" This profound discomfort with the idea of doing nothing, he argues, also underlies the shift in terminology in discourse on PSA screening from "watchful waiting" (i.e., doing nothing) to "expectant management" or "active surveillance." Finally, given the inherent uncertainties about how to apply overdiagnosis clinically, physicians seek to avoid what Aronowitz (2007, 269) calls "anticipated regret"—or the regret they anticipate having in the future if they do not act now and the patient has a negative outcome later. On the other side, however, as we have seen, skeptics argue that such emotional investments are at best irrelevant to the question of population screening guidelines, and at worst the source of problematic biases that distort such expert clinicians' ability to assess the relevant data fairly and accurately.

In the analysis presented in this chapter I approached the disagreement over mammography recommendations from the perspective of relevance and mental weighing. That is, I highlighted what for both the doctors and scientists and the patients I interviewed are the most salient benefits, harms, and forms of expertise applicable to the evaluation of mammography, and what is considered distracting, distorting, or simply less important, as well as how these applications of mental weight are deployed in the attentional conflict between interventionism and skepticism. This analytic approach does not seek to make a determination about which view is correct but rather to more deeply understand the basis on which each view is held, and the way that each applies emphasis to some details and ideas but not others. A comparative analysis of what is defined by interventionists and skeptics as "relevant" and "irrelevant" has the further benefit of flexibly demonstrating each framework's investments and constitutive exclusions. This provides a more complete understanding of the potentially relevant facts, as well as of the way a commitment to some is often attended by ignoring or downplaying others—identifying productive dissonances that could be used to increase each side's accountability for their own attentional exclusions. It also brings to light the way that hard data, statistical significance, and rationality are not always considered the appropriate measures of relevance. Rather than simply dismissing the evidence of emotion, intuition, and individual experience as unscientific and irrelevant, my analysis suggests that it may be better to acknowledge and evaluate these not-strictly-numeric ways decisions are being made. An important first step in this evaluation is to understand the underlying frameworks of relevance and corresponding patterns of attentional weight and linguistic emphasis.

Chapter 5

Mammography and Time

Disagreements over mammography are fundamentally about time: the optimal age to begin screening, how frequently to screen, how fast or slow tumors progress, and the necessity of early detection and swift treatment are all points of fierce debate between interventionists and skeptics. In his 2001 article, "Do Not Delay: Breast Cancer and Time, 1900–1970," Aronowitz describes two divergent understandings of the relationship between time and breast cancer that have consistently dominated the historical discourse on mammography. On the one hand, popular, public health, and medical writings since the beginning of the twentieth century have stressed the message of "do not delay" in seeking medical attention for any signs or symptoms of breast cancer. Aronowitz remarks on the "century-long stability to this core 'delay' message" (357). With the invention and popularization of mammography screening, "do not delay" shifted to "early detection"—moving the temporal line for action back in time and changing the focus from the symptomatic to the asymptomatic patient—but this did not fundamentally alter the temporal rule that *earlier is always better* when it comes to breast cancer detection and treatment. This push to find cancer as early as possible has been consistently accompanied, however, by a quieter, but persistent, temporal counterpoint of skepticism about early detection. This alternate temporal perspective emphasized that despite consistent campaigns for prompt treatment and then, once it was available, for mammography screening prior to any symptoms, breast cancer mortality rates have not changed (362). This clash of temporal perspectives, as Aronowitz points out, is among the most notable historical continuities in debates over breast cancer.

To understand the temporal foundations of the attentional battle over mammography, it is necessary to understand interventionism and skepticism as engaging different "temporal strategies" (Nowotny 1992, 432). These strategies include narrating the past to fit their perspectives and objectives in the present, as well as positing different intervals and temporal trajectories for both mammography guidelines and the biological progression of breast cancer. This chapter accordingly examines mammography as a *sociotemporal conflict*, drawing from the sociology of time, collective memory, and projectivity—particularly as these fields intersect with the sociology of attention—to highlight the key patterns of *temporal attention* at play.

Sociotemporality

The social nature of human time distinguishes it from other temporal orders, such as astronomical time or biological time (Nowotny 1992, 421; Zerubavel 1985, xii). Zerubavel (1985, xiv) describes the "sociotemporal order" as follows: "people clearly view time not only as a physico-mathematical entity, but also as an entity which is imbued with meaning." Such socially meaningful notions of time serve, importantly, to anchor our thinking and sense of reality, providing a "solid temporal ground against which the occurrence of certain events and the presence of particular persons and objects pass as 'normal' and unnoticeable" (21). Thus the *temporal patterns* of our *sociotemporal order* are essential elements of the cognitive scaffolding of our sense of normalcy and of default, taken-for-granted beliefs. Building on concepts such as *social time*, *temporal patterns*, and *temporal norms*, the sociology of time as a field examines "how [social time] is socially constituted, what leads to its emergence and change, which variations it exhibits between different kinds of societies or social groups, which social functions it serves and how societies cope with 'the problems of time'" (Nowotny 1992, 421–422).

The study of collective memory has been a powerful site for examining social time, since a key dimension of the sociotemporal order is how we remember and narrate the past and relate it to our mental filters in the present. Studies of such mnemonic work highlight the collective dimension of human memory, demonstrating how "entire communities, and not just individuals, remember the past" and documenting the "mnemonic battles" that ensue when these "mnemonic communities" construct divergent mental maps of history (Zerubavel 2003, 2, 4). The existence of multiple competing accounts of the past is an example of the multiplicity of sociotemporal orders, sometimes also referred to as "pluritemporalism": "the existence of a plurality of different modes of social time(s) which may exist side by side, and yet are to be distinguished from the time of physics or that of biology" (Nowotny 1992, 424). Thus, there are always "multiple pasts" (Zerubavel 2003, 32) that do not necessarily correspond with one another, leading to "temporal conflicts" (McGrath and Kelly 1992, 405)—but also to the solidification of group boundaries through shared norms of temporal attention.

In addition to competing accounts of the past, sociotemporality manifests in divergent reckonings of the "imagined future," as explored in Mische's (2009) work on the cultural sociology of projected futures, in which she points out that such projections are often manifestations of our social group memberships. Mische helpfully identifies several general characteristics sociologists can use to compare future projections, including "breadth" (are the possibilities imagined multiple or singular?) and "contingency," which she describes as "the degree to which future trajectories are imagined as fixed and predetermined versus flexible, uncertain, and dependent on local circumstances" (700). Also invoking the dimensions of flexibility and multiplicity in anticipated futures, Zerubavel (2003, 22) differentiates between unilinear temporal narratives, in which there is one possible future with a "clear course" that can be articulated in "general laws," and multilinear temporal narratives, which reflect a nonteleological, contingent understanding of the future. An additional, related aspect of imagined futures Mische (2009, 702) presents is "volition," or the extent to which it is believed that we can control or influence the future. Although future projections have been largely neglected in sociological theory and research relative to accounts of the past, she argues, analyzing them can deepen our understanding of beliefs and actions in the present.

The distinction between sociotemporal and biotemporal orders is essential for understanding debates about mammography. Conflicts around overdiagnosis, for example, are fundamentally about whether the sociotemporal order of screening schedules reflects the biotemporality of tumor growth. Implicit in these debates are also imagined futures for tumors which may or may not be singular or unilinear, contingent, or amenable to our volitional interventions in the present. These future projections differ between interventionists and skeptics (and manifest in different recommended actions in the present), with interventionists more likely to view the future as singular (such that intervening makes sense), whereas skeptics tend to view it as contingent, leading to hesitancy.

Furthermore, the distinction between sociotemporality and biotemporality is highly relevant to the debate over the age to begin screening, which, as we have seen, is the primary manifestation of the conflict between interventionists and skeptics at the institutional level and when translated into health policy.

Social definitions of age and age intervals always function to socially and temporally standardize biology, and they do not necessarily accurately reflect chronological age, let alone biological age. As Zerubavel (1991, 30–31) puts it: "society transforms mathematically negligible steps across conventional cutoff points in time into critical quantum leaps in 'age.' . . . The practical implications of such a manner of reckoning age can hardly be overstated, as evidenced by the way we actually cluster schoolchildren into discrete classes separated from one another by full-year gaps. A child born on January 1 must usually wait a full year longer than a child born only a couple of hours earlier, on December 31, before he or she can enter school." Not only do such "spasmodic" (Zerubavel 1991, 31) social definitions of age lump together people of different biological ages, but any possible cut points for such groupings are arbitrary social conventions. This can be seen in the way that different school districts actually use different cut points, with some breaking chronological age at September 1st for entry to school, for example, rather than January 1st.

In the mammography debates, the arbitrariness of age cut points is evident in the way that disagreement often revolves around decades (e.g., women age forty to forty-nine) rather than another, less socially tidy, even nondecimal number. Not only do age intervals socially standardize and group—and thereby distort—the continuum of chronological age, but the biological aging process, which is what is actually most relevant to the question of the necessity for mammography, certainly does not conveniently follow such social measurements of time. Clearly not all people of the same chronological age are the same "age" biologically, that is, in terms of their physical health. In this chapter I explore how the cognitive structure of these different sociotemporal orders and meanings in the mammography conflict is illuminated through a focus on the fundamental sociocognitive process of selective attention.

Sociotemporality and Attention

One of the cognitive functions of social groups is to perform temporal and mnemonic "synchronization" (Zerubavel 2003, 4); the resulting shared temporal norms and patterns, in turn, serve as an important basis for social differentiation and social solidarity (Zerubavel 1985, 67). This temporal synchronization is performed using the mental filters that cognitively unify members of social groups. Zerubavel describes the relationship between our sociomental filters and the synchronization of memory as follows: "remembering involves more than just recall of facts, as various mental filters that are quite independent of those facts nevertheless affect the way we process them in our minds . . . thus leading us to remember some more than others" (4). At this nexus of social cognition and collective memory lies the concept of *sociotemporal attention*.

The connection between mental filters held in the present and how we perceive time highlights the close ties between cognitive sociology and the sociology of time and collective memory (Beim 2007; Brekhus 2015, 147; Zerubavel 1985, 2003). As Brekhus (2015, 147) argues, "memory and perceptions of timing and time are important dimensions of our cognition," closely aligned with "key cognitive processes such as attention, frame, relevance, categorization, meaning, and identity." In keeping with the emphasis of this book on the sociology of attention, I will focus specifically on tracing the norms of temporal attention underlying the conflict between interventionists and skeptics, emphasizing the interrelatedness of patterns of attention and perceptions of time. Many prior works have demonstrated that *collective* memory is always also *selective* memory, and that mental weight is unevenly distributed in our recollections of history and perceptions of time (Brekhus 2015, 149, 155–159; Zerubavel 2003, 29). To return to the quote from Zerubavel, we inevitably remember some historical details more than others as a result of the mental filters we apply.

The observation that selection, reduction, and choice (although not always or even often conscious choice) form the basis for social time (Brekhus 2015, 149; Nowotny 1992, 433–434; Tabboni 2001, 9; Zerubavel 1985, 2003) highlights memory's fundamental connection with attention, which, as discussed previously, can be analogously defined as a process of mental selection in which certain details or dimensions of reality are designated for focus and emphasis while others are not selected and receive no attention. Zerubavel (2003, 27) explicitly connects attention and focus to the construction of sociotemporal order when he describes perceptions of the past as "a product of certain *norms of historical focusing* that dictate what we should mnemonically 'attend' and what we can largely ignore and thereby forget. It thus basically involves a fundamental distinction (closely resembling the one between 'figure' and 'ground') between what we regard as historically 'significant' and thus come to collectively remember, and what is considered 'irrelevant' and thereby essentially relegated to social oblivion."

Through such socially synchronized processes of *temporal attention*, groups construct historical narratives that in turn help support the validity of their cognitive filters and norms in the present. This process of narratively organizing temporality is what makes time human and gives it social meaning and intelligibility (Brekhus 2015, 148; Halbwachs 1950; Ricoeur 1984, 1988; Zerubavel 2003, 13). As alluded to already, one important function of such temporal narratives is to "construct a narrative past that fits with present understandings" (Brekhus 2015, 148; Nowotny 1992, 433). Zerubavel (2003, 13) elaborates on this process: "Indeed, it is through such emplotment (as well as reemplotment . . .) that we usually manage to provide both past and present events with historical meaning." Thus, narrating the past to fit with present aims and filters through attention and inattention is one "temporal strategy" used by cognitive and attentional communities to support currently held cognitive frameworks and to differentiate (and invalidate) other ways of thinking about time—as well as, by extension, the sociomental filters held by others in the present. Stated differently, the construction of temporal narratives can be understood as an attentional battle strategy in cultural contests over relevance. In addition to using present-time cognitive filters to narrate the past and to project the future, other strategies of temporal attention include "playing with and utilizing the interval" (Nowotny 1992, 444), as well as marking and unmarking historical periods or temporal units (Zerubavel 2003, 26). Temporal marking offsets some periods as temporal aberrations or "turning points," while other periods are unmarked and thus viewed as periods of continuity or of default temporal movement or progression (19).

Recognizing the attentional roots of such sociotemporal strategies, in this chapter I explore the temporal narratives associated with the attentional patterns of interventionism and skepticism. Having established in prior chapters the key characteristics of interventionism and skepticism as attentional types, here I extend this argument to connect the attentional patterns of each group with their use of temporal concepts, narratives, and strategies, drawing first from my interviews with doctors and scientists. Following this discussion, I address the temporal themes that emerged in my interviews with patients, highlighting the social meanings and temporal defaults that define their patterns of temporal attention to mammography.

Biological Time and Screening Schedules

As mentioned already, Aronowitz (2001) describes two temporal narratives competing consistently throughout the history of breast cancer diagnosis and treatment, both of which began well before mammography was even in use. "Do not delay" (and its later iteration of early detection) has been the dominant temporal narrative from the start, and forms one of the most stable historical continuities of breast cancer discourse. That being said, a competing skeptical temporal perspective has steadily appeared alongside the hegemonic narrative of early detection. This alternative temporal narrative takes shape primarily through bringing attention to the disjuncture between the biological temporality of breast cancer and the sociotemporal order defining early detection screening narratives. It is a lack of correspondence between the variable temporality of the molecular biology of tumors and the definitional sociotemporal regularity of screening and other temporal assumptions of early detection frameworks that is in large part responsible, mammography skeptics argue, for screening's lack of impact on breast cancer mortality rates. Examples from the contemporary academic literature on screening emphasizing the biotemporal diversity of conditions known as "disease," particularly cancer, include Moynihan, Henry, and Moons (2014, 2), Harris et al. (2011, 28), and Esserman, Thompson, and Reid (2013, 797), who describe the biotemporal diversity of cancer this way: "The word 'cancer' often invokes the specter of an inexorably lethal process; however, cancers are heterogeneous and can follow multiple paths, not all of which progress to metastases and death, and include indolent disease that causes no harm during the patient's lifetime." For skeptics, to take seriously this biotemporal diversity means that the goal should be not only to detect the mere presence of disease but also to identify those abnormalities whose biological temporality makes screening and treatment effective (Esserman, Thompson, and Reid 2013, 797; Harris et al. 2011, 28; Moynihan, Henry, and Moons 2014, 2). Esserman et al. (2013, 797) argue further for renaming those abnormalities without a linear, progressive biotemporality, reserving the term "cancer" for those with a high chance of lethal progression if left untreated.

The skeptic doctors and scientists I interviewed emphasized repeatedly and from a variety of perspectives this point that cancer's biological time is not reflected in the temporal assumptions about early detection that underlie mammography screening guidelines. Dr. Price, an oncologist, for example, describes how a reliance on pathologists to provide information about tumors has led to "a very static picture" that "turns out a crude measure of the dynamic process that is always going on in cancer." This has resulted, he explains, in the incorrect assumption that "a cancer is a cancer and all cancers progress" that underlies the logic of early detection. Dr. Jones, a radiologist, similarly states that the temporality of tumor growth is not progressive and linear:

> You can have—not a cancer that goes away, but you can have a cancer that's stable for many, many years and never harms anyone. You can also have a very small cancer that, you know, sizewise shouldn't metastasize and does. So I just think that in general it's not unique to breast that we are just at the forefront of figuring out what cancers, you know, how they behave biologically. . . . But it's true that cancers can be stable for many years and never metastasize, but I have also seen very low-grade cancers

that have not been seen on a mammogram or missed, that aren't in theory "growing in the breast," that have lymph node metastasis.

Dr. Raff, an academic medical researcher, likewise emphasizes that, although still poorly understood, the variable biological temporality of breast cancer is absolutely essential to attend and mentally weigh when determining the importance of early detection through screening. Using the example of DCIS, she explains that variation in tumor characteristics is the most likely reason why, despite increasing detection rates, the incidence of invasive breast cancer is not decreasing:

> Despite these high rates of DCIS detection, the incidence rates of invasive cancers don't go down; they just keep on climbing, and so it doesn't seem that we are really preventing invasive cancers by detecting and removing these DCIS lesions. So in my opinion, it's really important to consider when you discuss overdiagnosis, and it's important to bring us a better understanding of the natural history of breast cancer, which is actually much, much less understood than what most people think. The key thing with earlier detection of breast cancer of course is that you need to catch the cancer before it spreads. But breast cancer screening only changes the average tumor size from about 1.3 to about, uh, 0.8 centimeters in diameter. And when the—when the tumor is 0.8 centimeters in diameter, it has already gone through about 90 percent of its lifetime compared to when it's clinically detected. So do you then prevent the spreading? No one knows when these tumors spread. It likely varies. But if the tumor has already spread to the rest of the body before it becomes screen detectable, screening is unlikely to make any difference for the prognosis.

The biological temporality of tumors, as Dr. Raff expresses in these comments, is variable and poorly understood. Yet the sociotemporal logic of routine, annual mammography screening—to find tumors before they metastasize—assumes, incorrectly in her view, that tumors always metastasize only after they are large enough to be detectable by screening. Again, what these remarks all draw into focus and give attentional weight is a discordance between the biological temporality of breast cancer and the sociotemporal assumptions of early detection.

Dr. Freeman, a breast surgeon, argues that the same problematic temporal assumptions about cancer's progressive, linear, unidirectional development underlie not only the general idea of early detection but also our scientific and statistical models for assessing the effectiveness of mammography. As a result, the available data are distorted by this same mismatch between the biotemporality of cancer and the sociotemporality of mammography: "In the statistical models, you are . . . trying to simulate the natural history of breast cancer. But although the model is better doing this, they have to assume that there is a constant growth of the tumor; otherwise their models won't work. So by doing this, you are sort of disregarding the fact that some of these tumors found by mammography screening would not have been found without mammography screening. So they're not progressive and might even regress." In short, the skeptical participants collectively emphasize the point that the biological temporality of cancer is complex and nonlinear; it can progress via starts and stops, or metastasize while still tiny. It may not even be unidirectional, as expressed in Dr. Freeman's statement that it "might even regress."

The temporal mismatch between the biotemporality of breast cancer and the social timetable of screening recommendations is an example of "discrepancies between organic and mechanical periodicity" (Zerubavel 1985, 11), in which social and institutional timetables are out of sync with biological temporality. As the skeptical participants emphasize, it is inherently problematic to build a temporally regular screening program around the "biological time" of the tumor, which varies, is irregular, and is unknown. Indeed, at an even more macrohistorical level, the basic, foundational notion of a tumor's inevitable growth, which is the fundamental basis for any argument for early detection, reflects socially constructed understandings of time as unidirectional. Although now totally normalized and taken for granted, unidirectional concepts of time actually date to Benedictine and Utilitarian ideologies rejecting prior notions of the "eternal return" and other nonlinear temporal concepts. In reality, then, it was the Protestant Reformation that actually brought the notion of time as linear and finite to the modern era (54).

In contrast to the way the skeptical participants are attentive to and heavily weigh the disjuncture between the biological temporality of tumors and screening timetables, this point is largely considered irrelevant by interventionist scientists and medical researchers, who remain convinced of the inevitable growth of the tumor and the indispensability of early detection, embodying the historical continuity of "do not delay," Aronowitz describes.[1] These participants, exemplified here by Dr. Cashman, a radiologist, stress that, *even taking into account the variable biological progression of different tumors*, it is still *essential* to find them and treat them as early as possible, given the lack of certainty about the temporal characteristics of any specific tumor. Although interventionists sometimes recognize the variable biological temporality of breast cancer, in other words, their fundamental belief in early detection remains unshaken, with little weight given to this temporal disjuncture. As Dr. Cashman puts it, "even if you find a high-grade tumor that's small, that has the same survivability as a low-grade tumor of the same size. So even for these rapidly growing, more lethal cancers, particularly in younger women, if we find them small, we still interrupt the course of that cancer." In terms of attentional focus, what differentiates the temporal narratives of skeptics and interventionists on this point is that interventionists define the variable biological temporality of tumors as irrelevant—as something that can be "interrupted" or altered by early detection and treatment—maintaining focus on the importance of early detection *regardless of whether the timetables proposed for screening are incompatible with the biotemporality of the tumors being found*. Stated differently, in Mische's (2009) terms, for interventionists the imagined future of any cancer found is singular, noncontingent, and volitional. Skeptics, in contrast, organize their temporal narratives around the idea that it is *essential* to attend and adequately weigh the biological characteristics of cancer to understand whether early detection is relevant or not. Again applying Mische's terms, skeptics project a future for any possible tumor that reflects both greater breadth and contingency, and far less certainty about its amenability to our interventions. Several additional temporal themes emerge from these disagreements about early detection and the sociotemporal norms of screening as they relate to the biological temporality of tumor growth. One such temporal concept used by the participants in constructing either a skeptical or interventionist temporal narrative is "lead time."

"Lead Time Bias" versus "Sojourn Time": Temporal Defaults and Distortions

Dr. Freeman, the breast surgeon quoted above criticizing the way that statistical models always assume linear tumor growth, defines "lead time" as follows:

> Lead time is the time you put diagnosis forward by screening. So the whole point of mammography screening is that you are detecting breast cancer at an earlier stage, and then you can treat the breast cancer in an earlier stage and you can cure the patient. So what you do is that you shift from let's say a bad stage or from an aggressive stage to a less aggressive stage, and then you can treat the patient and the patient will survive. So this is really where you can get the effect on reducing mortality from breast cancer is that you move diagnosis forward in time. And this time is usually called lead time.

Skeptical participants concerned about the distorting effect on knowledge of ignoring the variable temporality of tumor growth often instead used the concept of "lead time *bias*" to explain that, while there is an *apparent* correlation between earlier detection (lead time) and prognosis, this does not account for variation in tumor biology. Lead time and lead time bias direct attention to either early detection and survival rates, in the case of lead time, or to biotemporal diversity and lack of improvement in mortality outcomes, in the case of lead time bias. The concept of lead time bias thus shifts the focus of attention away from the length of survival from the point of diagnosis, which is inevitably increased when diagnosis is moved earlier in time, to the question of whether earlier diagnosis actually improves life expectancy (see also Philipson et al. 2012, 668; Welch, Schwartz, and Woloshin 2011, 144). In so doing, lead time bias reframes the apparent relationship between early detection and increased life expectancy as likely due to mistaking the effect of *tumor selection* (again emphasizing biotemporal variability) for an effect of *lead time*, meaning that lead time is not relevant to mortality outcomes—it simply means that patients are aware of their cancer for longer without any change in the outcome. Dr. Raff, an academic medical researcher, explains this view:

> Of course it's very compelling, you know, when you see this curve with the correlation between tumor size at detection and then prognosis . . . It's fairly linear. The later you detect the disease, the poorer the prognosis. It's a very clear trend. But that doesn't necessarily mean that we change the prognosis by earlier detection. It might be just the selection of tumors. Those tumors that grow the fastest and are most aggressive are those that we detect when they're largest because they pop up and grow large before you find them. The slow-growing ones, I mean there's much more time to detect them. So the correlation might have nothing to do with early detection. It might be something that has to do with tumor biology.

Dr. Obermeyer, a professor of family medicine, similarly used the concept of lead time bias to emphasize that there is distortion in our understanding of early detection and the potential impact of altering the interval for mammography due to unknowns and variability in cancer's temporality:

> When we're talking about differences in our screening protocols going from one year to two years . . . that extra year that you miss that you might not have screened for the majority of cancers, the disease is not going to

progress that significantly that "early detection" a year earlier would have prevented any of the morbidity or the mortality. Um, and that's sort of, you know, what I referred to earlier as kind of that lead time bias that, you know, we picked up this cancer earlier. Did it really mean anything in the grand scheme of things?

In describing lead time as a source of "bias," skeptics are also clearly performing attentional discrediting through challenging traditionalists' norms of attentional weight, as discussed in chapter 4. In essence, their argument is that interventionists are overweighing rates of diagnosis and length of survival and underweighing the biological characteristics of cancer when determining the true importance of early detection.

In response to such arguments, interventionist proponents of early detection rhetorically reverse skeptics' evaluative judgment, rejecting the idea of lead time as a source of bias. They argue instead that lead time is actually *essential*, and some advocate for rebranding this period as the "sojourn time" of a cancer to normalize it and reduce any negative association. For example, Dr. Cashman, the radiologist I quoted earlier to illustrate interventionists' commitment to early detection regardless of biological variation in cancer's temporality, also argues that for mammography "you actually need lead time." Mammography is premised, he explains, on the notion that there is a temporal gap between when a cancer is detectable via screening and when it is clinically palpable. Thus, from his perspective, *lead time is a default norm* in cancer's temporality. As he puts it, "If the screen-detected cancer was detectable at the same time that it became clinically detectable, then why would you need a screen? You actually need lead time in order for mammography to actually work. We need a lead time between where it's not clinically apparent and to where it is. . . . And it's called the 'sojourn time' in the literature. It's the sojourn time of a cancer between the time that it becomes visible on a screen, a mammogram presumably, and when it becomes clinically palpable." Notably, in these comments, Dr. Cashman seems to be operating on the exact implicit assumption of a linear, unidirectional temporality for cancer that skeptics problematize, and thus he does not treat as relevant the more challenging critique they raise about the disconnect between screening's temporal assumptions and the complex and unpredictable, possibly even multidirectional, biological temporality of cancer. Rather, his temporal strategy is to use attentional reversal to emphasize the normative status of lead time and restore its default, taken-for-granted status in response to skeptics' claims of "lead time bias" (on such tactics of attentional subversion, see also Zerubavel 2018, 61–91).

Are We Finding Breast Cancer "Too Late"? ... or Maybe "Too Early"? The Significance of Treatment versus Early Detection

Debates about lead time bias are also interconnected with related temporal questions about whether advancements in treatment have changed or should change the threshold of what counts as "early" versus "delayed" detection and treatment. Skeptical doctors and scientists frequently argue that improvements in breast cancer treatment have made early detection significantly less urgent, shifting attention away from screening to bring more weight to the significance of treatment in the debates. Such reasoning belies a belief that there is a temporal limit to early detection; that is, their remarks imply that there is such a thing as a time "too early" to screen, given the tradeoff between the benefits and harms and the existence of increasingly effective therapies. In this same vein, some skeptics argue that moving the temporal line for detection later will have significantly less impact on mortality rates than the ideology of early detection suggests, challenging the idea that later detection is problematic. For example, Dr. Light, a professor of radiation medicine, says that, in his view, "the therapies have become so good that even if you detect it late ... it's curable in 90 plus percent of the time." Therefore, "letting it progress to a point where it's now a little more advanced ... we've still got therapy to cure it." Similarly, Dr. Malcolm, an epidemiologist and former breast surgeon, explains: "a rather reasonable interpretation of the evidence as it looks now is that cancers that 30–40 years ago could only be cured through advancement of diagnosis achieved through screening and detection before they became symptomatic, that some of those cancers can now be treated with modern adjuvant systemic treatments."

Dr. Franklin, a primary care physician and academic researcher, likewise emphasizes that it is essential to give attentional weight to improvements in treatment when assessing whether any temporal threshold for mammography is impactful. He explicitly connects this to the variability in cancer's biological temporality discussed already, dividing cancers into three biological trajectories, only one of which screening definitely helps: "Cancer is just a much more heterogeneous group of disorders, some of which really aren't going to be helped with screening, some of which are going to be overdiagnosed, and there's this middle group which are—it can be plausibly helped by screening. But as our treatments get better and better, it's much less advantageous to do so." Taken together, these remarks all emphasize the impact of treatment over early detection, suggesting that—due to treatment's greater contribution—there is less temporal urgency for mammography than early detection frameworks have suggested, and it is therefore not necessary to aggressively screen younger women.

While skeptics apply attentional weight to improved treatment, most interventionists did not waver at all in their commitment to the idea that *earlier detection is always better*, basically excluding from attention any independent contribution of treatment. Dr. Cashman offers perhaps the most extreme version of this resolute interventionist attentional commitment to early detection. Rhetorically sidestepping the question of whether it is treatment or early detection that is more responsible for improvements in outcomes, he substitutes the idea of "overtreatment" for "overdiagnosis" to argue that it is in actuality treatment, not detection, that causes *harm*: "I hate the term 'overdiagnosis' myself. I think we overtreat, and we're already learning how to treat less. And the main expense and the main mortality and the main harms of breast cancer is not in the diagnosis; it's in the treatment." Here Dr. Cashman draws attention to the harms of treatment, rather than the benefits of either treatment or early detection, to remove attention and weight from the harms of screening and the contributions of advances in treatment, maneuvering rhetorically to avoid any challenge to early detection.

Other interventionist participants acknowledge the benefits of improved therapies, but rather than using these improvements to justify pushing back the threshold for early detection or slowing the pace of screening, they tend to emphasize the idea that *treatment's efficacy is contingent on early detection*. Finding cancer as early as possible thus remains essential in their view, and there is no temporal limit to the benefit of early detection. In the following comments, for example, Dr. Shoumer, an oncologist, begins by acknowledging how improvements in treatment have reduced mortality from breast cancer 30 to 40 percent over the last several decades. However, rather than questioning whether this might lessen the urgency of early detection, he ends by emphasizing that early detection has been essential to treatment's impact: "So clearly the treatment of breast cancer has improved quite significantly. And just based on the efficacy of treatment, one could state that the mortality related to breast cancer has decreased probably by about a third to 40 percent over the past thirty to thirty-five years. So clearly that has contributed to it. At the same time, these two things are interconnected because our ability to cure breast cancer is much higher or much greater in patients with very small tumors than in patients with much larger tumors." Further supporting the point that early detection through mammography is responsible for any improvements in breast cancer outcomes, Dr. Shoumer immediately pivots in his remarks to focus on how much mammography has improved and how much earlier tumors are found now compared with earlier periods. Dr. Shoumer further argued that, in his view, because of these technological improvements in cancer detection—which occurred after the main clinical trials on which the data are based, and therefore are not reflected in most of the data used in research on mammography—the available research actually *underestimates* the benefits of early detection.

Dr. Adams, a radiologist and academic researcher, similarly focuses his comments on the positive impact of mammography rather than on improvements in treatment, arguing that improvements in therapy are relevant and effective only when cancer is found early: "Mammography is far from perfect. It does not find all cancers and does not find all cancers early enough to save all lives, but it is saving thousands of lives each year. The death rate from breast cancer had been unchanged for 50 years prior to the start of screening in the mid-1980s. As expected, the death rate began to decline in 1990. There are now more than 30 percent fewer women who die each year from breast cancer due to screening. Therapy has improved, but therapy saves lives when cancers are treated early." Note that, if anything, in Dr. Adams's view, the weakness of mammography is in *not finding enough cancers early enough*. This line of reasoning again disattends the key temporal question being raised by skeptics about the variable molecular biology of cancer. That is, from the perspective of overdiagnosis, some of the tumors found through mammograms were not going to grow linearly (or perhaps at all) during the screening interval under consideration and thus would have remained treatable even if the temporal line for their detection was pushed later.

"Unfair Endpoints"

Another example of temporal attention in debates about mammography has to do, not with the starting point for screening as in debates over "lead time" and the relative contributions of treatment and early detection, but with the correct endpoint to use when assessing mammography's effectiveness. The USPSTF's 2009 decision to push back their previously recommended starting point for routine mammography screening from forty to fifty years old was based on mammography's impact on the outcome of *mortality rates* from breast cancer. This is only one possible outcome or endpoint one could use, however. One could also focus on diagnosis rates, for example (e.g., Does mammography help find more cancers?). As Dr. Obermeyer, a professor of family medicine, explains, part of the debate over mammography thus emanates from the different camps "looking at the same evidence with actually different endpoints." In general, skeptics, like the USPSTF, advocate for using mortality rates over other possible measures such as diagnosis rates because most other measures are inflated by overdiagnosis, while mortality rates are not. Such "overdiagnosis bias" combines with "lead time bias" to artificially increase survival statistics (Welch, Schwartz, and Woloshin 2011, 145). Skeptics repeatedly pointed out that mortality rates have not meaningfully improved despite massive increases in participation in mammography screening, suggesting that mammography's main effect is to find tumors that would not ultimately go on to kill the person (i.e., most tumors are overdiagnosed). Again returning to the idea of projection or possible futures (Mische 2009), skeptics thus emphasize that there are multiple possible courses of development for any tumor found using mammography, and that volitional interventions made through screening and treatment only alter a subset. Dr. Samuels, a primary care physician, exemplifies this perspective: "when you see how many more cancers have been diagnosed and how the mortality hasn't really improved, it just makes me think that mammography isn't all it was cracked up to be." Dr. Bates, an academic medical researcher, similarly explains the connection between overdiagnosis and the lack of improvement in mortality rates, in this case using the example of DCIS, which she refers to as "stage 0" cancer—a term whose attentional effect is to invoke the temporal logic of early detection that "all cancers progress" as well as to gesture at the idea of biotemporal complexity by locating DCIS at a temporal point prior to any of that inevitable progression at "stage 0": "Many, many women have a story of their lives being saved by mammogram, even though as I read this, probably what the mammogram found was a stage 0 cancer, and then they became a cancer patient and it was treated as if it was cancer. Um, but that may have been what happened in those stories because the cancer mortality rate doesn't change. And that's a hard fact. That's a hard fact that the cancer mortality rate doesn't change." From the perspective of skepticism, then, the only legitimate measure of mammography's impact on breast cancer is mortality rates, since other measures inappropriately "count" such overdiagnosed tumors.

Dr. Freeman, a breast surgeon, is a partial exception to this characterization, as he is skeptical of mammography yet also critical of a too-narrow focus on mortality reductions. In his view, debates about mortality rates as an endpoint are becoming outmoded, shifting into a more useful conversation about the relative risks and benefits of screening: "Sometimes I am surprised to see that people are still really fighting over the relative reduction in mortality. Uh, which is for me personally, a little bit falsified because I don't think there are really big differences in . . . what the relative numbers are. So I think more and more we're shifting over to this discussion of the balance of the benefits and harms. And also the problems of overdiagnosis and how to study it and how to interpret the data that we are having." Importantly, however, Dr. Freeman still emphasizes that overdiagnosis is essential to take into consideration. This attention to overdiagnosis is what defines the skeptical perspective on how to validly determine mammography's impact. Thus, when skeptics advocate for using mortality rates, it is largely because they are the only statistical outcome measure that reflects the impact of overdiagnosis.

Interventionists, on the other hand, commonly argue that mortality rates are, as Dr. Mack, a breast surgeon, puts it, an "unfair endpoint" to use to evaluate screening's value. From her perspective, mortality is not the only "relevant" consideration to attend when determining the impact of screening: "When you find something small in a young woman and, had they not had that test, we wouldn't have found it until it was bigger. Um, while some people argue that some populations, that may not affect mortality, the type of treatment you get when you present with a larger tumor, . . . it often entails chemotherapy, whereas something very small, you may still get away without chemotherapy." Similarly advocating for refocusing attention away from mortality rates and using a broader notion of mammography's impact that considers the intensiveness and toxicity of treatment and other quality of life factors, Dr. Cashman wonders: "Do we have to use death as the one and only measure? Can we use quality of life? Can we use, you know, somewhat quantity of life?" In terms of attentional exclusions, traditionalists are pointing out that in restricting attention to mortality rates alone, skeptics are limited in their ability to recognize meaningful contingencies, especially relating to treatment, in mammography's impact on women's broader experience of breast cancer diagnosis and treatment.

While skeptics are insistent that because we cannot isolate the true impact of mammography unless we account for overdiagnosis, mortality rates are the only valid measure, interventionists argue that it is equally important to consider whether screening allows for less invasive treatment and thus improves patients' quality of life in the present. As we have seen throughout, this interventionist narrative disattends arguments about overdiagnosis. Indeed, acknowledging overdiagnosis would force interventionists to confront the possibility that improvements in "quality of life" or the ability to use less invasive treatment is equally as dependent upon the specific biological temporality of the tumors being found as it is on whether they are found earlier or later. At the same time, however, in their insistence on attentionally centering and heavily weighing overdiagnosis, skeptics may be underweighing the impact of early diagnosis on patients' experience of treatment, even if mortality outcomes remain the same with earlier or later diagnosis.

Temporal Ranges and Intervals: Arbitrary Age Cut Points and the Variable Meaning of a "Life Year"

While interventionists and skeptics dispute many temporal ideas, as we have seen, it is age that is the explicit focus of the institutional conflict over mammography guidelines. The different age recommendations should be familiar at this point: interventionists believe screening should begin at forty (if not earlier), and take place annually, while skeptics support delaying the starting age, as the USPSTF guideline does, to fifty or even later. A sociocognitive perspective on temporality posits that how each group parses the temporal continuum of age is equally arbitrary with respect to biological and astronomical time, reflecting instead their shared norms of attention, focus, and relevance. In addition, age distinctions or cut points are necessarily imbued with social meaning as opposed to strictly scientific or biological significance.

As previously established in the sociology of memory, "playing with and utilizing the interval" is one "temporal strategy" used by cognitive and attentional communities to support currently held beliefs and schemas and to differentiate (and invalidate) other ways of thinking about time—and thus the mental filters or schemas of those with rival perspectives (Nowotny 1992, 444). Participants on both sides of the mammography debates acknowledge that there is no "magical" or "actual" breaking point at age forty or fifty, or any other age, a claim that is also raised on both sides of debates over mammography in the academic literature (Kopans, Webb, and Cady 2014, 2794; Quanstrum and Hayward 2010, 1076). This may initially seem surprising given that age is such a central point of focus in the conflict. When acknowledging that any age line one could draw is at some level arbitrary, however, skeptics and interventionists apply this insight in totally different ways based on their underlying cognitive commitments with respect to early detection, overdiagnosis, and the risks of screening. Interventionists typically argue that, given that any age line is arbitrary, and given the benefits of early detection, there is no scientific reason not to start screening sooner. For example, Dr. Adams, an interventionist radiologist and academic researcher, argues that "the cancer detection rate changes gradually with increasing age ... and there is no sudden change at any age." He uses this point about the age continuum to bolster the idea that nothing "magical" happens at age forty, and in fact the only reason for not starting screening earlier than forty is that women under age thirty-nine were not included in clinical trials. Thus the reason screenings do not begin earlier than age forty, in his logic, is not that it is not beneficial or desirable to do so but that we do not have the data to support the benefit he believes is there, given that age is a continuum. He seems to view this as a technicality rather than a legitimate reason to wait until age forty: "The reason age forty is the threshold is that if you require scientific evidence, as do screening proponents, the randomized, controlled trials only included women age thirty-nine to seventy-four. Nothing magical happens at the age of forty, but we have always been science-based." These remarks clearly illustrate the use of the concept of an age continuum to support the defining interventionist commitment to as-early-as-possible detection, which Dr. Adams further narratively validates in this comment by framing it as the "science-based" perspective.

In contrast, Dr. Franklin, a primary care physician and academic researcher, while similarly recognizing the arbitrariness of age cut points, narratively frames his comments to support the opposing skeptical perspective that early detection needs to be questioned: "Well, here is one place I agree. Here is one place I agree with mammographers. There is no obvious place where to start. It's always arbitrary. . . . There's no obvious place to draw the line, so I can't get excited about the forty-versus-fifty thing." Rather than concluding, like Dr. Adams, that given that any starting point is arbitrary, there is no reason not to start earlier than age forty, he uses the idea that age is a continuum to argue that "it's as much a decision at fifty as it is at forty." As opposed to using the arbitrariness of any breaking point in the continuum of age to argue for making mammography recommendations more encompassing, then, skeptics suggest that this is a reason to limit recommendations to the patients most likely to benefit from screening. Given the biological and temporal heterogeneity of cancer, this requires attending to more clinically and biologically meaningful cut points than age. Thus, both Dr. Adams and Dr. Franklin argue that any temporal line one could draw is arbitrary, but their perspective vis-à-vis early detection, treatment, and the risks of screening, among other things, lead them to totally opposing rhetorical uses of that temporal observation.

Dr. Price, an oncologist, makes this connection between advocating for an earlier starting point and shorter interval for screening and being part of a cognitive community committed to early detection explicitly in the following:

> And, um, and the other is difference in perspectives. . . . You can usually anticipate a more encompassing recommendation for screening tests from the sub-specialists, and especially those that are involved in performing the tests, and in this case it's the radiology community. And from advocacy groups that have people who have been affected by the disease, as that changes perspective. Uh, so most of the breast cancer advocacy groups recommend starting at age 40. . . . So it—you can always anticipate

difference in perspectives are going to lead to differences in making recommendations based on the same evidence.

Likewise, skeptics' attention to overdiagnosis and the biological diversity of cancer lead them to advocate for less aggressive temporal intervals, or even more fitting, for the abandonment of temporal intervals entirely in favor of more biologically and clinically meaningful categories to structure screening guidelines. These observations highlight the defining connection between the sociocognitive frameworks of attentional groups and such temporal strategies as manipulating intervals.

In addition to altering temporal intervals to fit one's cognitive filters, the doctors' and scientists' narratives about age and screening also illustrate that age distinctions must be understood as "imbued with meaning" as part of a "sociotemporal order" as opposed to a strictly biotemporal order (Zerubavel 1985, xiv). Different ages and life stages are resonant with social meanings that shape the significance of different possible age cut points for screening guidelines. Dr. Price, the clinical oncologist quoted above, describes the social meanings that shape his feelings about excluding women under fifty: "I think what swayed me to this side [interventionism] is that, you know, when we say, 'It's 500 tests per life year gained' and you yourself look at a forty-year-old patient who walks in your door who just got diagnosed with breast cancer, that person looks a lot like me. You know, they have three young children, they have—they're working—you know what I mean?" Social meanings also color how Dr. Andrews, an ob-gyn and breast health specialist, understands what she calls "the value of a life year":

> Even if we look at the data and say, you know, "Clearly sixty-year-olds are getting much more bang for their buck. We only have to screen two hundred sixty-year-olds to find a breast cancer." (Laughs) Well, that's true. But was finding the breast cancer more important in that sixty-eight-year-old or was it more important in this forty-year-old? . . . And so I think that's why, you know, we're all looking at the same data; it's just like, you know, what's the value of that life? You know, I think that's what's kind of happened to me unfortunately and maybe it's unscientific, but I—I do kind of look at it and go, you know, I can't really say that I feel that a life year gained in the forties is the same as a life year gained in the eighties. I don't think that that's true.

Again, such sociotemporal meanings are distinct from temporal intervals based on astronomical time, or even biological risk or population mortality benefits, as Dr. Andrews acknowledges directly with the comment, "maybe it's unscientific."

The Attentional Topography of the Past

Although time flows continuously, "sociotemporal orders" arrange the past into discrete units through the attachment of social meaning to different periods and events, thus introducing "culturally based discontinuity into the otherwise even flow of natural time" (Zerubavel 1985, 111). This process of periodizing the past into socially meaningful "chunks," like defining age categories, occurs through the application of sociocognitive filters that always reflect "a particular mnemonic tradition often associated with a specific community" to the otherwise continuous stream of natural time (36). Cognitive communities thus use attention to shape collective memory, narrating the shape of the past and its relationship to the current time period in a manner that serves their perspectives and objectives in the present. "Groups arrange their memories of past events, highlighting, eliminating, and rearranging elements to construct a narrative past that fits with present understandings" (Brekhus 2015, 148). As suggested by the terms "highlighting" and "eliminating" in Brekhus's description, an important cognitive mechanism used to construct divergent narratives of the past is collective attention. Our thought communities construct the shape of historical narratives (e.g., progress or decline) as well as mentally segment "essentially continuous historical stretches into discrete 'periods'" by attending and disattending different details of the past in order to narrate either historical continuity or discontinuity (Zerubavel 2003, 7, 8). In addition to simple progress and decline narratives, such temporal narratives can take a zigzag structure that combines progress and decline to emphasize changes in historical trajectories (18). These zigzag narratives can take either a rise and fall or fall and rise form, but either way, "they always involve some dramatic *change of course*" (19).

In this section, I examine how interventionism and skepticism as attentional communities narrate the shape of the past in terms of temporal continuity and discontinuity, beginning with skeptics' claims of historical change, which they use to emphasize that while early detection was important in the past, that was at a time *very different* from the present in terms of both awareness and treatment. They use this claim of historical discontinuity to support the idea that early detection is not that important in the current period, even if it was in the past. Dr. Obermeyer, a professor of family medicine, is one example of someone who differentiates the present from the past based on improvements in treatment: "The early detection movement came out at a time very different from now with a lot of the treatments and sophistication of things available. So does early detection now provide the same benefits as early detection 10 years ago?" Dr. Thomas, also a primary care physician, similarly explains that "what happens in usual care now is very different than what happened in usual care when the screening studies were first done. So in fact there is a moving target a little bit and current treatments have really improved. And so the contribution of treatment to long-term survival has gotten much better than it did thirty years ago when we first started this stuff or forty years ago when the first screening studies were done." In these examples, both Dr. Obermeyer and Dr. Thomas create temporal discontinuity to narratively support a more limited role for early detection via mammography in the present. However, in other examples, historical *continuities* are invoked for similar ends; this is true, for example, when skeptics highlight the *consistent lack of change* in the mortality rate to show that early detection is not having an impact. This illustrates the way that attentional groups use a variety of (always selective, and sometimes conflicting) temporal strategies to construct a narrative past that fits with present understandings.

Illustrating the importance of attention patterns to fully understand such temporal constructions, both interventionists and skeptics at times portray the past in the identical schematic form of a progress narrative. However, members of each group select very different ideas and details to highlight as evidence for this upward trajectory, depending on what they define as "progress." For example, Dr. Shoumer, an oncologist with an interventionist orientation, highlights improvements in screening technology: "Since screening mammography was first implemented in the late 1960s until now, there has been marked progress in the technology of imaging of the breast, with much improved contrast, much improved detail and resolution and much reduction in the amount of radiation that is needed to deliver each test.... During the past forty years, thanks to mammography, the average time—the average size of breast cancers... has decreased dramatically from something like, 2.5 to 3 centimeters to about 1 centimeter or less."

In contrast, when skeptics construct progress narratives, they emphasize what they perceive as a growing scientific recognition of overdiagnosis and the limits of early detection as well as the transformative impact of improvements in treatment. For example, Dr. Raff, an academic medical researcher and expert on screening, reflects on the progress she perceives in acceptance of the idea of overdiagnosis in the following remarks:

> When I look back and try to recall what the debate was like when I first started, and when we wrote articles back then, we really had to argue that there was such a thing as overdiagnosis, and try to convince the editors

that this was a real problem—and we don't have to do that today. Today overdiagnosis is acknowledged as a—well, the most important harm of breast cancer screening, at least that's my impression. I mean it's a topic of all the top journals now from the *New England Journal of Medicine* to *JAMA* to *BMJ*. All of them publish articles on overdiagnosis in breast cancer screening and it's no longer a debate of whether there is overdiagnosis. It's more a debate of, you know, "What level are we talking about?" . . . But I think now there is a consensus at least in the scientific community that this is a problem, and it's something that we need to deal with. And that recognition was not there ten years ago to the same extent.

When Professor Markman, a professor of medicine and epidemiology, makes the case for historical progress, he similarly emphasizes that there has been growing recognition of the harms of screening:

I think there is more and more understanding that there really are some harms here. And that the idea is not just counting the benefits, but trying to balance benefits and harms. . . . So very subtly and over many years now the discussion I think has moved in a positive direction, such that the guidelines are not quite as strict as they were before. People are beginning to say, "Well, maybe there is an upper limit to screening. We really do need to talk to women. They really do need to make an informed decision." Um, and there is at least some understanding that every two years at least for some women is probably okay.

Thus, as opposed to using different narrative *forms* to describe the past in support of present aims and understandings, in this case the two groups are using the same narrative shape or formal structure to support very different aims in the present, simply by attentively selecting different details when constructing otherwise identical claims of, in this example, historical progress.

One additional temporal strategy used to scaffold interventionist and skeptic narratives is the definition of different turning points, or periods of historical change and anomaly versus continuity. Most obviously, interventionists typically mark the period since the USPSTF 2009 announcement as one of disruption, change, and anomaly from the early detection progress narrative that characterized the history of mammography prior to that point, as described previously. The period from 2009 to the present is defined by interventionists by unsettling efforts to "push back" the starting point for screening and "lengthen" the screening interval from one to two years. Note the way that such characterizations emphasize change and imply that the prior temporal schedule of annual screening for women age forty and over was a consistent recommendation and the default timeline prior to this turning point. Dr. Cashman exemplifies this temporal framing when he explains: "the most recent thing, at least in this country, would be the Task Force recommendations that came out [in 2009]. And they, as you know, changed the recommendations to not routinely screening women in their 40s and only screening every other year from fifty to seventy-four."

At the same time, however, rather than viewing age forty to fifty as the default and the 2009 USPSTF recommendation as a change, one can also parse the history of mammography guidelines in a manner totally compatible with the skeptical perspective. As discussed in the introduction, it is arguable that it has been *disagreement* over whether to screen women between forty and fifty, rather than agreement on the age forty recommendation, that has been most consistent throughout mammography's history. The USPSTF began to recommend screening women in their forties only in 2002, in fact. In light of this, another way to describe the different "eras" or "turning points" in the history of mammography screening recommendations is that disagreement over screening women age forty to fifty is the default, which defines the period leading up to 2002 as well as the period since 2009. It was only during the anomalous seven-year span between 2002 and 2009 that one can speak of any kind of "default" recommendation to screen women in their forties.

To this point in this chapter I have described some of the key temporal narratives and strategies used by the doctors and scientists I interviewed, arguing that, as attention structures in the present, interventionism and skepticism generate different accounts of the past and projected future, as well as of the relationship between screening's timetables and the biological time of cancer. These temporal narratives involve selective attention to concepts and details deemed salient within each attention structure and therefore fit within and help to support the validity of each perspective. At the same time, however, participants on both sides of the conflict generally agree that early detection has been a dominant cultural message for many decades, functioning as the hegemonic sociotemporal "truth" about breast cancer and mammography. Dr. Bates, an academic medical researcher, for instance, points out that, "'Early detection saves lives' has been a slogan for decades . . . it's been around a long, long time. So a whole generation of women grew up with that. And problematizing that is really tough, you know." Dr. Freeman, a breast surgeon, similarly describes what he calls "a massive campaign influencing women to undergo mammography screening." While skeptics may challenge the legitimacy of the sociotemporal norm of early detection, then, they also recognize that they are temporally and attentionally deviant, and early detection nonetheless functions as a dominant cultural discourse, with influence well beyond the medical and scientific communities directly involved in the mammography debates. In the next section, I take my examination of temporal attention outside of the medical realm to address how the patients I interviewed think about mammography and time. In their narratives, one can clearly see the impact of early detection as a hegemonic temporal framework.

Temporal Defaults, Autobiographical Alignment, and Anxious Waiting: How Patients Experience Mammography and Time

As discussed in chapter 2, only a handful of the patients I interviewed were actively following scientific disputes over mammography. Very few were aware of the USPSTF's age guideline change or the concept of overdiagnosis. Rather, for most, the hegemonic sociotemporal norm of early detection functioned as a default belief, which is why I refer to them as default interventionists. Allison, a fifty-year-old white professor who has had two or three mammograms, puts this most directly when she observes that "with every form of cancer, it's the same story: you need to catch it early. And I don't think I have ever heard inconsistency on that one." For other participants, the temporal logic of early detection was evident more indirectly in their belief that the body becomes increasingly at risk with aging. For example, Chyna, a Black forty-seven-year-old family services coordinator who has had at least six mammograms, explains: "the body changes so frequently . . . And I mean you just never know what could have occurred from one year to the other." Abby, a forty-four-year-old Black daycare worker who has had one prior mammogram, expresses a similar sentiment when she says, "I am at the age where you never know when it could just pop up. So I'm supposed to do it once a year. . . . You just don't know what's going on with your body after a certain age." In light of these fears about aging, preventive medical care undertaken as early as possible is understood as only and always beneficial. Rochelle, for example, who is forty-five, Black, and currently unemployed, explains that "If we take preventive measures in the beginning or as soon as possible, we won't have as many people having to do the aggressive treatment and that kind of thing." These remarks highlight the temporal dimension of default interventionism, namely the belief that earlier is always better and risk increases unilinearly with age; thus, while it is not possible to begin screening "too early," it is certainly possible to be "too late." There is no indication in default interventionism of weight or attention to alternative temporal ideas such as biotemporal diversity that challenge the temporal assumptions of early detection.

The hegemony of the temporal logic of early detection is further illustrated by Joanne, a conscious interventionist. Like most of the women I spoke with,

Joanne, a white, fifty-year-old technical writer and editor who has had at least six mammograms, does not question the logic of early detection. However, she is more conscious and self-reflexive about her reasons for screening and her belief in early detection than the default interventionists, in part because they stem from emotionally painful experiences with breast cancer diagnosed prior to age fifty in several friends. In chapter 4, Joanne very explicitly described how she mentally weighs the risks of screening against a significant default weight in favor of the benefits. As she explained, the evidence against early detection would have to be "overwhelming" and "almost double" for her to question the temporal norm of early detection, indicating that she weighs the value of early detection asymmetrically, giving it more mental weight than any evidence that could be measured against it.

Celeste agrees that early detection is the culturally dominant temporal logic, but for her, this is a negative—she disagrees with it but believes that she is socially deviant in questioning the temporality of early detection. Classified as a conscious skeptic, Celeste is forty-one, white, and works as an editor. She is one of the small number of patients I spoke with who were specifically conversant about debates about overdiagnosis, the harms of screening, and the lack of change in the mortality rate from breast cancer despite massive increases in rates of screening and diagnosis. Celeste has never had a mammogram and feels acutely that her skepticism of mammography is out of sync with dominant cultural beliefs about early detection, to the point that expressing her views causes interpersonal conflict with loved ones. This was a consistent theme among the skeptical patients I interviewed. In other words, patients critical of mammography and early detection illustrate the continued hegemony of the temporal logic of early detection by expressing how poignantly aware they are of the social deviance of their own beliefs. Celeste explains: "I think I am counter-normative. I think that most of the people around me are probably still feeling like they need to go get their mammograms early and often. And that possibly contributes to the fact why I don't really want to talk about it. . . . I don't want to have that kind of fight." Early detection thus clearly functioned as a hegemonic temporal default among the patients I interviewed, regardless of whether they challenged it and experienced social resistance like Celeste, or presumed its validity like Joanne.

Often what seemed to most powerfully dictate how patients responded to the temporal norm of early detection was their autobiographical experiences. Prior experiences with breast cancer and screening created patterns of autobiographical attention and weight that patients had to reconcile with the default norm of early detection in a process of autobiographical alignment. What they considered "early" or "late," in other words, depended on what they had previously experienced or observed among family and friends—or in some cases in their professional roles—even if such experiences are always also set against the dominant temporal background of early detection. Their concepts of screening and time are thus doubly *socio*temporal, reflecting both broad cultural norms and more proximate interpersonal meanings and interactions. The significance of biographical experiences in shaping patients' perceptions of breast cancer's temporality exemplifies the necessity of analyzing the coordination of personal and sociotemporal meanings in a process DeGloma (2015, 160) refers to as "mnemonic alignment." Patients' perceptions of mammography and time are thus the result of a process of attentively reconciling and aligning autobiographical experiences with broad sociotemporal norms such as early detection.

For instance, Nicole, who is forty-six, white, and has had at least six mammograms, sometimes cares for young women dying of breast cancer in her work as a hospice nurse. In addition, her mother and several aunts have had breast cancer. For Nicole, her family history and what she observes in her work with hospice patients makes forty feel much too late to begin getting screened. Yet despite her family history, she has struggled with her insurance company to get coverage for her own mammograms prior to age forty. She describes her sentiments about mammography and age in the following comments:

> I have had some women as young as twenty-nine die with metastatic breast cancer, and I had a young lady—she was my age. She was six months older than me. Um, she died about a month ago. And that was terrifying to see her in hospice. And she had been diagnosed at age thirty-eight or thirty-nine. So, I think there needs to be really liberal exceptions, too, with family history . . . It does feel like a ticking time bomb when you have, you know, all of this family and it's like that they, you know, "They don't—they don't want me to do this. They don't want to start it until forty-five."

Similarly illustrating how understandings of "early" or "late" detection depend on community-based experiences and observations, both Joanne and Nancy talk about friends who were diagnosed with breast cancer prior to age fifty, and how those experiences led them to feel that fifty is "too late" to begin screening:

> I guess like everything, you look at your own personal experience. And it's funny because I am actually at [name of local cancer center] today. I bring a friend here for chemo. Uh, this is her second—she has metastatic

breast cancer and she just turned fifty. Her first occurrence was when she was forty-one years old. And I have two other friends that both—now the one it was in situ, and so it wasn't—hadn't spread but, you know, of the many women I know who have breast cancer, three of them had their first cases at—before they were fifty. (Joanne, age fifty, white, technical writer/editor, six or more mammograms)

I can think of another person I knew, and she is dead from breast cancer, was in her forties and had two young girls at home. . . . I think fifty is too late and it—it does need to start sooner. (Nancy, forty-six, white, counselor, four or five mammograms)

The widely shared experience of personally knowing women diagnosed with breast cancer prior to age fifty thus powerfully reinforces for many of the interview participants the importance of early detection and their sense that "earlier is better," and fifty is "too late." Thus, part of the process of becoming conscious interventionists through autobiographical alignment is to take on the temporal norms associated with early detection.

For a few participants, however, personal experiences knowing young women with breast cancer lead instead to skepticism about the value of early detection, particularly when loved ones or acquaintances died despite early detection and treatment. In these cases, watching someone endure painful treatment and die anyway reinforces the idea that sometimes early detection just means living longer with the disease and enduring more toxic treatment, with no ultimate benefit to mortality. Thus some autobiographical experiences lead women to question the default norm of early detection, becoming conscious skeptics rather than conscious interventionists. Christina's experience is illustrative of this autobiographically motivated shift to conscious skepticism:

On the personal side, I had a friend. I worked with her. I started working in that office when I was twenty-two and she was thirty-eight, and I started that position as a temp and I was filling in for her because she was going out the next day to have a mastectomy and she was pregnant at the time. And they hired me and I worked with her for the next three and a half years. And I watched how much she suffered, and she actually died six months after I left there and we had stayed in touch. And I went to visit her in the hospital multiple times when she was in the hospital and again, even after I left, so I have seen someone suffer up close and personal. And who knows what the, you know, chemotherapy that she had right after her daughter was born, and the radiation, and all that. Who knows how long that prolonged her life? But it didn't save it.

She died at forty-two, which is the age I am now. And, you know, I don't want to go through that. And I mean I know there—I know there is another side of it. I know some women survive it. You know, my—my great-aunt is, what, ninety-two or ninety-three now and she—she survived post-menopausal breast cancer. But not the kind you get when you're around my age. And I know that it's worse for young women and if I have something growing in me that they're going to catch, it's probably the worst kind. And I know how few women's lives are saved by what they do catch and how invasive those procedures are. And I don't want to go through years of suffering for those if two cases in however many lives might be saved by it.

For Christina, although she also had a great-aunt who survived breast cancer later in life, the experience of watching her friend and coworker die despite early detection and treatment takes on greater attentional weight in defining her understanding that the societal quest to find breast tumors in younger and younger women has actually pushed the threshold for what is helpful "too early." Although basically the inverse in terms of the meanings taken from such experiences compared with the conscious interventionists discussed previously, Christina's vision of the appropriate timeframe for mammography is nonetheless similarly shaped by her social and interactional experiences set against the hegemonic sociotemporal default of early detection. Generally speaking, what emerges in each of these examples is participants' negotiation of sociotemporal frames as they resonate or fail to resonate with their biographical experiences. It is only in this process of sociotemporal attentional alignment that the difference between a recommendation of age forty or fifty as a starting point becomes truly meaningful. In part, this process of alignment involves the projection of imagined futures in which the observed biographies of friends and loved ones become models or scripts for possible futures for oneself that may or may not support the dominant sociotemporal norm of early detection and treatment.

In addition to using the observed biographies of friends and loved ones as temporal scripts, another dimension of the significance of autobiographical experience in shaping patients' thinking about screening recommendations was their phenomenal and affective experiences of "anxious waiting." Recall that 70 percent ($N = 16$) of the twenty-three interview participants who had had at least one prior mammogram had to return for additional screening or testing. Tania, for example, who is fifty, white, a contingent faculty member, and has had at least six mammograms, describes being routinely recalled for further screening and evaluation following her screenings:

> Several times I have had to, like, wait six months for more testing, and then it's fine. I think it's been pretty consistent. Um, I don't think every time. You know, I'd have to look back at the records and I kind of block it out, but the ones I remember of course are the ones where there was, you know, the waiting and everything. It feels like the narrative has built up for me, which I don't want to be cavalier about, is that, you know, I go to the doctor and they always need to do more tests and it's always fine. So on one hand you'd think, "Well, I can just go through this again," but it is always that waiting. I think because there's so much fear around death, basically.

For Tania, these intense periods of anxious waiting for her results have become a "narrative" that has "built up" such that her temporal experience of mammography is now defined by worried waiting. Regardless of whether she in fact had this experience with each and every mammogram, as she explains, these are the instances that have taken on more attentional weight and thus define her temporal and affective experience of mammography. Jocelyn, who at age forty-seven has had three mammograms, similarly finds screening very stressful, as illustrated in the following anecdote about her first mammogram, which was followed by a terrifying month of follow-up testing before she learned she had benign variation in her anatomy.

> I remember I had actually got my first mammogram when I was thirty-nine. I was just about to turn forty, so they were like, "Well, it's your annual. Go. You're turning forty." Um, and it, you know, it was—it was terrible. I mean I waited, you know, four weeks for a repeat testing, and I ended up having an anomaly that's not cancerous. I have lymph nodes that are in the wrong places, so it looks odd on a mammogram. But so, you know, so I don't find testing to be soothing.

Even when the outcome is ultimately not a cancer diagnosis, as in both of these examples, screening is described as an extremely stressful experience of waiting by the majority of the women I spoke with who had ever been recalled for further testing. It bears repeating in this context that anxiety was one of the harms emphasized in the skeptic attention type's expansive concept of the harms of screening, the "screening cascade," discussed in chapter 4 (and one of the harms excluded from interventionists' more narrow definitions). In this context, however, my point is to highlight the temporal experience of screening from the patient's perspective, particularly the way autobiographical experiences with screening and cancer diagnoses get connected with the background hegemonic temporal framework of early detection, often resulting in a looming temporal fear ("Am I too late?").

My focus in this chapter has been to illustrate the many ways that disagreements over breast cancer are fundamentally about time, whether "official" disputes over age recommendations, or more foundational temporal concepts and beliefs such as early detection, lead time, and overdiagnosis. When describing these debates, the interventionist and skeptic doctors and scientists I interviewed used "temporal strategies" and "temporal narratives" to highlight the particular details of scientific data and history deemed relevant by, and offering support for, their attentional filters. Further, as perspectives, skepticism and interventionism are themselves fundamentally temporal, oriented as they are around either support for or skepticism of the hegemonic temporal norm of early detection. At the most basic level, then, interventionists construct temporal narratives that support early detection, while skeptics attend selectively to details that bring the cultural weight granted to early detection into question. In short, mining the intersections of attention and temporality reveals the significance of temporal meanings in the cultural conflict between interventionists and skeptics. Both groups deploy temporal strategies and narratives to support their cognitive filters and to invalidate the relevance structures of the other. More generally, these different temporal constructions illustrate the defining connection between attention as a cognitive process and the social reckonings of time and history that underlie cultural conflicts, including those situated in such seemingly objective, value-free fields as science and medicine.

For the patients I interviewed, most of whom are default interventionists and not specifically aware of the ongoing debates in medicine, early detection is clearly the dominant temporal framework for their thinking about mammography. I observed only a few cases of specific cognizance of the details skeptics use to construct their temporal critiques, and they were clustered among conscious skeptic patients whose knowledge of ideas like overdiagnosis led them to challenge the taken-for-granted temporality of early detection. However, these patients explicitly understand both themselves as temporal deviants and early detection as the dominant temporal norm in their social circles and the broader culture. Finally, perhaps the most salient temporal meaning of mammography for patients is the cycle of "anxious waiting" that defines their experience of being recalled for further testing following routine mammograms. Sociotemporal meanings are central to patients' thinking about mammography. It is only in the interplay between their sociobiographical experiences and the culturally hegemonic temporal narrative of early detection that patients' concepts of what constitutes "early" or "late" screening take shape. In terms of their affective, phenomenal experience of mammography, for the many patients who experience being recalled following routine mammograms for further testing, these sociotemporal meanings come together in a painful experience of anxious waiting and worried wondering whether their mammogram was in fact "early enough."

Conclusion

Attentional Flexibility

> Breast cancer, like almost all other diseases, has been and will continue to be transformed by what we believe about it and how we respond to it.
>
> —Aronowitz, *Unnatural History: Breast Cancer and American Society*

My use throughout the book of the sociology of attention as a lens to analyze cultural and scientific debates over mammography has had three primary aims: first, to offer a sociological perspective on the conflict, which was previously almost totally absent from the conversation both within and outside of the academy; second, to demonstrate that the sociology of attention can offer a valuable set of concepts and theories for medical sociologists, both in general and particularly for scholars working on the construction of scientific knowledge, and also for analysts of cultural conflicts more generally; third, to provide an empirical case study in the sociology of attention, which to this point has been developing predominantly as a theoretical perspective.

I began to seriously engage with attention processes in my first book, *Blind to Sameness* (2013), where I developed and applied the analytic approach of "filter analysis," first outlined in my collaborative work with Tom DeGloma (DeGloma and Friedman 2005). My specific focus in *Blind to Sameness* was to show how taken-for-granted beliefs about the self-evidence of bodily sex difference function as a "sociomental filter" through which we selectively perceive only those details of human bodies that indicate sex, ignoring any ambiguous or similar physical features. I argued that this focus on attentional patterns, particularly the identification of normatively inattended biological sameness among all human bodies, allowed for new ways of imagining the relationships among sex, gender, and the body that could provide a fresh perspective on decades-long tensions surrounding how to incorporate an analysis of the sexed body into the interdisciplinary field of gender studies.

Attention has since seen significant theoretical development in cognitive sociology (Schroer 2019; Zerubavel 2015, 2018). Although sometimes treated as but one of a series of equally important cognitive processes studied by sociologists—as illustrated, for example, when Brekhus (2015, 147) lists the "key cognitive processes" as "attention, frame, relevance, categorization, meaning, and identity"—there seems to be an emerging recognition of the uniquely fundamental social role of attention processes. For instance, it is arguable that attention actually unifies many of these other "key cognitive processes" as a common underlying mechanism. In any case, it is evident that there is growing interest in the sociology of attention as an area of study in its own right, with several recent works developing attention concepts and reflecting on the importance of attention as a focus for sociological analysis. Brekhus argues that cognitive sociology can be productively applied to nearly any area of interest to sociologists (193). I agree, and I would add that this is particularly the case for an analysis of patterns of attention. Despite this, and despite the notable recent theoretical and conceptual developments in the field, there exist few empirical illustrations of the sociology of attention's analytic insights and generative potential as a tool for sociologists working in areas not normally considered to be "about cognition."

With this in mind, I conceived this project in part as an empirical case study in the sociology of attention. For this purpose, my empirical case is actually largely irrelevant; the point is to illustrate the unique insights available through taking attention as an analytical focus when analyzing any substantive topic. That being said, I chose to analyze the case of mammography because I believe the mammography debates can specifically benefit from a sociological analysis of patterns of attention. Mammography is the subject of one of the most entrenched and rancorous medical conflicts in recent history. Disagreement among experts has stagnated around largely the same issues for decades, without any real indication that the discourse is evolving productively or that a mutually satisfactory resolution to the conflict is any closer. As discussed in the introduction, this disagreement is particularly polarized in the United States. This likely reflects, among other factors, a broader healthcare culture of overuse and prominent specialist organizations in the context of a for-profit, managed care system, combined with a largely unerring faith in screening and early intervention. Further, sociologists have not yet established a clear voice in these debates, allowing the conflict to play out in medicine and politics without the benefits of a sociological perspective. I suggest that the sociology of attention provides a promising framework for this missing sociological contribution to the mammography debates by offering a perspective and set of concepts that facilitate mining the medical discourse to reveal its deeper meanings and patterns. This presses beyond the observation *that* medical knowledge is socially constructed to examine *how* it is constructed. In addition, because the focus of an analysis in terms of attention is how knowledge and conflicts are constructed, rather than evaluative or normative claims about which side is correct, such analysis may offer the possibility of previously unexplored paths to dialogue in the mammography conflict. It may also bring awareness to a new perspective for sociologists to apply, not just to this case, but to other analyses of the social construction of medical knowledge, as well as to cultural and political conflicts outside of medicine.

Uncertainty and Selective Attention

One of the guiding ideas of cognitive sociology is that reality is always more vague, messy, and continuous than the world of clear distinctions (objects, time periods, and so on) that we consciously experience. I have a long-standing interest in the interpretive processes through which social actors reduce this complexity, cognitively and perceptually organizing the blurred continuousness of time and the constant flow and flux of sensory stimuli into recognizable, meaningful social units. Any resulting account or perception of this complex, unruly stream of stimuli is of course necessarily selective; thus, attention is an important cognitive process through which social actors manage such complexity. The attentional filters we learn to apply through socialization in our attentional communities tell us how to "properly" apply rules of relevance to interpret and attend this "disorder" or "flux" such that it is attentionally transformed and stabilized (and through this process inevitably reduced and simplified) into an ordered, socially shared reality, one that reflects collective systems of meaning and can be used for intersubjective communication and validation.

Medicine as a field is no exception to this fundamental complexity, although "uncertainty" is the more common term in the medical literature. Most decisions and errors of interpretation in medicine are known to be made in situations of incomplete information (Bosk 1979, 23). Indeed, "radical uncertainty in medicine is a constant" (Hunter 1991, 32). Most of the time, the scientific and medical reality of the body's health or disease is at least somewhat ambiguous, and it is the work of doctors to create a clear narrative out of this messiness to reassure both patients and themselves that they are "doing everything they can" (Hunter 1991, 32). Welch, Schwartz, and Woloshin (2011, 164) call this "intolerance of uncertainty." New forms of medical technology, including screening technologies such as mammography, function in part as tools to help reduce this inherent uncertainty. At times, however, the desire to provide certainty can lead to excessive use of such technologies without actually providing clarity (Hunter 1991, 38). In addition, new technologies can sometimes generate additional, unanticipated forms of anxiety and uncertainty (Welch, Schwartz, and Woloshin 2011, 166). The sociology of screening literature, for example, documents that the information available through screening results in new illness identities and concepts of risk based on asymptomatic "proto illnesses" (Casper and Morrison 2010; Gillespie 2015; Willis 1998). Uncertainty is also created whenever population screening alters concepts of disease previously taken for granted (Timmermans and Buchbinder 2010). Although often perceived as highly accurate, population screening is "inherently probabilistic" (Davison, Macintyre, and Smith 1994, 343). In genetic screening, for instance, just having a particular allelic pattern or chromosomal abnormality does not necessarily mean one will go on to develop the disease. Another downside to pursuing diagnostic certainty, of course, is the possibility of overdiagnosis, which, as I highlighted throughout the book, is never fully knowable due to its counterfactuality. For these reasons and more, uncertainty is likely to remain an intrinsic feature of population screening. Despite its clear, documented prevalence in medicine, however, uncertainty remains underexamined (Hunter 1991, 20).

As a population screening test, mammography is no exception to the reality of uncertainty in medicine. Several factors make the actualities of mammography messier even than other population screening tests, and certainly more complex than either interventionists' or skeptics' accounts acknowledge. For one, the existing randomized controlled trials were based on older versions of the technology and therefore cannot fully represent current standards of mammography—and it seems highly unlikely that any future trials will be introduced, given that this would require a control group of participants who cannot receive mammography screenings. This would provoke cultural and medical discomfort at best but would more likely be deemed unethical or even illegal. There is also the legitimate conundrum of how to weigh the overdiagnosis that is inevitable with routine mass mammography (although this is true of other screenings as well). Do we "count" (attend, weigh) overdiagnosis when determining the benefits of mammography, even though it is a population data phenomenon and not possible to observe or measure on the level of clinical care of specific patients? Or do we dismiss it as a necessary and acceptable byproduct of a process (medical screening) that is otherwise essential? If we ignore overdiagnosis, we accept the unnecessary treatment of some patients with surgery and toxic drugs, and we also distort the statistics on the prevalence of breast cancer and the effectiveness of mammography and treatment. On the other hand, again, it is not currently possible to apply overdiagnosis clinically, since we do not know in the case of any individual woman whether a tumor will metastasize. Finally, there is the problem that mammography screening has never, not from the start, only been about the science. Breast cancer is politicized, monetized, and intertwined with powerful cultural beliefs about gender and sexuality (King 2008; Sledge 2021; Sulik 2010). A significant technological and financial industry has also grown up around mammography screening that now includes many people who have built their lives and careers around its value and validity.

The reality is that mammography is ambiguous. Interventionists and skeptics resolve this uncertainty through emphasizing different facts, ideas, problems, and details to create a "clear" standpoint out of the messiness. Again, we see how selective attention is a principal cognitive mechanism for the resolution of uncertainty. Each attentional group, however, is only attending and describing part of the story, like the parable of the blind men and the elephant, in which very different descriptions of an elephant result from touching just one part of its body.

Considering this, a *symmetrical analysis* of the patterns of attention underlying differing interpretations of mammography is both revelatory of and necessary for accessing the underlying messiness that no singular narrative reflects. I define a symmetrical analysis of attention as one that compares the attention patterns of multiple perspectives, without treating one as more correct than the others, and then uses the resulting variations in what is considered relevant to generate a more robust understanding of the multiple interpretive possibilities. Such an analysis also attends symmetrically to both attention and inattention. Again, this is accomplished through generating multiple contrasting interpretive possibilities that comparatively reveal the others' nodes of inattention without defining one as more correct than others. This generous, "diffractive" analytical work of cataloging inattention is of particular sociological importance, as the inattended is by definition difficult for anyone to recognize from within a singular cognitive paradigm or filter. In addition, analytically pursuing such productive dissonances creates more accountability for our own exclusions (Barad 2007). Indeed, like most mental filters, skepticism and interventionism are characterized by a rigid adherence to the norms of relevance and attention that maintain their distinctive narratives, making their own patterns of inattention into cognitive occlusions. A symmetrical analysis in terms of attention and inattention is expressly intended to break down any such singular, rigid account of relevance by creating awareness, humility, and an attentional pause to recognize other possible relevance systems. At the same time, I also recognize that this can be more complex to achieve than it may sound; for example, all perspectives and ideas are not equally prominent or available for symmetrical consideration, especially in the face of clearly dominant ideas like early detection. In such cases, a truly symmetrical consideration may require more effortful focus on nondominant perspectives to bring them into equal, productively dissonant tension with hegemonic beliefs. I address this point more fully below in the section on early detection as a hegemonic attention norm.

Professional Filters and Interpretation

It is tempting to make the case that interventionism and skepticism are essentially professional disciplinary attention filters, such that secondary socialization in radiology, for example, would be the source of an interventionist filter. Indeed, we know that "attention patterns . . . differ from one profession to another" and it is "partly through learning their profession's specialized vocabulary that members come to acquire its distinctive attentional habits" (Zerubavel 2015, 66–67). In the specific context of the mammography conflict, Norris et al. (2012) offer support for the role of professional filters in shaping perspectives on mammography; they find that the medical specialty of the panelists on the USPSTF correlated with whether they favored or were opposed to routine annual screening of women age forty to forty-nine, which the authors attribute to what they call "intellectual interest." My findings also support the idea that certain disciplinary norms and practices interrelate with an interventionist viewpoint, most notably treating individual patients with cancer in a clinical setting, which seems to strongly influence one's thinking to minimize the harms and amplify the benefits of screening. It is also undeniable that the defining ideas of medical training within specific disciplines may sit more easily with either a skeptic or interventionist viewpoint. Radiologists, for example, spend their careers perfecting the art of seeking and finding things in the body that are not otherwise visible or felt, such that ideas like "go in search" and "early detection" fit quite naturally. Other disciplines, of course, have different orienting ideas that may not naturalize early detection quite as effectively. Indeed, in my sample, more radiologists and cancer specialists who work daily with patients diagnosed with breast cancer were categorized as interventionists, and more academic researchers, epidemiologists, and primary care doctors were categorized as skeptics. However, there were also exceptions to these generalizations, and I suggest it is actually more illuminating to think of interventionism and skepticism in terms of their organizing beliefs and patterns of attention than as something that doctors in specific medical disciplines are socialized to hold.

In light of this, I argue that the attention types underlying disagreements over mammography are not specific or limited to medical discipline but do at times align with the secondary socialization into professional norms of relevance associated with different disciplines. More precisely, it is early detection that organizes the mental filters most salient to the mammography conflict. Thus, while radiologists are more likely to put a great deal of faith in early detection because it is the basis of their practice, it is the idea, not the medical discipline, that best clarifies the attentional structure of the mammography conflict.

Early Detection as a Hegemonic Attentional Norm

While I endeavored to treat interventionism and skepticism totally symmetrically in my analysis—focusing equally on the attentional patterns of each—it was difficult to avoid the reality that early detection is a culturally hegemonic, taken-for-granted idea, while skepticism of early detection is significantly more culturally marginal. That is, while these two perspectives may equally organize the scientific conflict, they are not equivalent in their broader societal influence or acceptance. This is another reason why it is important to think of interventionism not as limited to particular medical disciplines but instead as a set of ideas that determine patterns of attention and inattention in support of a belief in early detection and medical intervention more generally. Given that early detection is a hegemonic cultural norm, however, symmetrical analysis could not mean totally equal analytical focus in this case, as combatting the hegemony and reification of early detection required somewhat more emphasis. Rather, the symmetry of my analysis is in equally revealing the attention structure of each side and examining both the norms of attention and inattention in each case.

Bearing this in mind, I further consider it one of the contributions of this work to bring greater awareness to skeptical ideas about early detection, which are typically culturally marginalized and can even be difficult to cognitively process when the culture of early detection is so familiar. The skeptic interview participants made this point repeatedly when describing challenges to mammography as difficult for people to recognize and accept due to the ingrained logic of early detection. As a hegemonic cultural norm, early detection is difficult to problematize because it seems so intuitive. Given the social marginality of skepticism, we lack a widely recognized, compelling counternarrative to early detection that might provide access to an interpretive alternative in the face of this self-evidence.

The destabilization of such taken-for-granted social norms is a hallmark of sociological analysis. This kind of work is both intellectually fascinating and socially essential to combat *reification*, understood as the belief that a social convention is actually real or inevitable. The contribution of the sociology of attention to such efforts is to emphasize the importance of comparing different patterns of attention to generate awareness of attentional alternatives. What raising awareness of attentional alternatives uniquely offers as an approach to combatting reification is a way to help us recognize *inattention*, or what we must be unaware of to perceive things as we do. These inattended alternative ideas and beliefs are often no less empirically correct given the messy complexity of reality; rather, they are simply defined as "irrelevant" or "invalid" by our attentional filters, and we are therefore unable to recognize them without some sort of intellectual, affective, or attentional provocation. One of my aims in systematically bringing equal focus to the attentional patterns of interventionism and skepticism is to generate "data" for such a provocation that can broaden our sense of the potentially relevant "facts" in the mammography debates.

Interventionism and Skepticism as Attention Filters

Rather than comparing professional disciplinary groups, I have understood interventionism and skepticism as the two ideal-typical patterns of attention that organize the conflict over mammography. I refer to interventionism and skepticism as ideal types because, while individual actors may not always hold precisely one view or the other, these two patterns of attention best capture the elements of most consequence to understanding the disagreement. As with all ideal types, then, the value is not in their comprehensiveness but in how effectively they expose what is most salient to the topic under consideration. It is in this spirit that I focused this book on the ideal types of interventionism and skepticism; I propose that these two categories capture the most significant elements of the conflict over mammography and thus provide a deeper understanding of the attentional organization of the disagreement as a whole.

While not the only important point of dispute, early detection is centrally important to the patterns of focus defining each side of the conflict. Each viewpoint is *attentionally anchored* by a position on early detection that in turn serves as the foundation for a constellation of other ideas and beliefs. Early detection thus organizes the *attentional relationships* and patterns of *attentional weight* among the different aspects of interventionist and skeptic narratives.

Collectively, these beliefs create *norms of relevance* that in turn organize the patterns of attention and inattention around which the disagreement revolves. Thus, fundamentally, debates over mammography can be understood as an *attentional conflict* anchored by two contrasting views of early detection. Stated another way, *early detection* functions as a *foundational attentional filter* that shapes the overall pattern of attention and relevance within each perspective. The metaphor of a filter is based on blockages and holes, which here represent attention and inattention (Friedman 2013). Thus, the participants' positions on early detection provides the shape of the filter and the number, arrangement, and size of its holes, organizing what details they select (and the details to which they are inattentive) with respect to other points of disagreement. The result is a network of interlinked beliefs and perceptions created through attention that logically coheres around one's view of early detection.

Summarized briefly, the interventionist pattern of attention is defined by a belief in the validity of the concept of early detection and a focus on the benefits of screening. Earlier is always better than later when it comes to cancer detection from the interventionist perspective; there is no sense that there is a possibility of screening "too early." In keeping with this, interventionists dismiss or inattend overdiagnosis as a largely theoretical, rather than real, problem, and minimize the other possible harms of screening as insignificant compared with the risk of *not* screening, which they in some cases rhetorically equate with death. As such, interventionists are critical of the USPSTF recommendation to delay mammograms until age fifty and reduce the frequency of screening from annual to biennial. They are also critical of the composition of the Task Force for not including enough clinical experts in breast cancer, whom they believe are the appropriate source of medical authority to decide this question.

Skeptics, in contrast, are fundamentally supportive of the USPSTF's recommendation. They are, as a rule, not fully persuaded of mammography screening's effectiveness and are more concerned than interventionists about the negative repercussions of screening. Their patterns of attention are therefore organized around questioning early detection. They believe there is a limit to mammography such that it can be "too early" and show us "too much," resulting in overdiagnosis and increases in the other possible harms of screening. They also conceptualize the harms of screening in a more expansive way than interventionists in that they include not just the physical harms of potential follow-up testing and unnecessary treatment due to overdiagnosis but also the psychological harm of the often-needless stress faced by the many patients who are recalled for further evaluation following routine mammograms, which frequently involves a lengthy period of anxious waiting. Finally, they focus attention on the importance of improvements in breast cancer treatment, which they argue make early detection less essential and therefore further tip the balance in favor of the risks rather than the benefits of mammography.

As mentioned already, one benefit of conceptualizing interventionism and skepticism as mental filters is that it allows for the identification of both "positively" held beliefs associated with each perspective and what each inattends or treats as "irrelevant." Analytically, this involves symmetrical analysis of both sides of the conflict, as well as of both attention and inattention. By definition, recognizing and analyzing what one does not attend poses a challenge. In general, it is more difficult to notice absence than presence (Zerubavel 2018, 9). Lacking positive evidence for those things we do not perceive is therefore the first obstacle to acknowledging such attentional exclusions (Zerubavel 2015, 7). One of the analytic benefits of filter analysis is that it is explicitly conceived to provide access to this information, shifting the boundaries of consciousness to bring awareness to the previously inattended.

One of the clearest examples of inattention in the mammography conflict is the way a belief in early detection restricts interventionists' ability to acknowledge overdiagnosis or to think in new ways about treatment beyond the approach of always seeking out more and smaller cancers. Interventionists thus have trouble cognitively integrating an acknowledgment of the flaws skeptics find in the conceptual model of cancer that underlies the theory of early detection—that is, that cancer is always progressive. They also often misattribute to early detection benefits that may actually be the result of improvements in treatment. Fundamentally, they are resistant to the idea of the harms of screening and are recalcitrant in their commitment to the essentialness of early detection.

On the other side, a commitment to questioning early detection limits skeptics' ability to give full attention to other potentially important dimensions of breast cancer diagnosis and treatment, such as the possible impact of delaying treatment on a patient's treatment experience and quality of life. In focusing attention on overdiagnosis, then, skeptics may not be giving adequate weight to the realities of clinical medicine. Perhaps most significantly, this means the inability to know, in the case of any individual patient, whether their particular tumor has been overdiagnosed. But it also includes the reality of face-to-face interactions with patients who may not be convinced that overdiagnosis is real, or that early detection has been oversold. As Dr. Blakely, a primary care doctor, puts it, and I think many people can relate to this sentiment, "It's a terribly hard sell. If someone's got a cancer, they want it out," and "they're willing to go through an unnecessary biopsy if it means that they're going to, you know, rule out that it's cancer."

While my data and analysis focus on revealing the attentional organization of disagreement over mammography, I also recognize that interventionism and skepticism as generic attentional types are relevant to other cases within medicine, particularly in the context of the broader U.S. healthcare culture of overuse and overmedicalization. These include most obviously other medical screenings but also potentially conflicts between midwifery and medical models of understanding pregnancy and childbirth, or naturopathic or functional medicine approaches as contrasted with traditional allopathic western medicine. In each case, interventionists and skeptics differ over now-familiar questions, such as whether abnormalities always develop in a predictable way to cause harm, the likelihood of treatment causing more harm than good, whether knowing about something as soon as possible is intrinsically beneficial or potentially harmful, and more generally whether rapid, high-intensity responses to finding and treating "abnormalities" is always beneficial to health. For example, a midwifery perspective questions the medicalization of pregnancy and childbirth, including the necessity of early detection of abnormalities through fetal screening and ultrasound. This skeptical perspective also emphasizes the harms of fetal monitoring during labor and the use of pharmaceutical drugs to accelerate labor, and it challenges the belief that medicalized hospital births are "safer" than home birth (Markens, Browner, and Press 1999; Martin 2001; Rapp 1999; Rothman 1986, 1991). A naturopathic or herbalist approach to health similarly questions the necessity and benefit of pharmaceutical interventions to manage illness. That interventionism and skepticism are relevant to a wide range of examples in medicine is further illustrated in Welch, Schwartz, and Woloshin's *Overdiagnosed: Making People Sick in the Pursuit of Health* (2011), which can be understood in this context as essentially a book-length critique of interventionism touching on hypertension, diabetes, and various forms of cancer screening, including prostate cancer, lung cancer, and thyroid cancer in addition to breast cancer.

It is important to point out, however, that there is no intrinsic political or ideological alignment of interventionism or skepticism. For example, in the context of COVID-19, skepticism appears to best reflect the underlying attention structure of an anti-masking or anti-vaccination perspective (McKelvey 2020; Stewart 2020). Alternately, taking the interventionist/skeptic typology outside of medicine entirely and applying it to economics, skepticism might be associated with laissez-faire approaches, contrasted with more interventionist perspectives that call for governmental regulation—whether in making corrections for the market or through income redistribution. What unifies all of these otherwise very different examples is certain common formal features of the structure of attention, rather than the particular content or the political alignment or implications of the perspective. Beyond interventionism and skepticism, the general point is that such formal attentional maps of cultural conflicts can be revealed through a sustained, cross-contextual focus on cognitive structure to identify the relevant attentional types as well as through applying the related concept of attentional battle.

Attentional Battles and Battle Strategies

Beyond laying out the two attentional types that define the structure of the mammography debates, I also described how interventionists and skeptics actively engage in attentional warfare by using their incommensurable matrices of attention to discredit and marginalize one another. As discussed in chapter 3, where I illustrated this attentional work of differentiation, marginalization, and discrediting, the concept of *attentional battle* further usefully connects attentional filters to the elevated emotions of cultural conflicts.

Two key attentional battle strategies are *mental weighing*, discussed in chapter 4, and the *construction of temporal narratives*, discussed in chapter 5. The strategy of mental weighing has to do with the application of incompatible value schemas to ideas about mammography, including different default mental weights and notions of importance or relevance. Thus, mental weighing highlights what each side of the conflict considers the most salient benefits, harms, and forms of expertise applicable to the evaluation of mammography, and what is considered distracting, distorting, or simply less important. Chapter 5 examines mammography as a *sociotemporal conflict*, illustrating the use of *temporal strategies* as another tool in the attentional battle over mammography. Temporal concepts and concerns are fundamental to mammography, as exemplified in debates over age guidelines as well as concepts like "early" detection. Importantly, as I argued, such sociotemporal conflicts are also *attentional* conflicts, involving temporal strategies rooted in patterns of attention. For example, how each group parses the temporal continuum of age is equally arbitrary with respect to biological and astronomical time, reflecting instead their shared norms of attention, focus, and relevance.

Further, as alluded to already, by analyzing the conflict as an attentional *battle*, one of the contributions the sociology of attention can offer to the mammography debates is to help clarify what underlies the elevated emotions of the conflict. Examining this emotion through the lens of attention, and specifically the concept of attentional battles and battle strategies, reveals some of what fuels the high emotions of the debate, offering new opportunities for deeper mutual understanding and more effective communication—perhaps ultimately even a path toward resolution to the conflict, despite the high emotion involved.

In addition to providing insight into the connection between attention and the elevated emotion of cultural conflicts, the concept of attentional battle offers a number of additional analytical benefits. Perhaps most significantly, as an intrinsically comparative perspective focused on the analysis of competing attentional types, attentional battle as a focus effectively challenges the reification of attention and promotes attentional flexibility. In addition, the distinction I propose between *battles for attention* and *battles over attention* highlights the way that analysis of the organization of attention *within* each competing perspective in a cultural conflict is at least as important as (and in fact deepens understanding of) the competing claims in any framing contest. This focus on analyzing the *intra-* rather than only the *inter-*perspectival organization of attention in cultural conflicts can not only hone our understanding of the specific source of differences between polarized positions but also reveal formal similarities between attention filters that otherwise appear totally opposed. Thus, while my focus throughout the book has been to use the concept of attentional battle to draw out aspects of the conflict over mammography that have not been foregrounded in prior work, and my primary intervention is accordingly with that case, I also aim to advance the general proposition that there is a need for more analysis of patterns of attention in cultural conflicts. My analysis thus pushes beyond the case of mammography both by demonstrating how this type of analysis might be conducted and by providing a conceptual vocabulary for this work.

Patients' Attention in/to Mammography

Arguably the most fundamental tenet of the sociology of attention is the existence of attentional diversity. From a sociological perspective, such variations are essential to illustrating that attention is neither biological nor universal. Comparing attentional alternatives also serves to powerfully dereify taken-for-granted notions of relevance and irrelevance. Recognizing the importance of capturing attentional variation, I did not limit my analysis to interventionism and skepticism. While these are the two dominant attentional types that organize medical and scientific debates, they certainly do not exhaust the attentional possibilities. It is in this spirit that I examined the patterns of attention and relevance present in patients' narratives of mammography alongside those of scientific experts. Although the conflict over mammography is ostensibly about women age forty to fifty, I took as an open question whether the debates among experts, and their organizing attentional norms of interventionism and skepticism, can also capture patients' patterns of attention. Examining the ways that patients' attention patterns intersect and diverge with interventionism and skepticism allowed me to move beyond a strictly binary conception in which two polarized positions offer the only attentional alternatives. At the same time, it revealed the broader influence of hegemonic ideas like early detection on patterns of patients' attention, even when their specific knowledge of the disagreement among experts was low.

In keeping with the idea that support for early detection is culturally hegemonic, interventionists "claim" patients as allies who share their beliefs, arguing that women "just want their screening" and are not interested in delaying mammography or questioning early detection. In one sense, skeptics agree with this characterization, arguing that early detection has been such a consistent point of cultural emphasis that patients are totally steeped in its attentional logic. However, when skeptics make this point, they are generally trying to frame patients as suffering from a limiting *overbelief* in early detection. In this manner, how patients are portrayed by both skeptics and interventionists is yet another *attentional strategy* in the mammography wars.

As such, these competing characterizations of patients are more illustrative of the rhetorical strategies used in the attentional battle between skeptics and interventionists than they are a reflection of patients' actual beliefs. My in-depth interviews with thirty women age forty to fifty, which were the focus of chapter 2 and also discussed in chapter 4 on mental weighing and chapter 5 on temporality, suggest that early detection as a hegemonic attentional norm does seem to broadly shape most patients' sense of relevance. It may take the form of a taken-for-granted, default idea, as is the case with default interventionists, or it may be actively recognized as a broadly shared cultural norm that they attentionally deviate from in a conscious way, as in the case of conscious skeptics. Patients also emphasized other concerns about mammography that were not always foregrounded in medical and scientific debates, however, such as their embodied experience of mammograms, or surprise insurance bills for diagnostic follow-up mammograms. In addition, and counter to any claims that the disagreement among experts is confusing patients or suppressing participation in mammography, most of the patients I interviewed were not specifically aware that there was any significant disagreement about mammography in the medical profession, and even among those who had some knowledge of the conflict, I did not find significant evidence of patients avoiding mammograms as a result of being influenced by skeptics' arguments. Indeed, even some of the most well-informed and critical patients I spoke with still participate in screening, which is why I developed the category of conflicted skeptics.

In conjunction with the dominant cultural narrative of early detection, what was most influential in shaping patients' sense of relevance and concern with respect to mammography were their social experiences, whether of friends and family members who have had breast cancer or of their own prior screening experiences (both with mammograms and other forms of screening). This finding illustrates the fundamental idea of attention's social roots, as well as the importance of understanding the relationship between such autobiographical experiences and other relevant sociotemporal norms and frameworks such as early detection or screening timetables. Patients' perspectives on medical recommendations are best understood as the result of a process of attentionally aligning their biographical experience with the available sociotemporal norms and guidelines.

This biographical alignment is also what underlies patients' affective responses to mammography. For instance, many patients were highly fearful of breast cancer, often connecting their fear to one or more friends or relatives with breast cancer diagnoses. As suggested by the idea of the *screening paradox*, the reality is that many such "survivors" of breast cancer may have been overdiagnosed. Regardless, the effect of this experience is typically to increase women's fear and motivate more active screening, as captured with the category of conscious interventionists, whose process of autobiographical alignment with dominant early detection narratives and sociomedical debates over mammography recommendations shifted them cognitively out of a position of default interventionism into more deliberative, active awareness about mammography. However, depending on the patient's prior biographical experiences—for example, whether a loved one survived as a result of medical intervention or died despite it, or whether prior screening experiences resulted in an upsetting false-positive result—it is possible to understand different fear responses as a result of the autobiographical alignment process. In the case of conflicted and conscious skeptics, for example, mammography was typically perceived as increasing rather than allaying anxiety.

These observations about attentional diversity and the social and biographical origins of patients' sense of relevance and patterns of attention further illustrate the attentional roots, not just of the conflict among experts, but of tensions between doctors and patients. As mentioned already, some of the most prominent concerns expressed by the patients I interviewed were excluded from medical debates. One of these themes was feeling cynical and mistrustful of doctors. At times the interview participants tied this to the idea that patients, specifically patients as women, are not being considered appropriately in the debates, but they also expressed feeling attentionally out of sync more generally with their doctors. Somewhat surprisingly, this was articulated both by consciously interventionist patients, who were typically seeking more mammograms, and skepticism-aligned patients, who were seeking fewer, although the participants most likely to say that they experience dissonance with their doctors and feel more broadly socially marginal in their views were those who are the most skeptical of mammography. These patients often reported feeling socially isolated, unable to share their feelings about mammography with friends and family. Some also expressed that they find it difficult to locate a doctor who is open to their skepticism and follows the USPSTF guidelines, further illustrating the cultural hegemony of early detection. Dissonance between doctors' and patients' patterns of relevance and attention is an important source of patient dissatisfaction, which I touched on in chapter 1 (e.g., Hesse-Biber 2014; Hunter 1991; Silverman et al. 2001; Timmermans and Berg 2003, 71).

Among many of the patients I interviewed, although for different reasons depending on whether they were conscious interventionists or conflicted or conscious skeptics, there was a clear sentiment that their doctors' patterns of attention were out of sync with their own wishes and concerns. This suggests that the sociology of attention offers a potential framework for medical sociologists seeking to better understand the source of such breakdowns in communication. One implication is that it may be helpful for practitioners to create a brief *attentional pause* to actively seek out such dissonances in attention and become aware of attentional alternatives that may be heavily weighed by their patients before making a recommendation. If undertaken with humility, such an attentional pause could also create valuable accountability for their own attentional exclusions. It bears pointing out in this context that such explicit consideration of patient perceptions and preferences is already emphasized in the USPSTF recommendation for mammography for women age forty to fifty. Given that the balance of risks and benefits is insufficiently clear for this age group, they recommend "a conversation with women to ensure a realistic understanding of the limited absolute benefit of screening in the face of potential harms" and "discussions to elicit patient preferences" as opposed to a blanket recommendation in favor of screening (Sheridan, Harris, and Woolf 2004, 57).

Cultivating Attentional Flexibility

Cognitively, socialization is always a process of narrowing focus and reducing attentional alternatives through applying socially shared frameworks of relevance (Zerubavel 2015, 72–73). This reduced awareness is essential to protect us from being mentally overwhelmed by the immense complexity of the stimuli we could potentially attend at any given moment. Indeed, being unable to attend to our environment in such a selective manner can be a symptom of mental illness (73). At the same time, however, "our ability to attend to the world in a selective manner also blinds us to everything else that might have otherwise 'entered' our mind" (74). Our focused attention on one set of ideas, in other words, often makes it extremely cognitively difficult for us to conceive of alternative understandings or solutions to a problem. The inevitable attentional "constriction" of socialization, then, literally results in "narrow-mindedness" and mental rigidity (74–75). One of the results of this narrowing and rigidifying of our attention is that we tend to reify our own frameworks of relevance (8).

One significant benefit of both filter analysis as an analytical approach and the sociology of attention as a theoretical framework is that they quite intentionally facilitate symmetrical analysis of both attention and inattention. In so doing, they also challenge mental rigidity by revealing attentional alternatives. Analyzing attention patterns thus intrinsically de-essentializes relevance by revealing the inattended messiness and complexity that is normally blocked out of our simplified, rigid perceptions. Within this complexity made manifest through an analysis of inattention is the attentional evidence that could be available to legitimate other interpretations and meanings. Thus, rather than narrowing, a symmetrical analysis of attention provokes the recognition of productive dissonances that expand attention and increase awareness of alternative interpretive possibilities. Stated differently, rather than rigidity and reification, attentional analysis can create more mental flexibility and openness to alternative systems of relevance. In the medical literature, uncertainty and ambivalence are often portrayed negatively, as barriers to care or adherence to recommendations that need to be overcome. For example, O'Neill et al. (2012) highlight ambivalence as a barrier to mammography and other screening. However, if rather than adherence, the goal is recognizing and becoming accountable for attentional exclusions, heightened uncertainty and ambivalence might instead be understood positively as mental flexibility. Indeed, the literal meaning of ambivalence is simply the coexistence of two contradictory meanings or feelings, which is arguably a desirable state, particularly when considering the risks and benefits of a medical test or procedure. This positive take on ambivalence also resonates with Heath's (2014, np) reframing of uncertainty in medicine: "The basis of scientific creativity, intellectual freedom, and political resistance is uncertainty. We should nurture it and treasure it and teach its value, and not be afraid of it. . . . What we need is the courage to always consider the timely, the concrete, the local, and the particular when we care for each individual patient and, if necessary, the courage to disregard the rules."

Heath's words also remind us that the generative potential of uncertainty lies not simply in recognizing the inevitability of contradiction and ambiguity, but in digging into the specifics of different perspectives, situations, and structures of attention. This is also part of Barad's (2007, 205) point when she argues that the power of diffractive consideration of differences and contradictions is in "insisting on accountability for the *particular* exclusions that are enacted" (emphasis added) in any given conception of reality. Attentional analysis embraces ambiguity from a similar perspective—with a goal of cultivating attentional diversity, mental flexibility, and accountability for exclusions instead of fear. While intentionally pursuing uncertainty and ambivalence can feel uncomfortable, that discomfort is potentially generative rather than merely negative (Broom and Kenny 2021, 481).

In addition to analytically facilitating such generative ambivalence, another great virtue of the sociology of attention is that—as a set of concepts and theories—it is applicable to almost any topic or field, bringing new questions and lines of inquiry to ongoing debates. My focus throughout the book has been to illustrate this potential in the data-driven arena of population science and medical guidelines, using the example of ongoing disputes surrounding mammography screening. While the social construction of medical knowledge is well documented (Arksey 1994; Berg 1992; De Vries and Lemmens 2006; Fleck 1979; Hunter 1991; Kuhn 1962; Scheff 1963; Wendland 2007), this perspective has not previously been applied to mammography, and the sociology of attention is not currently a recognized theoretical framework in the field.

Social actors do not simply perceive scientific data. Rather, they perceive data through frameworks of meaning and attention. The same is true of how research studies are designed and concepts are operationalized. The history of mammography demonstrates this point very clearly. Despite decades of data, interventionists and skeptics are unable to come to agreement on mammography. This is likely not because there are not enough data, but because they are interpreting the data that exist through different frameworks of meaning: one that supports early detection and one that questions it. Reflecting the mental rigidity of each side, interventionists are afraid to acknowledge any limitations or risks of mammography, while skeptics resist any idea that adds to what they perceive as an already overly bloated cultural sense of mammography's benefits. More data alone will not change the fundamental fault lines of this disagreement, and the perennial debates about whether to screen women in their forties do not get at the heart of the conflict. In fact, as I discussed in chapter 5, many skeptics and interventionists actually agree that any potential age lines are arbitrary. Some scholars have further questioned whether mammography screening should even be a focus of research and debate in breast cancer at all (Sulik 2015).

In light of this, what is needed is a new analytic approach to bring out the deeper roots of disagreement in the mammography conflict so that they can be better understood and acknowledged. This requires addressing how the different epistemic cultures and associated mental filters of interventionists and skeptics—especially foundational beliefs such as early detection, population screening, and clinical authority—restrict the way they, and all of us, really, are able to think about mammography. I believe, and I have endeavored to demonstrate throughout this book, that the sociology of attention is a powerful tool for such an analysis. Although my primary focus has been to show why such an analytic approach is of value to the sociological study of mammography, and by extension science and medicine more broadly, at the most general level, my analysis also points to the productivity of looking at cultural conflicts in other arenas of social life as "attentional battles," or contests over what one should attend as relevant (Zerubavel 2015, 57). With this in mind, one of the intended contributions of my treatment of mammography is to provide a model for this type of analysis and to further develop some of the existing conceptual tools, particularly *attentional types* and *attentional battles*. Analysis in terms of attentional types emphasizes the form rather than the specific content of competing perspectives in a cultural or political disagreement. This focus on form drives focus to the most salient, defining attentional patterns of each perspective and encourages the development of generic attentional types that can be applied beyond one's particular case. Attentional battle, as an intrinsically comparative perspective focused on the analysis of competing attentional types, effectively challenges the reification of attention through promoting attentional flexibility. It can also help identify the attentional relationships between seemingly totally opposed attentional types within a conflict as well as between attentional battles in totally different contexts.

Appendix

Methodological Note

Accountability, Analytic Exclusions, and Autobiographical Alignment

Given that the researcher is the primary instrument of qualitative research (Ravitch and Carl 2020, 14), and in the spirit of accountability for one's own attentional exclusions, emphasized as a benefit of the sociology of attention throughout the book, I would like to begin this methodological note with a reflection on some of the topics I have *not* addressed with my analysis due to my professional socialization in sociology—specifically cognitive sociology—and my prior screening experiences as a patient.

In the broadest sense, as a sociologist, I have been trained to think about phenomena in terms of how they are influenced by their social and cultural contexts as well as their effects on the social world. What this means is that what primarily stood out to me as relevant and deserving of attention and emphasis as a researcher is the social and cultural aspects of mammography as opposed to more strictly biomedical details and concerns, although these foci are certainly not always totally distinct. Accordingly, I have attempted to tease out sociological aspects of a number of biomedical ideas throughout the book, including early detection, lead time, overdiagnosis, and more. Along with the broad perspective of sociology, a key emphasis of my training and the focus of much of my prior research is cognitive sociology, which has sensitized me to notice and attach significance to the influence of thought collectives and social patterns of thought. These are the foundational perspectives, concepts, and theories—the interpretive filters and norms of attention—that I brought to this analysis of the mammography conflict.

While these particular attentional sensitizations have allowed me to make a number of unique and hopefully useful observations about a conflict of perspectives that is otherwise largely deadlocked, my narrow focus on patterns of cognition, like all interpretations, can only exist given other attentional exclusions. For example, the political economy of the U.S. healthcare system in general, and of breast cancer screening in particular, are unquestionably relevant to why efforts to reduce mammography screening are met with such impassioned resistance. King (2008), for example, has written about the culture of private breast cancer philanthropy, in which corporations engage in market-driven efforts to "cure" breast cancer that are often more publicly recognizable than public health prevention efforts, analyzing the implications of consumer-based philanthropy for medical research, patients' experiences of the disease, and how political and medical institutions approach breast cancer in general. While I have alluded to some connections to economic considerations throughout the book, I only directly addressed financial motivations and impacts as they emerged as significant in my participants' patterns of attention. Similarly, I only examined gender to the extent that it was relevant to the patterns of attention exemplified by my participants; a more wholistic application of a gendered analysis would reveal and emphasize dimensions of mammography that I failed to fully address here. Indeed, the manifestations and impacts of "pink ribbon culture"—the intersection of hegemonic gender ideologies with breast cancer discourse, diagnosis, funding, and treatment—has been a significant focus of prior analyses (e.g., Broom 2001; Clarke 1999; Ehrenreich 2001; Fosket 2000; Johansen et al. 2013; Lupton 1994; Montini 1996; Sledge 2021; Sulik 2010). These are of course only a fraction of the insights excluded by my attention to attention.

In addition to the analytic focus and attendant exclusions resulting from my interest in patterns of attention and cognition, I recognize that my own screening experiences as a patient have also shaped my patterns of attention and mental weight in the same process of autobiographical alignment I describe among my interviewees. For most of my twenties, every time I had a pap smear it found "atypical" cells. The nature of the abnormality (not disease, as I had no symptoms) was never formally diagnosed despite multiple colposcopies (a procedure to visualize the cervix) and biopsies. Sometimes human papillomavirus (HPV) can be a cause of abnormal pap smears, and even cervical cancer, but my repeated tests for HPV were always negative. Eventually, after many years of increased frequency of pap smears, all of which had atypical results, one finally came back normal, and my pap results have been normal ever since. One doctor's (untestable) theory is that I had a strain of HPV that the available test did not include (there are more than one hundred types, and only a handful that are known to be high risk are included in the test). Eventually, my body had managed to fight off the virus on its own, which was the reason my pap screenings no longer came back with abnormal results. Regardless, the experience was stressful and time consuming, filled with anxious waiting for results and medical procedures that provided no answers.

Although the physical risks of the increased screening—and even the multiple colposcopies and biopsies—were minimal, the argument by skeptics that the harms of screening must be conceptualized more broadly than just physical risks certainly resonated with me on a personal level. In addition, just prior to this period, a very close friend's mother died of cervical cancer in her forties, which added significant additional fear and anxiety to the cycles of repeated screenings and rescreenings, in my case making me more of a conscious interventionist than a skeptic—although after many years of testing and screening without any real answers, I definitely began to have some doubts.

In my thirties, when pregnant with twins, a totally routine prenatal screening—a nuchal scan and associated bloodwork—led to a terrifying rush to further diagnostic testing and several agonizing days of waiting to learn whether one or both of the fetuses I was carrying had a potentially life-threatening chromosomal abnormality. My husband and I arrived at the appointment for the twelve-week scan, as most expectant parents do, excited to learn more about how the twins were developing and hoping to catch a glimpse of them on the ultrasound and hear their heartbeats again. Shortly after the scan, a genetic counselor grimly delivered the news that our results indicated a statistically significant risk of a serious genetic condition in both fetuses and recommended that we have another test immediately that same afternoon to seek a definitive diagnosis. The test was a chorionic villus sampling (CVS), in which a sample of chorionic villi (part of the placenta) is removed for testing using a large needle, in my case inserted through the abdominal wall. In addition, because I was carrying twins, each with their own placenta, I had to have the procedure twice in a row. In the end, I actually had to endure the procedure three times that day, because one of the samples was inadequate for testing. The CVS test carries some risk of infection and miscarriage, and even fourteen years later I remember it as extremely painful, even physically traumatic in the moment. And of course, emotionally, we were extremely worried, and had to sit with that fear while we waited for the results for several days. When the patients I interviewed described their experiences of "anxious waiting" and in some cases their fear of screening itself, I again found personal resonance with those ideas. In the end, we were lucky. Our developing fetuses did not have any of the genetic conditions the screening results had flagged as an elevated risk. In fact, it turned out that one component of my bloodwork was very statistically unusual (although not dangerous) and that was throwing off the statistical calculations of the entire screening test. I walked away from the experience feeling more than a little mistrustful of the results of screening and, like some of the skeptical patients I interviewed, as a result, for me there is now more to the question of whether to get screened than questions like "Why not?" and "What's the harm?" suggest.

I am currently forty-seven years old, and I imagine the reader might be wondering whether I have annual mammograms or have had even one mammogram yet, given my prior experiences with screening and my research for this book. I actually began working on this project in 2014 when I was forty years old, the very age that mammography recommendations become most contested. I did not have a mammogram that year. In fact, I did not have my first mammogram until after I submitted the first draft of this manuscript to the publisher for review in 2020 at age forty-six. The reasons I waited as long as I did were the following: (1) I had steeped myself in the details of the conflict and was at least somewhat persuaded by the idea that early detection is such a deeply taken-for-granted belief that it can be cognitively difficult to perceive and weigh the benefits and harms of mammography accurately; (2) Medical sociology is one of my areas of interest, so I had prior knowledge of and teach regularly about our culture of overuse and overmedicalization. I therefore had some mistrust and fear of screening due to this background knowledge, which was emotionally intensified by my prior personal experiences with "false-alarm" pap and prenatal screenings; (3) Socially, I had several good friends who found themselves in a cycle of constantly receiving suspicious mammography results and being recalled for further screening and even biopsies, none of which turned out to be cancer. I was also fortunate that at that time no one in my closest circle of friends or family had had breast cancer. If anything, then, the skeptical perspective resonated with my autobiographical experiences, and I chose not to get screened in my early forties. At some point during my forty-fifth year, however, I decided to have a mammogram after I completed and submitted the first draft of this manuscript, which I did, as I mentioned, in early fall 2020. This was in part because I decided that I wanted to have experienced my own mammogram before publishing a book on mammography, but at the same time, if I ended up having a negative experience, or if I was diagnosed with breast cancer, I did not want that to color my analysis too strongly (thus the decision to wait until after the book was under review).

My first mammogram was in some ways a very different experience than most, largely because of the doctor and facility I very intentionally chose. Knowing that there was a high likelihood that I would have to have follow-up imaging, I decided to see a local practitioner I had heard about who reads your mammogram on the spot and then calls you into her office to give you the results at the same appointment. So there is no anxious waiting—no waiting at all, really—for the results. In addition, if she determines that you require another mammogram or other diagnostic imaging to further investigate something, she will complete that testing at the very same appointment, before you leave the office, and inform you of the results. While in this specific sense my experience is somewhat unique, in other ways my experience is just like many other women's. In my case, the initial screening mammogram revealed what she suspected to be a cyst in one breast and some calcification in another area. She ordered a second mammogram, and when that did not clarify things adequately, she immediately took me into another room of the office and performed an ultrasound of my breasts. At that point, satisfied that the cyst was indeed a cyst and the calcification was not currently a problem either, she asked me to come back for another mammogram in six months (so, sooner than even the most aggressive screening guidelines recommend). Her reasoning was that she wanted to see if the calcification changed, since she did not have a prior mammogram for comparison and had no way of knowing if it was new or something long-standing and stable. Six months later, I had that follow-up mammogram, which was again followed by a diagnostic ultrasound, and luckily nothing had changed.

I am scheduled to return for my next regular mammogram, six months after the second, in a few months. On the one hand, in less than a year, I have had three mammograms and two ultrasounds, and realistically I expect to have more of each when I return for my next visit. That feels like a lot of testing. Even more significantly, I could not help but imagine what it would have felt like to have all of that testing in a more typical facility, where at each stage I would have to return home and wait for the results. What for me was an hour-long appointment each time would have turned into weeks or months of scheduling and attending appointments and waiting anxiously for the results. Given my research, I was also very cognizant that the follow-up testing would be billed to my insurance as diagnostic testing rather than preventive screening and would therefore most likely be paid out differently by my insurer. I had not confirmed ahead of time my specific coverage for diagnostic mammography and breast ultrasound, so I knew there was a good possibility that I would receive a "surprise bill" (which would not be a surprise for me because of my research, but I think would be for many women and certainly was for many of the patients I interviewed). Although I was already aware of the distinction between how screening and diagnostic mammograms are paid by insurers, when I sat to wait for the doctor to review my mammogram, I noticed the following two announcements displayed prominently on a bulletin board in the waiting room:

> "Our policy: Please note that if you come in for a *screening* mammogram, but additional views and/or an ultrasound are done, your insurance form will be submitted as a *diagnostic* mammogram."
>
> "To all my patients: It is my job to do a complete and thorough mammogram on all of you. This often results in additional images to clear areas that look different from previous years. As a result of this, your mammogram will be coded as *diagnostic*. I will not practice any other way. If you choose not to allow additional views, I will abide by your wishes, however, your mammogram will be incomplete. In other words, I will not be able to rule out a small cancer. Please consider this carefully before we do your mammogram."

In short, I was highly sensitized to the potential risks and harms of mammography before making my first appointment. As such, it was very clear to me that the practice I chose had taken measures to institutionally mitigate or eliminate some of them—the routinization of anxious waiting between screening mammograms, results, and additional diagnostic testing; the surprise of an unexpected insurance charge for a follow-up mammogram, even if not the bill itself; and so on. That being said, I did experience—in an accelerated timeframe, and therefore without nearly as much stress—the hamster wheel of a mammogram, followed by additional testing, followed by a negative result but a request to return on an intensified schedule for another cycle of the same. My personal experience with mammography did not inform the analysis I have presented in this book (again, I did not have a mammogram until it was submitted), although, as mentioned already, my prior screening experiences likely did contribute to piquing my interest in the debates over mammography, particularly the critiques of screening offered by mammography skeptics. In addition, writing this book clearly shaped my experience of my own mammogram, providing a framework that, among other things, brought into stark attentional relief how my experience converged with and diverged from the accounts shared with me by the patients I interviewed.

Sampling, Recruitment, and Data Analysis

In this book I engage three different types of empirical data to triangulate ideas about mammography and identify productive dissonances in perspective: interviews with doctors and scientists, interviews with women age forty to fifty, and content analysis of media coverage of mammography. In what follows I describe in more specific detail than I was able to include in the body of the manuscript how I went about recruiting my participants, the focus of my interviews and content analysis, and my approach to analyzing the data I collected. Each of the three study protocols was reviewed and approved by the institutional review board for the protection of human subjects in research at the University of Delaware.

Interviews with Doctors and Scientists

When I initially decided to study the mammography conflict, what most interested me about it was the official, institutionalized deadlock of perspectives and the high emotion of the discourse among professional experts. Given my background in cognitive sociology, I thought it could be interesting to approach analyzing the disagreement as a cognitive conflict and to map the patterns of thought underlying the arguments proffered on each side. While such an analysis could be approached through a content analysis of academic journals and/or popular media, I also knew that I wanted to capture nuanced, specific details of the different understandings at play, and I wanted to be able to probe for more information about particular ideas and reactions, since very little was available in the way of qualitative analysis of the finer details of the contrasting beliefs about mammography.

I ultimately conducted in-depth interviews with twenty-nine physicians, medical researchers, and leaders of both government-sponsored and private medical organizations in 2014 and early 2015. All but five participants were U.S.-based; the remaining five resided in Europe at the time of the interview but considered themselves experts on U.S. guidelines and were contributors to the research literature on mammography. My sampling strategy was two-pronged: I actively sought participants I thought would be knowledgeable about mammography (e.g., contributors to the scholarly literature, directors of leading cancer centers), but I also included clinicians who were not directly involved in debates about mammography but were more likely to interact with the "typical" low-risk patient making decisions about whether and how often to be screened. My goal was to capture a balance of different specialties and perspectives. I recruited participants through professional organizations' membership lists and direct emails to clinics and medical school departments. I also contacted experts on screening quoted in the media and listed on government websites. While a few interviews generated additional referrals, there were rarely more than two connected participants.

Among the disciplines represented in the final sample were radiology, oncology, surgery, internal medicine, and public health. The interview participants' professional roles also varied and included clinicians, medical and public health researchers, and leaders of government and professional organizations. (See table 1.1 in chapter 1 for additional sample details.) As a result, the sample should have captured a broad range of professional perspectives, although this also introduced variation in how the participants interact with mammography professionally that may have been significant in shaping their views. Another limitation of the sample is that, across specializations, those with a specific interest in mammography were likely overrepresented. This has the benefit of providing access to significant expertise but is limiting in terms of generalizability to the broader population of primary care physicians, for instance. It could also explain why the sample included more skeptical than interventionist participants ($N = 16$ vs. 10), which at first glance may appear to contradict my claim that early detection still remains largely unquestioned as a cultural and medical norm. I suspect that more skeptics were drawn to the study precisely because they view themselves as both experts and attentional deviants, and were therefore motivated to participate in the interviews as a way to generate more cultural recognition of the harms of early detection. Another limitation is that I failed to recruit a diverse sample in terms of race and ethnicity (all participants in this sample identified as white). This may have influenced discussion of racial disparities in mammography screening, among other things, which were not a significant part of the interviews despite being an area of focus in research on adherence to mammography recommendations (Corcoran et al. 2012; Dean et al. 2014; Tejeda et al. 2009).

The interview guide, designed to elicit experts' views and opinions, addressed current mammography guidelines in the United States, perceptions of disagreement/consensus about these recommendations, perceptions of patients' beliefs and behaviors, and the strengths and limitations of mammography as a tool. All but two interviews were conducted over the phone, with one in person and one via email at the participant's request. Oral interviews were audio recorded and transcribed by a professional transcriptionist. Deidentified transcripts were imported into NVivo qualitative analysis software for coding.

I coded the interviews using a combination of thematic pattern, descriptive, and interpretive/analytic codes (Miles and Huberman 1984; Saldana 2013), including two rounds of open coding and a third round of more focused coding to identify patterns within codes. In the first round of coding I captured broad themes and in vivo codes; initial in vivo codes included the following: skeptics, true believers, early detection, fatigue, individualist perspective, and numerator-denominator problem. Other codes I used at this stage included rhetorical moves, harms of screening, overdiagnosis, and treatment. As I initially coded each transcript, I also created memos summarizing each participant's overall perspective, noting preliminary connections and differences among the participants and making notes about emerging themes.

The following is an excerpt from one of these early memos from November 2014, in which I first began to describe the polarized perspectives I ultimately called skepticism and interventionism:

> One of the interesting ideas is that there seems to be a contrast between an "individualist" perspective that is associated with "true believers" and those who "work directly with women with cancer"—so radiologists, breast surgeons, oncologists. The "skeptics" tend to take a more "population" or "evidence-based medicine" perspective and tend to be statisticians, primary care people, etc. There are exceptions, certainly, especially to the disciplinary division (i.e., there are radiologists who are skeptics), but I have noticed a clear pattern and this has come up a few times in the interviews. Related to this, there seems to be a different emphasis on whether you emphasize "saving" an individual woman, or whether you emphasize the number of women who must be screened (along with overdiagnosis and treatment) to do so. The "pro-screening" folks are afraid to acknowledge any of the limitations and negatives of mammography. The "skeptics" are afraid to acknowledge any of the benefits.
>
> "early detection": is this always important? Does it actually save lives?
> "go in search": seeing more is always better
>
> These are two points on which the two groups also differ. From an individual perspective, catching something early seems like a good thing. From a population perspective, it is totally unclear whether it helps save lives to "go in search" rather than wait until it grows.

A later round of coding focused in much greater depth on a set of codes I initially grouped as exemplifying what I, at the time, called "rhetorical moves and cognitive processes" (I did not yet recognize that attention would be the focus of my analysis) to identify and refine subthemes, variations, and contradictions and to begin to develop concepts. In this analysis I tracked how the participants characterized the different perspectives in the debate, as well as a number of ideas that had begun to emerge as central to the conflict, focusing on the nuances of the language used and the classification processes underlying their narratives. Some of these themes will be very familiar to the reader at this point because they ultimately became major points of focus in the book, such as evidence vs. values; the natural history of breast cancer; overdiagnosis; the screening paradox; expertise; characterizations of the USPSTF; and the harms of screening. This particular round of analysis examined a total of twenty-eight codes, noting for each what variations and subthemes were present. I also pulled representative quotations and tracked which participants best illustrated which perspective. What emerged from this analysis were the two attentional types—skepticism and interventionism—and a rough map of the rhetorical and cognitive structure of each perspective. This analysis was completed prior to initiating data collection for the second set of interviews and therefore inevitably shaped to some extent how I perceived the patients' narratives.

Interviews with Patients

As I discussed in detail in chapter 2, during the first round of interviews, the doctors and scientists made a lot of claims, often delivered with great certainty, about what women believe and how they behave in reaction to the conflict over mammography. Given these strongly worded claims about women's beliefs and behaviors, I wanted to analyze patients' perspectives directly, particularly women who fell in the age range about which experts disagree, forty to fifty. There is a sense in which, while the conflict is about these women, theirs are not the primary voices in the discourse.

Most prior research addressing women's knowledge about and reactions to the USPSTF guideline change, which I reviewed in chapter 2, primarily focuses on the effects of the guideline change on frequency of screening and takes as a given that early detection is valid and regular mammography is beneficial. It does not provide an in-depth understanding of how patients think about mammography guidelines or how they interpret the disagreement among experts. In addition, most of the existing literature on patients' reactions to the mammography conflict is quantitative survey-based research and thus is limited in its ability to explore the nuances of patients' beliefs and behaviors. Using thirty in-depth interviews, I explore in much more depth than this prior work the frameworks of belief and attention structuring patients' responses to the mammography conflict. Because I had already completed the interviews with doctors and scientists and identified the broad contours of interventionism and skepticism, I specifically wanted to understand whether the conflict among experts was relevant to how women thought about mammography or their decisions about whether to get screened in their forties. Thus, there was a deductive element to the second analysis, given the findings of the prior interviews, but I was also interested in patients' intrinsic patterns of emphasis, which I captured inductively and ultimately used to illustrate the idea of attentional diversity in chapter 2. This second round of interviews took place in 2016 and 2017.

To recruit the patient participants, I began by using personal networks and posting notices in my local community. I shared information about the study in community Facebook groups of which I am a member (e.g., parenting groups, yard sale groups), and posted paper flyers in local laundromats, coffee shops, grocery stores, and libraries. I also asked a friend living in a different state to post notices in similar locations in her local community. In an effort to ensure socioeconomic diversity in my sample of patients, I also targeted local organizations that address socioeconomic inequalities, including community centers, food banks, affordable housing organizations, and social service agencies (e.g., women's resource centers, domestic abuse support organizations). I visited some of these in person and requested to post a flyer, and I called and mailed flyers to others. Finally, I reached out to several primary care practices located in predominantly nonwhite, low-income urban neighborhoods. After speaking with the research coordinator at one of these practices and receiving approval from their Quality Improvement Committee, who reviewed a project proposal and my IRB protocol, I ultimately received approval to recruit participants in their waiting room. It was a very large, urban, primary care group practice with over fifty providers, including primary care physicians, nurse practitioners, dentists, ob-gyns, and social workers. I visited the busy waiting room of this practice approximately weekly from June until August of 2017, ultimately recruiting nine participants there for on-the-spot interviews.

The final sample of thirty women was 63 percent white and 33 percent Black, with one participant who identified as Hispanic or Latina. Eighty percent of the participants were employed, and 77 percent had at least a college degree, with 43 percent having a graduate degree. See table 2.1 in chapter 2 for a summary of the sample characteristics. Eighteen of the interviews took place over the phone, and twelve were completed in person, with nine of the in-person interviews taking place on site at the medical practice. All interviews were audio recorded with the participant's prior consent. The substantive focus of the interviews was to learn what the participants knew about mammography, what their prior experiences with mammograms were like, what kinds of interactions they had had with their doctors about mammography or the conflict, and their reactions to the conflict. I began by asking about current mammography guidelines to capture what they already knew about the conflict, which, as discussed in chapter 2, was often very little. I then asked about their prior mammography experiences, how they decided whether to get a mammogram, and what conversations they had had about mammograms with their medical providers, if any. Finally, I described the different guidelines to them and asked for their response to the disagreement among experts.

I took the same approach to coding these interviews as I used when I coded the interviews with doctors and scientists, conducting two rounds of open coding followed by a third round of more focused coding of a smaller set of themes that emerged as particularly salient during the initial rounds of coding to identify subthemes and counterexamples. These codes included different forms of fear, social beliefs/cultural climate, and feelings of dismissal by doctors. As mentioned already, I also specifically looked for evidence of the two attention types I had previously developed based on my analysis of the interviews with doctors and scientists, interventionism and skepticism. For each of the six codes included in this more focused analysis, I wrote a memo that summarized the theme, including variations and subthemes, pulled representative quotations, and noted which participants illustrated which perspective.

Content Analysis of News Stories

The doctors and scientists I interviewed made many claims and accusations, often contradicting one another, about how mammography in general and the conflict over guidelines specifically has been covered by the media. Media is also influential in shaping broad cultural discourses, including the beliefs about the value of early detection that are so central to questions about mammography. In light of this, the third and final form of empirical data I included in the book was the complete set of articles written about mammography from 2002 through 2015 in the four U.S. newspapers with the highest circulation: *The New York Times*, *The Los Angeles Times*, *The Wall Street Journal*, and *USA Today*. I determined which publications had the highest circulation using an article from the Poynter Institute identifying the top U.S. newspapers by circulation as of 2014 (Beaujon 2014). As discussed in chapter 3, this generated a total initial sample of 589 articles mentioning mammography, all of which were exported as pdf files for content analysis. The sample was reduced to 341 articles after removing duplicates and articles that mentioned mammography in passing but did not provide enough content for substantive analysis.

I developed a coding instrument with a mix of free response and fixed choice items based on the questions generated by my interviews with doctors and scientists. The goal was to capture whether and how media coverage had been biased toward either the skeptic or traditionalist viewpoint as well as whether and how the harms of screening were discussed in the media. Together with an undergraduate research assistant, I pilot tested the coding instrument on a total of forty stories, making minor revisions to questions that were unclear or difficult to answer before coding the entire sample. Once finalized, the coding instrument was entered into Qualtrics survey software, which we used to code the 341 articles and generate descriptive statistics. The undergraduate assistant coded one publication, and I coded the other three and spot-checked her coding for consistency with my own. I also conducted crosstabulations using Excel and coded text-based responses by hand.

Feedback and Revision Process

My initial draft of the manuscript presented each data source separately, devoting one chapter each to the interviews with doctors and scientists, the interviews with patients, and the content analysis. Although the sociology of attention was already present as my analytical framework in this early draft, the book was not yet organized thematically around different attention concepts such as attentional diversity, attentional battles, attentional weight, and temporal attention. Inspired by feedback from two early readers, I radically overhauled the structure of the manuscript, instead using each chapter to highlight a concept from the sociology of attention. This change allowed me to develop more fully several conceptual contributions to the sociology of attention and to bring the different data sources into conversation rather than treating them in isolation. The reviewers assigned upon submission of the manuscript to Rutgers University Press provided additional suggestions that led me to situate my arguments more fully in relation to the U.S. healthcare system as a whole and to further refine the categories and concepts used to capture attentional diversity, specifically the concepts of autobiographical attention and alignment, and the attentional distinctions among default and conscious interventionists and conflicted and conscious skeptics.

Acknowledgments

This book was developed over many years with the support of a great number of people—editors, reviewers, mentors, colleagues, students, interview participants, friends, and family. At Rutgers University Press, I would especially like to acknowledge Peter Mickulas and the two reviewers, whose enthusiasm for the project and constructive suggestions helped propel me to the finish line. I am also grateful for feedback provided by academic colleagues at various stages, including Joanna Kempner, Piper Sledge, Ann Bell, and Tammy Anderson. Charlotte Shreve, then an undergraduate student at University of Delaware, helped with coding the news data. Thanks also to Angel Butts for her assistance with editing and proofreading. Tom DeGloma's careful, generous reading of an early draft pushed me to articulate the broader applications of interventionism and skepticism more forcefully. He also suggested the relevance of the concept of *mnemonic alignment*. As ever, I owe the deepest debt of gratitude to Eviatar Zerubavel for encouraging me to be creative and courageous with my ideas. His feedback was instrumental in helping me to recognize and commit to the ultimate structure and focus of the book. I also could not have told this story without the doctors, scientists, and patients who generously gave of their time and attention during the interviews. Finally, I thank my friends and family for their loving support and welcome distraction from work, especially my husband, Jeremy, and our sons, Finn and Sawyer.

Notes

Introduction

1. I am borrowing this term from Quanstrum and Hayward (2010) as well as adapting the title of Barron Lerner's (2003) book, *The Breast Cancer Wars*.
2. Prior to 2002 the USPSTF also did not recommend screening women under fifty.

Chapter 1   Skepticism and Interventionism as Attentional Types

1. All names are pseudonyms.
2. Note that some of the interviews took place in 2014 before the American Cancer Society 2015 guideline changing their recommendation from age forty to age forty-five, which is why some participants described the ACS as aligned with the American College of Radiology guidelines and in opposition to the USPSTF.
3. Sometimes considered a "precancer" or "stage zero" cancer, ductal carcinoma in situ (DCIS) refers to abnormal cells that are confined to the milk duct in the breast. Although it accounts for 25 percent of all breast cancer diagnoses, because it is unlikely to spread beyond the breast, it is often highlighted as an example of likely overdiagnosis and overtreatment (van Seijen et al., 2019).

Chapter 2   Attentional Diversity

1. Although most official guidelines differentiate women age forty to forty-nine from those age fifty and over, I opted to include fifty-year-olds in my sample on the logic that, having recently shifted from one category to the other, they might have an interesting perspective on the disagreement.
2. I should mention here that just under a third of the interview participants were recruited from the waiting room of the same medical group (see the methodological appendix for further details about each of the different recruitment strategies I used), which may be responsible for some of the uniformity in these findings. That being said, this was an extremely large and multidisciplinary practice with over fifty providers, including many primary care and ob-gyn doctors as well as dentists and social workers. In addition, of the nine patients recruited at this practice, several were there waiting for someone else and were not themselves patients of the practice. In at least a few additional cases, participants recruited at this practice also discussed their interactions with doctors other than those at the practice during the interview.

Chapter 3   Attentional Battles over Mammography

1. Relatedly, in the context of debates over PSA screening in the 1990s, Aronowitz (2021) mentions Kolata's role in exposing conflicts of interest in the marketing and promotion of prostate-specific antigen (PSA) tests.

Chapter 4   Attentional Weight

1. For example, according to the American Cancer Society, having two relatives with the disease increases your likelihood of a personal diagnosis threefold ("Breast Cancer Risk Factors" 2021).

2. The research cited in a National Public Radio report suggests that the recall rate can be up to 50 percent (Hobson 2015).

Chapter 5 Mammography and Time

1. Aronowitz (2021) points out that dominant views of prostate screening share this same "a cancer is a cancer" mindset.

References

Adami, Hans-Olov, Mette Kalager, Unnur Valdimarsdottir, Michael Bretthauer, and John P. A. Ioannidis. 2019. "Time to Abandon Early Detection Cancer Screening." *European Journal of Clinical Investigation* 49 (3): e13062. https://doi.org/10.1111/eci.13062.

Alac, Morana. 2008. "Working with Brain Scans: Digital Images and Gestural Interaction in fMRI Laboratory." *Social Studies of Science* 38 (4): 483–508. https://doi.org/10.1177/0306312708089715.

Allegra, Carmen J., Denise R. Aberle, Pamela Ganschow, Stephen M. Hahn, Clara N. Lee, Sandra Millon-Underwood, Malcom C. Pike, Susan D. Reed, Audrey F. Saftlas, Susan A. Scarvalone, Arnold M. Schwartz, Carol Slomski, Greg Yothers, and Robin Zon. 2009. "NIH State-of-the-Science Conference Statement: Diagnosis and Management of Ductal Carcinoma in Situ (DCIS)." *NIH Consensus and State-of-the-Science Statements* 26 (2): 1–27.

Allen, Summer V., Lise Solberg Nes, Mary L. Marnach, Kristen Polga, Sarah M. Jenkins, Julia A. Files, Ivana T. Croghan, Karthik Ghosh, and Sandhya Pruthi. 2012. "Patient Understanding of the Revised USPSTF Screening Mammogram Guidelines: Need for Development of Patient Decision Aids." *BMC Women's Health* 12 (36). https://doi.org/10.1186/1472-6874-12-36.

American Academy of Family Physicians. 2017. "Summary of Recommendations for Clinical Preventive Services." Leawood, KS: American Academy of Family Physicians.

American College of Radiology. 2021. "Mammography Guidelines." Accessed November 16, 2021. https://www.acraccreditation.org/mammography-saves-lives/guidelines.

Anderson, Britta L., Renata R. Urban, Mark Pearlman, and Jay Schulkin. 2014. "Obstetrician-Gynecologists' Knowledge and Opinions about the United States Preventive Services Task Force (USPSTF) Committee, the Women's Health Amendment, and the Affordable Care Act: National Study after the Release of the USPSTF 2009 Breast Cancer Screening Recommendation Statement." *Preventive Medicine* 59: 79–82. https://doi.org/10.1016/j.ypmed.2013.11.008.

Arana-Chicas, Evelyn, Avat Kioumarsi, Amy Carroll-Scott, Philip M. Massey, Ann C. Klassen, and Michael Yudell. 2020. "Barriers and Facilitators to Mammography among Women with Intellectual Disabilities: A Qualitative Approach." *Disability & Society* 35 (8): 1290–1314. https://doi.org/10.1080/09687599.2019.1680348.

Arksey, Hilary. 1994. "Expert and Lay Participation in the Construction of Medical Knowledge." *Sociology of Health & Illness* 16 (4): 448–468. https://doi.org/10.1111/1467-9566.ep11347516.

Arleo, Elizabeth Kagan, R. Edward Hendrick, Mark A. Helvie, and Edward A. Sickles. 2017. "Comparison of Recommendations for Screening Mammography Using CISNET Models." *Cancer* 123 (19): 3673–3680. https://doi.org/10.1002/cncr.30842.

Armstrong, David. 2012. "Screening: Mapping Medicine's Temporal Spaces." *Sociology of Health & Illness* 34 (2): 177–193. https://doi.org/10.1111/j.1467-9566.2011.01438.x.

Armstrong, Natalie. 2021. "Overdiagnosis and Overtreatment: A Sociological Perspective on Tackling a Contemporary Healthcare Issue." *Sociology of Health & Illness* 43 (1): 58–64. https://doi.org/10.1111/1467-9566.13186.

References

Armstrong, Natalie, and Helen Eborall. 2012. "The Sociology of Medical Screening: Past, Present and Future." *Sociology of Health & Illness* 34 (2): 161–176. https://doi.org/10.1111/j.1467-9566.2011.01441.x.

Aronowitz, Robert A. 2001. "Do Not Delay: Breast Cancer and Time, 1900–1970." *The Milbank Quarterly* 79 (3): 355–386. https://doi.org/10.1111/1468-0009.00212.

———. 2007. *Unnatural History: Breast Cancer and American Society*. New York: Cambridge University Press.

———. 2021. "Prostate Cancer: People Transforming a Diagnosis, A Diagnosis Transforming People." *Science, Technology and Society* 26 (1): 41–63. https://doi.org/10.1177/0971721820960254.

Aschwanden, Christie. 2015. "Science Won't Settle the Mammogram Debate." *FiveThirtyEight*. Accessed October 15, 2018. https://fivethirtyeight.com/features/science-wont-settle-the-mammogram-debate/.

Bailar, John C. 1976. "Mammography: A Contrary View." *Annals of Internal Medicine* 84 (1): 77–84. https://doi.org/10.7326/0003-4819-84-1-77.

Banaji, Mahzarin R., and Anthony G. Greenwald. 2013. *Blindspot: Hidden Biases of Good People*. New York: Delacorte Press.

Barad, Karen. 2007. *Meeting the Universe Halfway: Quantum Physics and the Entanglement of Matter and Meaning*. Durham, NC: Duke University Press.

Barker, Kristin K. 1998. "A Ship upon a Stormy Sea: The Medicalization of Pregnancy." *Social Science & Medicine* 47 (8): 1067–1076. https://doi.org/10.1016/S0277-9536(98)00155-5.

Barker, Kristin K., and Tasha R. Galardi. 2011. "Dead by 50: Lay Expertise and Breast Cancer Screening." *Social Science & Medicine* 72 (8): 1351–1358. https://doi.org/10.1016/j.socscimed.2011.02.024.

Beaujon, Andrew. 2014. "USA Today, WSJ, NYT Top U.S. Newspapers by Circulation." *Poynter*. Accessed November 12, 2021. https://www.poynter.org/reporting-editing/2014/usa-today-wsj-nyt-top-u-s-newspapers-by-circulation/.

Beckfield, Jason, Sigrun Olafsdottir, and Benjamin Sosnaud. 2013. "Healthcare Systems in Comparative Perspective: Classification, Convergence, Institutions, Inequalities, and Five Missed Turns." *Annual Review of Sociology* 39 (1): 127–146. https://doi.org/10.1146/annurev-soc-071312-145609.

Beim, Aaron. 2007. "The Cognitive Aspects of Collective Memory." *Symbolic Interaction* 30 (1): 7–26. https://doi.org/10.1525/si.2007.30.1.7.

Bell, Ann V. 2009. "'It's Way out of My League': Low-Income Women's Experiences of Medicalized Infertility." *Gender & Society* 23 (5): 688–709. https://doi.org/10.1177/0891243209343708.

———. 2010. "Beyond (Financial) Accessibility: Inequalities within the Medicalisation of Infertility." *Sociology of Health & Illness* 32 (4): 631–646. https://doi.org/10.1111/j.1467-9566.2009.01235.x.

Benford, Robert. 1987. "An Insider's Critique of the Social Movement Framing Perspective." *Sociological Inquiry* 67 (4): 409–430. https://doi.org/10.1111/j.1475-682X.1997.tb00445.x.

Benford, Robert D., and David A. Snow. 2000. "Framing Processes and Social Movements: An Overview and Assessment." *Annual Review of Sociology* 26 (1): 611–639. https://doi.org/10.1146/annurev.soc.26.1.611.

Berg, Marc. 1992. "The Construction of Medical Disposals Medical Sociology and Medical Problem Solving in Clinical Practice." *Sociology of Health & Illness* 14 (2): 151–180. https://doi.org/10.1111/j.1467-9566.1992.tb00119.x.

Berry, Donald A. 2014. "Failure of Researchers, Reviewers, Editors, and the Media to Understand Flaws in Cancer Screening Studies: Application to an Article in Cancer." *Cancer* 120 (18): 2784–2791. https://doi.org/10.1002/cncr.28795.

Best, Joel. 2017. "Typification and Social Problems Construction." In *Images of Issues: Typifying Contemporary Social Problems*, edited by Joel Best, 3–11. New York: Routledge.

Bleyer, Archie. 2015. "Screening Mammography: Update and Review of Publications since Our Report in the New England Journal of Medicine on the Magnitude of the Problem in the United States." *Academic Radiology* 22 (8): 949–960. https://doi.org/10.1016/j.acra.2015.03.003.

Bleyer, Archie, and H. Gilbert Welch. 2012. "Effect of Three Decades of Screening Mammography on Breast-Cancer Incidence." *New England Journal of Medicine* 367 (21): 1998–2005. https://doi.org/10.1056/NEJMoa1206809.

Block, Lauren D., Marian P. Jarlenski, Albert W. Wu, and Wendy L. Bennett. 2013. "Mammography Use among Women Ages 40–49 after the 2009 U.S. Preventive Services Task Force Recommendation." *Journal of General Internal Medicine* 28 (11): 1447–1453. https://doi.org/10.1007/s11606-013-2482-5.

Bloor, Michael. 1995. *The Sociology of HIV Transmission*. London: SAGE.

Bosk, Charles L. 1979. *Forgive and Remember: Managing Medical Failure*. Chicago: University of Chicago Press.

Bradley, Cathy J., Charles W. Given, and Caralee Roberts. 2002. "Race, Socioeconomic Status, and Breast Cancer Treatment and Survival." *Journal of the National Cancer Institute* 94 (7): 490–496. https://doi.org/10.1093/jnci/94.7.490.

"Breast Cancer Risk Factors You Cannot Change." 2021, December 16. https://www.cancer.org/cancer/breast-cancer/risk-and-prevention/breast-cancer-risk-factors-you-cannot-change.html.

"Breast Cancer Screening with Mammography in Women Aged 40–49 Years." 1996. Organizing Committee and Collaborators, Falun Meeting, Falun, Sweden, March 21–22. *International Journal of Cancer* 68: 693–699. https://doi.org/10.1002/(SICI)1097-0215(19961211)68:6<693::AID-IJC1>3.0.CO;2-Z.

Brekhus, Wayne. 1998. "A Sociology of the Unmarked: Redirecting Our Focus." *Sociological Theory* 16 (1): 34–51. https://doi.org/10.1111/0735-2751.00041.

———. 2003. *Peacocks, Chameleons, Centaurs: Gay Suburbia and the Grammar of Social Identity*. Chicago: University of Chicago Press.

———. 2015. *Culture and Cognition: Patterns in the Social Construction of Reality*. Malden, MA: Polity Press.

Brekhus, Wayne H., David L. Brunsma, Todd Platts, and Priya Dua. 2010. "On the Contributions of Cognitive Sociology to the Sociological Study of Race." *Sociology Compass* 4 (1): 61–76. https://doi.org/10.1111/j.1751-9020.2009.00259.x.

Brewer, Noel T., Tayla Salz, and Sarah E. Lillie. 2007. "Systematic Review: The Long-Term Effects of False-Positive Mammograms." *Annals of Internal Medicine* 146 (7): 502–510. https://doi.org/10.7326/0003-4819-146-7-200704030-00006.

Broom, Alex, and Katherine Kenny. 2021. "The Moral Cosmology of Cancer: Making Disease Meaningful." *Sociological Review* 69 (2): 468–483. https://doi.org/10.1177/0038026120962912.

Broom, Dorothy. 2001. "Reading Breast Cancer: Reflections on a Dangerous Intersection." *Health* 5 (2): 249–268. https://doi.org/10.1177/136345930100500206.

Brubaker, Sarah Jane. 2007. "Denied, Embracing, and Resisting Medicalization: African American Teen Mothers' Perceptions of Formal Pregnancy and Childbirth Care." *Gender & Society* 21 (4): 528–552. https://doi.org/10.1177/0891243207304972.

References

Carter, Kimbroe J., Frank Castro, and Roy N. Morcos. 2018. "Insights into Breast Cancer Screening: A Computer Simulation of Two Contemporary Screening Strategies." *AJR. American Journal of Roentgenology* 210 (3): 564–571. https://doi.org/10.2214/AJR.17.18484.

Carter, Stacy M. 2021. "Why Does Cancer Screening Persist Despite the Potential to Harm?" *Science, Technology and Society* 26 (1): 24–40. https://doi.org/10.1177/0971721820960252.

Casper, Monica J., and Daniel R. Morrison. 2010. "Medical Sociology and Technology: Critical Engagements." *Journal of Health and Social Behavior* 51 (1) (supp.): S120–S132. https://doi.org/10.1177/0022146510383493.

Cerulo, Karen A., ed. 2002. *Culture in Mind: Toward a Sociology of Culture and Cognition*. New York: Routledge.

Clarke, Juanne. 1999. "Breast Cancer in Mass Circulating Magazines in the USA and Canada, 1974–1995." *Women and Health* 28 (4): 113–130. https://doi.org/10.1300/J013v28n04_07.

Committee on Practice Bulletins—Gynecology. 2017. "Breast Cancer Risk Assessment and Screening in Average-Risk Women." Acog.org. Accessed June 8, 2022. https://www.acog.org/clinical/clinical-guidance/practice-bulletin/articles/2017/07/breast-cancer-risk-assessment-and-screening-in-average-risk-women.

Conrad, Peter. 2005. "The Shifting Engines of Medicalization." *Journal of Health and Social Behavior* 46 (1): 3–14. https://doi.org/10.1177/002214650504600102.

Conrad, Peter, and Kristin K. Barker. 2010. "The Social Construction of Illness: Key Insights and Policy Implications." *Journal of Health and Social Behavior* 51 (1) (supp.): S67–S79. https://doi.org/10.1177/0022146510383495.

Corbelli, Jennifer, Sonya Borrero, Rachel Bonnema, Megan McNamara, Kevin Kraemer, Doris Rubio, Irina Karpov, and Melissa McNeil. 2014. "Physician Adherence to U.S. Preventive Services Task Force Mammography Guidelines." *Women's Health Issues: Official Publication of the Jacobs Institute of Women's Health* 24 (3): e313–e319. https://doi.org/10.1016/j.whi.2014.03.003.

Corcoran, Jacqueline, Meghan Crowley, Holly Bell, Andrea Murray, and Lauren Grindle. 2012. "U.S. Latinas' Knowledge and Attitudes toward Mammography: Meta-Synthesis." *Journal of Human Behavior in the Social Environment* 22 (6): 671–689. https://doi.org/10.1080/10911359.2012.655959.

Cox, Susan M., and William McKellin. 1999. "'There's This Thing in Our Family': Predictive Testing and the Construction of Risk for Huntington Disease." *Sociology of Health & Illness* 21 (5): 622–646. https://doi.org/10.1111/1467-9566.00176.

Davidson, AuTumn S., Xun Liao, and B. Dale Magee. 2011. "Attitudes of Women in Their Forties toward the 2009 USPSTF Mammogram Guidelines: A Randomized Trial on the Effects of Media Exposure." *American Journal of Obstetrics and Gynecology* 205 (1): 30.e1–7. https://doi.org/10.1016/j.ajog.2011.04.005.

Davis, Murray. 1983. *Smut: Erotic Reality/Obscene Ideology*. Chicago: University of Chicago Press.

Davison, Charlie, Sally Macintyre, and George Davey Smith. 1994. "The Potential Social Impact of Predictive Genetic Testing for Susceptibility to Common Chronic Diseases: A Review and Proposed Research Agenda." *Sociology of Health & Illness* 16 (3): 340–371. https://doi.org/10.1111/1467-9566.ep11348762.

De Vries, Raymond, and Trudo Lemmens. 2006. "The Social and Cultural Shaping of Medical Evidence: Case Studies from Pharmaceutical Research and Obstetric Science."

Social Science & Medicine 62 (11): 2694–2706. https://doi.org/10.1016/j.socscimed.2005.11.026.

Dean, Lorraine, S. V. Subramanian, David R. Williams, Katrina Armstrong, Camille Zubrinsky Charles, and Ichiro Kawachi. 2014. "The Role of Social Capital in African-American Women's Use of Mammography." *Social Science & Medicine* 104: 148–156. https://doi.org/10.1016/j.socscimed.2013.11.057.

DeGloma, Thomas. 2015. "The Strategies of Mnemonic Battle: On the Alignment of Autobiographical and Collective Memories in Conflicts over the Past." *American Journal of Cultural Sociology* 3 (1): 156–190. https://doi.org/10.1057/ajcs.2014.17.

DeGloma, Thomas E., and Asia May Friedman. 2005. "Thinking with Socio-Mental Filters: Exploring the Social Structuring of Attention and Significance." Paper presented at the annual meeting of the American Sociological Association, Philadelphia, August 2005.

Dehkordy, Soudabeh Fazeli, Kelli S. Hall, Allison L. Roach, Edward D. Rothman, Vanessa K. Dalton, and Ruth C. Carlos. 2015. "Trends in Breast Cancer Screening: Impact of U.S. Preventive Services Task Force Recommendations." *American Journal of Preventive Medicine* 49 (3): 419–422. https://doi.org/10.1016/j.amepre.2015.02.017.

DiMaggio, Paul. 1997. "Culture and Cognition." *Annual Review of Sociology* 23 (1): 263–287. https://doi.org/10.1146/annurev.soc.23.1.263.

Douglas, Mary. 1966. *Purity and Danger: An Analysis of Concepts of Pollution and Taboo*. London: Routledge/Keegan Paul.

Dumit, Joseph. 2004. *Picturing Personhood: Brain Scans and Biomedical Identity*. Princeton, NJ: Princeton University Press.

Ebell, Mark H., Thuy Nhu Thai, and Kyle J. Royalty. 2018. "Cancer Screening Recommendations: An International Comparison of High Income Countries." *Public Health Reviews* 39 (7). https://doi.org/10.1186/s40985-018-0080-0.

Ehrenreich, Barbara. 2001. "Welcome to Cancerland: A Mammogram Leads to a Cult of Pink Kitsch." *Harpers Magazine* (November): 43–53.

Eibich, Peter, and Léontine Goldzahl. 2020. "Health Information Provision, Health Knowledge and Health Behaviours: Evidence from Breast Cancer Screening." *Social Science & Medicine* 265: 113505. https://doi.org/10.1016/j.socscimed.2020.113505.

Epstein, Cynthia Fuchs. 1988. *Deceptive Distinctions: Sex, Gender, and the Social Order*. New Haven, CT: Yale University Press.

Esserman, Laura J., Ian M. Thompson, Jr., and Brian Reid. 2013. "Overdiagnosis and Overtreatment in Cancer: An Opportunity for Improvement." *JAMA* 310 (8): 797–798. https://doi.org/10.1001/jama.2013.108415.

Farr, Deeonna E., Heather M. Brandt, Daniela B. Friedman, Swann Arp Adams, Cheryl A. Armstead, Jeanette K. Fulton, and Douglas M. Bull. 2020. "False-Positive Mammography and Mammography Screening Intentions among Black Women: The Influence of Emotions and Coping Strategies." *Ethnicity & Health* 25 (4): 580–597. https://doi.org/10.1080/13557858.2019.1571563.

Faulkner, Alex. 2012. "Resisting the Screening Imperative: Patienthood, Populations and Politics in Prostate Cancer Detection Technologies for the UK." *Sociology of Health & Illness* 34 (2): 221–233. https://doi.org/10.1111/j.1467-9566.2011.01385.x.

Feagin, Joe R. 2010. *The White Racial Frame: Centuries of Racial Framing and Counter-Framing*. New York: Routledge.

Fine, Gary Alan. 2012. *Sticky Reputations: The Politics of Collective Memory in Midcentury America*. New York: Routledge.

Finney Rutten, Lila J., Jon O. Ebbert, Debra J. Jacobson, Linda B. Squiers, Chun Fan, Carmen Radecki Breitkopf, Véronique L. Roger, and Jennifer L. St. Sauver. 2014. "Changes in U.S. Preventive Services Task Force Recommendations: Effect on Mammography Screening in Olmsted County, MN 2004–2013." *Preventive Medicine* 69: 235–238. https://doi.org/10.1016/j.ypmed.2014.10.024.

Fleck, Ludwik. 1979. *Genesis and Development of a Scientific Fact*. Chicago: University of Chicago Press.

Food and Drug Administration. 2022. "MQSA National Statistics." Accessed February 7, 2022. https://www.fda.gov/radiation-emitting-products/mqsa-insights/mqsa-national-statistics.

Fosket, Jennifer. 2000. "Problematizing Biomedicine: Women's Constructions of Breast Cancer Knowledge." In *Ideologies of Breast Cancer: Feminist Perspectives*, edited by Laura Potts, 15–36. London: Macmillan.

———. 2004. "Constructing 'High-Risk Women': The Development and Standardization of a Breast Cancer Risk Assessment Tool." *Science, Technology, & Human Values* 29 (3): 291–313. https://doi.org/10.1177/0162243904264960.

Friedman, Asia. 2013. *Blind to Sameness: Sexpectations and the Social Construction of Male and Female Bodies*. Chicago: University of Chicago Press.

———. 2016. "'There Are Two People at Work That I'm Fairly Certain Are Black': Uncertainty and Deliberative Thinking in Blind Race Attribution." *The Sociological Quarterly* 57 (3): 437–461. https://doi.org/10.1111/tsq.12140.

———. 2019. "Cultural Blind Spots and Blind Fields." In *The Oxford Handbook of Cognitive Sociology*, edited by Wayne H. Brekhus and Gabe Ignatow, 467–482. Oxford: Oxford University Press.

Friedman, Erica B., Jennifer Chun, Freya Schnabel, Shira Schwartz, Sidney Law, Jessica Billig, Erin Ivanoff, Linda Moy, Deborah Axelrod, and Amber Guth. 2013. "Screening Prior to Breast Cancer Diagnosis: The More Things Change, the More They Stay the Same." *International Journal of Breast Cancer* 2013: 327567. https://doi.org/10.1155/2013/327567.

Garfinkel, Harold. 1967. *Studies in Ethnomethodology*. Englewood Cliffs, NJ: Prentice-Hall.

Genuis, Stephen J., and Shelagh K. Genuis. 2004. "Resisting Cookbook Medicine." *BMJ* 329 (7458): 179. https://doi.org/10.1136/bmj.329.7458.179.

Gifford, Sandra M. 1986. "The Meaning of Lumps: A Case Study of the Ambiguities of Risk." In *Anthropology and Epidemiology: Interdisciplinary Approaches to the Study of Health and Disease, Culture, Illness, and Healing*, edited by Craig R. Janes, Ron Stall, and Sandra M. Gifford, 213–246. Dordrecht: Springer Netherlands.

Gillespie, Chris. 2015. "The Risk Experience: The Social Effects of Health Screening and the Emergence of a Proto-Illness." *Sociology of Health & Illness* 37 (7): 973–987. https://doi.org/10.1111/1467-9566.12257.

Goffman, Erving. 1961. *Encounters: Two Studies in the Sociology of Interaction*. Indianapolis: Bobbs-Merrill.

———. 1963. *Stigma: Notes on the Management of Spoiled Identity*. Englewood Cliffs, NJ: Prentice Hall.

———. 1974. *Frame Analysis: An Essay on the Organization of Experience*. Cambridge, MA: Harvard University Press.

Goldzahl, Léontine. 2017. "Contributions of Risk Preference, Time Orientation and Perceptions to Breast Cancer Screening Regularity." *Social Science & Medicine* 185: 147–157. https://doi.org/10.1016/j.socscimed.2017.04.037.

References

Gøtzsche, Peter C., and Ole Olsen. 2000. "Is Screening for Breast Cancer with Mammography Justifiable?" *Lancet* 355 (9198): 129–134. https://doi.org/10.1016/S0140-6736(99)06065-1.

Grant, Linda, Kathryn B. Ward, and Xue Lan Rong. 1987. "Is There an Association between Gender and Methods in Sociological Research?" *American Sociological Review* 52 (6): 856–862. https://doi.org/10.2307/2095839.

Green, Eileen E., Diane Thompson, and Frances Griffiths. 2002. "Narratives of Risk: Women at Midlife, Medical 'Experts' and Health Technologies." *Health, Risk & Society* 4 (3): 273–286. https://doi.org/10.1080/1369857021000016632.

Greenberg, Daniel S., and Judith E. Randal. 1977. "The Questionable Breast X-Ray Program." *Washington Post*, May 1. http://www.washingtonpost.com/archive/opinions/1977/05/01/the-questionable-breast-x-ray-program/dad02766-e48b-43af-8e1e-df5661d7dec6/?tid=ss_mail.

Griffiths, Frances, Eileen Green, and Gillian Bendelow. 2006. "Health Professionals, Their Medical Interventions and Uncertainty: A Study Focusing on Women at Midlife." *Social Science & Medicine* 62 (5): 1078–1090. https://doi.org/10.1016/j.socscimed.2005.07.027.

Halbwachs, Maurice. 1950. *On Collective Memory*. Chicago: University of Chicago Press.

Hankin, Janet R., and Eric R. Wright. 2010. "Reflections on Fifty Years of Medical Sociology." *Journal of Health and Social Behavior* 51 (1) (supp.): S10–S14. https://doi.org/10.1177/0022146510383840.

Haraway, Donna. 1988. "Situated Knowledges: The Science Question in Feminism and the Privilege of Partial Perspective." *Feminist Studies* 14 (3): 575–599. https://doi.org/10.2307/3178066.

———. 1992. "The Promises of Monsters: A Regenerative Politics for Inappropriate/d Others." In *Cultural Studies*, edited by Lawrence Grossberg, Cary Nelson, and Paula Treichler, 295–337. New York: Routledge.

Hardesty, Lara A., Kimberly E. Lind, and Eric J. Gutierrez. 2016. "Compliance with Screening: Mammography Guidelines after a False-Positive Mammogram." *Journal of the American College of Radiology: JACR* 13 (9): 1032–1038. https://doi.org/10.1016/j.jacr.2016.03.016.

Harris, Russell, George F. Sawaya, Virginia A. Moyer, and Ned Calonge. 2011. "Reconsidering the Criteria for Evaluating Proposed Screening Programs: Reflections from 4 Current and Former Members of the U.S. Preventive Services Task Force." *Epidemiologic Reviews* 33 (1): 20–35. https://doi.org/10.1093/epirev/mxr005.

Harris, Russell P., Timothy J. Wilt, and Amir Qaseem. 2015. "Screening for Cancer: Advice for High-Value Care from the American College of Physicians." *Annals of Internal Medicine* 162 (10): 718–725. https://doi.org/10.7326/M14-2327.

He, Xiaofei, Karen E. Schifferdecker, Elissa M. Ozanne, Anna N. A. Tosteson, Steven Woloshin, and Lisa M. Schwartz. 2018. "How Do Women View Risk-Based Mammography Screening? A Qualitative Study." *Journal of General Internal Medicine* 33 (11): 1905–1912. https://doi.org/10.1007/s11606-018-4601-9.

Heath, Iona. 2014. "Role of Fear in Overdiagnosis and Overtreatment: An Essay by Iona Heath." *BMJ* 349: g6123. https://doi.org/10.1136/bmj.g6123.

Hejduková, Pavlína, and Lucie Kureková. 2017. "Healthcare Systems and Performance Evaluation: Comparison of Performance Indicators in V4 Countries Using Models of Composite Indicators." *Economics & Management* 20 (3): 133–146. https://doi.org/10.15240/tul/001/2017-3-009.

Hendrick, R. Edward, and Mark A. Helvie. 2011. "United States Preventive Services Task Force Screening Mammography Recommendations: Science Ignored." *AJR. American Journal of Roentgenology* 196 (2): W112–116. https://doi.org/10.2214/AJR.10.5609.

Hersch, Jolyn, Jesse Jansen, Alexandra Barratt, Les Irwig, Nehmat Houssami, Kirsten Howard, Haryana Dhillon, and Kirsten McCaffery. 2013. "Women's Views on Overdiagnosis in Breast Cancer Screening: A Qualitative Study." *BMJ* 346: f158. https://doi.org/10.1136/bmj.f158.

Hesse-Biber, Sharlene. 2014. *Waiting for Cancer to Come: Women's Experiences with Genetic Testing and Medical Decision Making for Breast and Ovarian Cancer*. Ann Arbor: University of Michigan Press.

Hicks, Lisa K. 2015. "Reframing Overuse in Health Care: Time to Focus on the Harms." *Journal of Oncology Practice* 11 (3): 168–170. https://doi.org/10.1200/JOP.2015.004283.

Hill Collins, Patricia. 2009. *Black Feminist Thought: Knowledge, Consciousness, and the Politics of Empowerment*. 2nd ed. New York: Routledge.

Hinz, Erica K., Rashmi Kudesia, Renee Rolston, Thomas A. Caputo, and Michael J. Worley. 2011. "Physician Knowledge of and Adherence to the Revised Breast Cancer Screening Guidelines by the United States Preventive Services Task Force." *American Journal of Obstetrics and Gynecology* 205 (3): 201.e1–5. https://doi.org/10.1016/j.ajog.2011.04.025.

Hobson, Katherine. 2015. "Called Back After a Mammogram? Doctors Are Trying to Make It Less Scary." *National Public Radio*, October 15. https://www.npr.org/sections/health-shots/2015/10/15/448888415/called-back-after-a-mammogram-doctors-are-trying-to-make-it-less-scary.

Hoffmann, Tammy C., and Chris Del Mar. 2015. "Patients' Expectations of the Benefits and Harms of Treatments, Screening, and Tests: A Systematic Review." *JAMA Internal Medicine* 175 (2): 274–286. https://doi.org/10.1001/jamainternmed.2014.6016.

Hofmann, Bjorn. 2014. "Diagnosing Overdiagnosis: Conceptual Challenges and Suggested Solutions." *European Journal of Epidemiology* 29 (9): 599–604. https://doi.org/10.1007/s10654-014-9920-5.

House, James S. 2002. "Understanding Social Factors and Inequalities in Health: 20th Century Progress and 21st Century Prospects." *Journal of Health and Social Behavior* 43 (2): 125–142. https://doi.org/10.2307/3090192.

Howard, David H., and E. Kathleen Adams. 2012. "Mammography Rates after the 2009 US Preventive Services Task Force Breast Cancer Screening Recommendation." *Preventive Medicine* 55 (5): 485–487. https://doi.org/10.1016/j.ypmed.2012.09.012.

Howard, David H., Lisa C. Richardson, and Kenneth E. Thorpe. 2009. "Cancer Screening and Age in the United States and Europe." *Health Affairs* 28 (6): 1838–1847. https://doi.org/10.1377/hlthaff.28.6.1838.

Howson, Alexandra. 1999. "Cervical Screening, Compliance and Moral Obligation." *Sociology of Health & Illness* 21 (4): 401–425. https://doi.org/10.1111/1467-9566.00164.

Hunter, Kathryn. 1991. *Doctors' Stories: The Narrative Structure of Medical Knowledge*. Princeton: Princeton University Press.

Independent UK Panel on Breast Cancer Screening. 2012. "The Benefits and Harms of Breast Cancer Screening: An Independent Review." *The Lancet* 380 (9855): 1778–1786. https://doi.org/10.1016/S0140-6736(12)61611-0.

Iwase, Madoka, Hiroko Tsunoda, Kanako Nakayama, Emiko Morishita, Naoki Hayashi, Koyu Suzuki, and Hideko Yamauchi. 2017. "Overcalling Low-Risk Findings: Grouped Amorphous Calcifications Found at Screening Mammography Associated with Minimal Cancer Risk." *Breast Cancer* 24 (4): 579–584. https://doi.org/10.1007/s12282-016-0742-z.

References

Jakobson, Roman, and Linda R. Waugh. 1979. *The Sound Shape of Language*. Boston: De Gruyter Mouton.

Jiang, Miao, Danny R. Hughes, and Richard Duszak. 2015. "Screening Mammography Rates in the Medicare Population before and after the 2009 U.S. Preventive Services Task Force Guideline Change: An Interrupted Time Series Analysis." *Women's Health Issues: Official Publication of the Jacobs Institute of Women's Health* 25 (3): 239–245. https://doi.org/10.1016/j.whi.2015.03.002.

Johansen, Venke, Therese Andrews, Haldis Haukanes, and Ulla-Britt Lilleaas. 2013. "Symbols and Meanings in Breast Cancer Awareness Campaigns." *NORA—Nordic Journal of Feminist and Gender Research* 21 (2): 140–155. https://doi.org/10.1080/08038740.2013.797024.

Joyce, Kelly. 2008. *Magnetic Appeal: MRI and the Myth of Transparency*. Ithaca, NY: Cornell University Press.

Kadivar, Hajar, Barbara A. Goff, William R. Phillips, C. Holly A. Andrilla, Alfred O. Berg, and Laura-Mae Baldwin. 2012. "Nonrecommended Breast and Colorectal Cancer Screening for Young Women: A Vignette-Based Survey." *American Journal of Preventive Medicine* 43 (3): 231–239. https://doi.org/10.1016/j.amepre.2012.05.022.

———. 2014. "Guideline-Inconsistent Breast Cancer Screening for Women over 50: A Vignette-Based Survey." *Journal of General Internal Medicine* 29 (1): 82–89. https://doi.org/10.1007/s11606-013-2567-1.

Keating, Nancy L., and Lydia E. Pace. 2015. "New Guidelines for Breast Cancer Screening in US Women." *JAMA* 314 (15): 1569–1571. https://doi.org/10.1001/jama.2015.13086.

Keen, John D. 2010. "Promoting Screening Mammography: Insight or Uptake?" *Journal of the American Board of Family Medicine: JABFM* 23 (6): 775–782. https://doi.org/10.3122/jabfm.2010.06.100065.

Kessler, Suzanne, and Wendy McKenna. 1978. *Gender: An Ethnomethodological Approach*. Hoboken, NJ: John Wiley and Sons.

Khuri, Fadlo R. 2015. "What We Know and What We Think We Know: An Editor's Perspective on a Charged Debate." *Cancer* 121 (1): 4–5. https://doi.org/10.1002/cncr.29080.

Kikuzawa, Saeko, Sigrun Olafsdottir, and Bernice A. Pescosolido. 2008. "Similar Pressures, Different Contexts: Public Attitudes toward Government Intervention for Health Care in 21 Nations." *Journal of Health and Social Behavior* 49 (4): 385–399. https://doi.org/10.1177/002214650804900402.

King, Samantha. 2008. *Pink Ribbons, Inc.: Breast Cancer and the Politics of Philanthropy*. Minneapolis: University of Minnesota Press.

Kiviniemi, Marc T., and Jennifer L. Hay. 2012. "Awareness of the 2009 US Preventive Services Task Force Recommended Changes in Mammography Screening Guidelines, Accuracy of Awareness, Sources of Knowledge about Recommendations, and Attitudes about Updated Screening Guidelines in Women Ages 40–49 and 50+." *BMC Public Health* 12 (24 Oct.): 899. https://doi.org/10.1186/1471-2458-12-899.

Klawiter, Maren. 2008. *The Biopolitics of Breast Cancer: Changing Cultures of Disease and Activism*. Minneapolis: University of Minnesota Press.

Knaapen, Loes. 2014. "Evidence-Based Medicine or Cookbook Medicine? Addressing Concerns over the Standardization of Care." *Sociology Compass* 8 (6): 823–836. https://doi.org/10.1111/soc4.12184.

Kopans, Daniel B. 2010. "The 2009 US Preventive Services Task Force (USPSTF) Guidelines Are Not Supported by Science: The Scientific Support for Mammography Screening." *Radiologic Clinics of North America* 48 (5): 843–857. https://doi.org/10.1016/j.rcl.2010.06.005.

References

———. 2013. "Point: The *New England Journal of Medicine* Article Suggesting Overdiagnosis from Mammography Screening Is Scientifically Incorrect and Should Be Withdrawn." *Journal of the American College of Radiology* 10 (5): 317–319. https://doi.org/10.1016/j.jacr.2013.01.024.

———. 2014. "Mammograms Save Lives." *Wall Street Journal*, May 22. https://www.wsj.com/articles/daniel-b-kopans-mammograms-save-lives-1400800454.

Kopans, Daniel B., Matthew L. Webb, and Blake Cady. 2014. "The 20–Year Effort to Reduce Access to Mammography Screening: Historical Facts Dispute a Commentary in Cancer." *Cancer* 120 (18): 2792–2799. https://doi.org/10.1002/cncr.28791.

Kuhn, Thomas S. 1962. *The Structure of Scientific Revolutions.* Chicago: University of Chicago Press.

Lakoff, George, and Mark Johnson. 1980. *Metaphors We Live By.* Chicago: University of Chicago Press.

Lee, Carol H., D. David Dershaw, Daniel Kopans, Phil Evans, Barbara Monsees, Debra Monticciolo, R. James Brenner, Lawrence Bassett, Wendie Berg, Stephen Feig, Edward Hendrick, Ellen Mendelson, Carl D'Orsi, Edward Sickles, and Linda Warren Burhenne. 2010. "Breast Cancer Screening with Imaging: Recommendations from The Society of Breast Imaging and the ACR on the Use Of Mammography, Breast MRI, Breast Ultrasound, and Other Technologies for the Detection of Clinically Occult Breast Cancer." *Journal of the American College of Radiology* 7 (1): 18–27. https://doi.org/10.1016/j.jacr.2009.09.022.

Lehoux, Pascale, Jean-Louis Denis, Melanie Rock, Myriam Hivon, and Stephanie Tailliez. 2010. "How Medical Specialists Appraise Three Controversial Health Innovations: Scientific, Clinical and Social Arguments." *Sociology of Health & Illness* 32 (1): 123–139. https://doi.org/10.1111/j.1467-9566.2009.01192.x.

Lerner, Barron. 2003. *The Breast Cancer Wars: Hope, Fear, and the Pursuit of a Cure in Twentieth-Century America.* New York: Oxford University Press.

Lewin, Alana A., Yiming Gao, Leng Lin Young, Marissa L. Albert, James S. Babb, Hildegard K. Toth, Linda Moy, and Samantha L. Heller. 2018. "Stereotactic Breast Biopsy with Benign Results Does Not Negatively Affect Future Screening Adherence." *Journal of the American College of Radiology* 15 (4): 622–629. https://doi.org/10.1016/j.jacr.2017.12.034.

Lewis, Caroline. 2020. "Why Some Breast Cancer Screenings Come with Unexpected Costs." *Gothamist*, February 18. https://gothamist.com/news/why-some-breast-cancer-screenings-come-unexpected-costs.

Light, Donald W. 2004. "Introduction: Ironies of Success: A New History of the American Health Care 'System.'" *Journal of Health and Social Behavior* 45 (Extra Issue: Health and Health Care in the United States: Origins and Dynamics): 1–24. http://www.jstor.org/stable/3653821.

Link, Bruce G., and Jo C. Phelan. 1995. "Social Conditions as Fundamental Causes of Disease." *Journal of Health and Social Behavior*, Extra Issue: Forty Years of Medical Sociology: The State of the Art and Directions for the Future: 80–94. https://doi.org/10.2307/2626958.

Lupton, Deborah. 1994. "Femininity, Responsibility, and the Technological Imperative: Discourses on Breast Cancer in the Australian Press." *International Journal of Health Services* 24 (1): 73–89. https://doi.org/10.2190/1B6J-1P5R-AXCR-MRNY.

Mack, Arien, and Irvin Rock. 1998. *Inattentional Blindness.* Boston: MIT Press.

Markens, Susan, Carole H. Browner, and Nancy Press. 1999. "'Because of the Risks': How US Pregnant Women Account for Refusing Prenatal Screening." *Social Science & Medicine* 49 (3): 359–369. https://doi.org/10.1016/s0277-9536(99)00097-0.

References

Martin, Brian. 2004. "Dissent and Heresy in Medicine: Models, Methods, and Strategies." *Social Science & Medicine* 58 (4): 713–725. https://doi.org/10.1016/S0277-9536(03)00223-5.

Martin, Emily. 2001. *The Woman in the Body: A Cultural Analysis of Reproduction*. Boston: Beacon Press.

Martinelli, Mauro, and Giuseppe Alessandro Veltri. 2021. "Do Cognitive Styles Affect Vaccine Hesitancy? A Dual-Process Cognitive Framework for Vaccine Hesitancy and the Role of Risk Perceptions." *Social Science & Medicine* 289: 114403. https://doi.org/10.1016/j.socscimed.2021.114403.

Masuda, Takahiko, and Richard E. Nisbett. 2001. "Attending Holistically versus Analytically: Comparing the Context Sensitivity of Japanese and Americans." *Journal of Personality and Social Psychology* 81 (5): 922–934. https://doi.org/10.1037//0022-3514.81.5.922.

McCaffery, Kirsten J., Jesse Jansen, Laura D. Scherer, Hazel Thornton, Jolyn Hersch, Stacy M. Carter, Alexandra Barratt, Stacey Sheridan, Ray Moynihan, Jo Waller, John Brodersen, Kristen Pickles, and Adrian Edwards. 2016. "Walking the Tightrope: Communicating Overdiagnosis in Modern Healthcare." *BMJ* 352: i348. https://doi.org/10.1136/bmj.i348.

McGrath, Joseph E., and Janice R. Kelly. 1992. "Temporal Context and Temporal Patterning: Toward a Time-Centered Perspective for Social Psychology." *Time & Society* 1 (3): 399–420. https://doi.org/10.1177/0961463X92001003005.

McKelvey, Tara. 2020. "Coronavirus: Why Are Americans so Angry about Masks?" *BBC News*, July 20. https://www.bbc.com/news/world-us-canada-53477121.

Mechanic, David. 2001. "The Managed Care Backlash: Perceptions and Rhetoric in Health Care Policy and the Potential for Health Care Reform." *Milbank Quarterly* 79 (1): 35–54. https://doi.org/10.1111/1468-0009.00195.

———. 2004. "The Rise and Fall of Managed Care." *Journal of Health and Social Behavior* 45 (Extra Issue: Health and Health Care in the United States: Origins and Dynamics): 76–86. https://doi.org/10.1111/1468-0009.00195.

Mechanic, David, and Donna D. McAlpine. 2010. "Sociology of Health Care Reform: Building on Research and Analysis to Improve Health Care." *Journal of Health and Social Behavior* 51 (1) (supp.): S147–S159. https://doi.org/10.1177/0022146510383497.

Mechanic, David, and David A. Rochefort. 1996. "Comparative Medical Systems." *Annual Review of Sociology* 22: 239–270. https://doi.org/10.1146/annurev.soc.22.1.239.

Meißner, Hanna. 2016. "New Material Feminisms and Historical Materialism: A Diffractive Reading of Two (Ostensibly) Unrelated Perspectives." In *Mattering: Feminism, Science, and Materialism*, edited by Victoria Pitts-Taylor, 43–57. New York: NYU Press.

Miles, Matthew B., and A. Michael Huberman. 1984. *Qualitative Data Analysis: A Sourcebook of New Methods*. Beverly Hills: Sage Publications.

Miller, Brittany C., Jennifer M. Bowers, Jackelyn B. Payne, and Anne Moyer. 2019. "Barriers to Mammography Screening among Racial and Ethnic Minority Women." *Social Science & Medicine* 239: 112494. https://doi.org/10.1016/j.socscimed.2019.112494.

Mische, Ann. 2009. "Projects and Possibilities: Researching Futures in Action." *Sociological Forum* 24 (3): 694–704. https://doi.org/10.1111/j.1573-7861.2009.01127.x.

Mishra, Shiraz I., Bruce DeForge, Beth Barnet, Shana Ntiri, and Laura Grant. 2012. "Social Determinants of Breast Cancer Screening in Urban Primary Care Practices: A Community-Engaged Formative Study." *Women's Health Issues: Official Publication of the Jacobs Institute of Women's Health* 22 (5): e429–438. https://doi.org/10.1016/j.whi.2012.06.004.

References

Missinne, Sarah, Elien Colman, and Piet Bracke. 2013. "Spousal Influence on Mammography Screening: A Life Course Perspective." *Social Science & Medicine* 98: 63–70. https://doi.org/10.1016/j.socscimed.2013.08.024.

Missinne, Sarah, Karel Neels, and Piet Bracke. 2014. "Reconsidering Inequalities in Preventive Health Care: An Application of Cultural Health Capital Theory and the Life-Course Perspective to the Take-up of Mammography Screening." *Sociology of Health & Illness* 36 (8): 1259–1275. https://doi.org/10.1111/1467-9566.12169.

Montini, Theresa. 1996. "Gender and Emotion in the Advocacy for Breast Cancer Informed Consent Legislation." *Gender and Society* 10 (1): 9–23. https://doi.org/10.1177/089124396010001002.

Moore, Sarah. 2010. "Is the Healthy Body Gendered? Toward a Feminist Critique of the New Paradigm of Health." *Body & Society* 16 (2): 95–118. https://doi.org/10.1177/1357034X10364765.

Moudatsou, Maria M., George Kritsotakis, Athanasios K. Alegakis, Antonios Koutis, and Anastasios E. Philalithis. 2014. "Social Capital and Adherence to Cervical and Breast Cancer Screening Guidelines: A Cross-Sectional Study in Rural Crete." *Health & Social Care in the Community* 22 (4): 395–404. https://doi.org/10.1111/hsc.12096.

Moynihan, Ray, Jenny Doust, and David Henry. 2012. "Preventing Overdiagnosis: How to Stop Harming the Healthy." *BMJ* 344: e3502. https://doi.org/10.1136/bmj.e3502.

Moynihan, Ray, David Henry, and Karel G. M. Moons. 2014. "Using Evidence to Combat Overdiagnosis and Overtreatment: Evaluating Treatments, Tests, and Disease Definitions in the Time of Too Much." *PLoS Medicine* 11 (7): e1001655. https://doi.org/10.1371/journal.pmed.1001655.

Mullaney, Jamie L. 1999. "Making It 'Count': Mental Weighing and Identity Attribution." *Symbolic Interaction* 22 (3): 269–283. https://doi.org/10.1525/si.1999.22.3.269.

Myers, Evan R., Patricia Moorman, Jennifer M. Gierisch, Laura J. Havrilesky, Lars J. Grimm, Sujata Ghate, Brittany Davidson, Ranee Chatterjee Montgomery, Matthew J. Crowley, Douglas C. McCrory, Amy Kendrick, and Gillian D. Sanders. 2015. "Benefits and Harms of Breast Cancer Screening: A Systematic Review." *JAMA* 314 (15): 1615–1634. https://doi.org/10.1001/jama.2015.13183.

National Institutes of Health Consensus Development Panel. 1997. "National Institutes of Health Consensus Development Conference Statement: Breast Cancer for Women Ages 40–49, January 21–23, 1997." *Journal of the National Cancer Institute* 14: 1019.

Nisbett, Richard E. 2003. *The Geography of Thought: How Asians and Westerners Think Differently . . . and Why*. New York: Free Press.

Noe, Alva. 2004. *Action in Perception*. Cambridge, MA: MIT Press.

Norris, Susan L., Brittany U. Burda, Haley K. Holmer, Lauren A. Ogden, Rongwei Fu, Lisa Bero, Holger Schünemann, and Richard Deyo. 2012. "Author's Specialty and Conflicts of Interest Contribute to Conflicting Guidelines for Screening Mammography." *Journal of Clinical Epidemiology* 65 (7): 725–733. https://doi.org/10.1016/j.jclinepi.2011.12.011.

Nowotny, Helga. 1992. "Time and Social Theory: Towards a Social Theory of Time." *Time & Society* 1 (3): 421–454. https://doi.org/10.1177/0961463X92001003006.

O'Neill, Suzanne C., Isaac M. Lipkus, Jennifer M. Gierisch, Barbara K. Rimer, and J. Michael Bowling. 2012. "It's the Amount of Thought That Counts: When Ambivalence Contributes to Mammography Screening Delay." *Women's Health Issues* 22 (2): e189–e194. https://doi.org/10.1016/j.whi.2011.08.008.

Oeffinger, Kevin C., Elizabeth T. H. Fontham, Ruth Etzioni, Abbe Herzig, James S. Michaelson, Ya-Chen Tina Shih, Louise C. Walter, et al. 2015. "Breast Cancer Screening for

Women at Average Risk: 2015 Guideline Update from the American Cancer Society." *JAMA* 314 (15): 1599–1614. https://doi.org/10.1001/jama.2015.12783.

Omi, Michael, and Howard Winant. 1986. *Racial Formation in the United States*. New York: Routledge/Taylor & Francis Group.

Pace, Lydia E., Yulei He, and Nancy L. Keating. 2013. "Trends in Mammography Screening Rates after Publication of the 2009 US Preventive Services Task Force Recommendations." *Cancer* 119 (14): 2518–2523. https://doi.org/10.1002/cncr.28105.

Parker, Lisa, Lucie Rychetnik, and Stacy Carter. 2015. "Values in Breast Cancer Screening: An Empirical Study with Australian Experts." *BMJ Open* 5 (5): e006333. https://doi.org/10.1136/bmjopen-2014-006333.

Patel, Samir B. 2018. "Estimated Mortality of Breast Cancer Patients Based on Stage at Diagnosis and National Screening Guideline Categorization." *Journal of the American College of Radiology* 15 (9): 1206–1213. https://doi.org/10.1016/j.jacr.2018.04.010.

Pathirana, Thanya, Justin Clark, and Ray Moynihan. 2017. "Mapping the Drivers of Overdiagnosis to Potential Solutions." *BMJ* 358: j3879. https://doi.org/10.1136/bmj.j3879.

Pescosolido, Bernice A., and Jennie J. Kronenfeld. 1995. "Health, Illness, and Healing in an Uncertain Era: Challenges from and for Medical Sociology." *Journal of Health and Social Behavior*, Extra Issue: Forty Years of Medical Sociology: The State of the Art and Directions for the Future: 5–33. https://doi.org/10.2307/2626955.

Phelan, Jo C., Bruce G. Link, and Parisa Tehranifar. 2010. "Social Conditions as Fundamental Causes of Health Inequalities: Theory, Evidence, and Policy Implications." *Journal of Health and Social Behavior* 51 (1) (supp.): S28–S40. https://doi.org/10.1177/0022146510383498.

Philipson, Tomas, Michael Eber, Darius N. Lakdawalla, Mitra Corral, Rena Conti, and Dana P. Goldman. 2012. "An Analysis of Whether Higher Health Care Spending in the United States versus Europe Is 'Worth It' in the Case of Cancer." *Health Affairs* 31 (4): 667–675. https://doi.org/10.1377/hlthaff.2011.1298.

Power, Michael. 1999. *The Audit Society: Rituals of Verification*. Oxford: Oxford University Press.

Prasad, Amit. 2005. "Making Images/Making Bodies: Visibilizing and Disciplining through Magnetic Resonance Imaging." *Science, Technology and Human Values* 30 (2): 291–316. https://doi.org/10.1177/0162243904271758.

Qaseem, Amir, Jennifer S. Lin, Reem A. Mustafa, Carrie A. Horwitch, and Timothy J. Wilt. 2019. "Screening for Breast Cancer in Average-Risk Women: A Guidance Statement from the American College of Physicians." *Annals of Internal Medicine* 170 (8): 547–560. https://doi.org/10.7326/M18-2147.

Quadagno, Jill. 2010. "Institutions, Interest Groups, and Ideology: An Agenda for the Sociology of Health Care Reform." *Journal of Health and Social Behavior* 51 (2): 125–136. https://doi.org/10.1177/0022146510368931.

Quanstrum, Kerianne H., and Rodney A. Hayward. 2010. "Lessons from the Mammography Wars." *New England Journal of Medicine* 363 (11): 1076–1079. https://doi.org/10.1056/NEJMsb1002538.

Raftery, James, and Maria Chorozoglou. 2011. "Possible Net Harms of Breast Cancer Screening: Updated Modelling of Forrest Report." *BMJ* 343: d7627. https://doi.org/10.1136/bmj.d7627.

Railton, Kevin. 2015. "'Dual Process' Models of the Mind and the 'Identifiable Victim Effect.'" In *Identified versus Statistical Lives: An Interdisciplinary Perspective*, edited by I. Glenn Cohen, Norman Daniels, and Nir Eyal, 24–41. Oxford: Oxford University Press.

Rapp, Rayna. 1999. *Testing Women, Testing the Fetus: The Social Impact of Amniocentesis in America*. New York: Routledge.

Raspberry, Kelly, and Debra Skinner. 2011. "Enacting Genetic Responsibility: Experiences of Mothers Who Carry the Fragile X Gene." *Sociology of Health & Illness* 33 (3): 420–433. https://doi.org/10.1111/j.1467-9566.2010.01289.x.

Ravitch, Sharon M, and Nicole Mittenfelner Carl. 2020. *Qualitative Research: Bridging the Conceptual, Theoretical, and Methodological*, 2nd ed. Beverly Hills, CA: Sage Publications.

Ray, Kimberly M., Bonnie N. Joe, Rita I. Freimanis, Edward A Sickles, and R. Edward Hendrick. 2018. "Screening Mammography in Women 40–49 Years Old." *American Journal of Roentgenology* 201 (2): 264–270. https://doi.org/10.2214/AJR.17.18707.

Reed, Kate. 2009. "'It's Them Faulty Genes Again': Women, Men and the Gendered Nature of Genetic Responsibility in Prenatal Blood Screening." *Sociology of Health & Illness* 31 (3): 343–359. https://doi.org/10.1111/j.1467-9566.2008.01134.x.

Reibling, Nadine, Mareike Ariaans, and Claus Wendt. 2019. "Worlds of Healthcare: A Healthcare System Typology of OECD Countries." *Health Policy* 123 (7): 611–620. https://doi.org/10.1016/j.healthpol.2019.05.001.

Reynolds, Handel. 2012. *The Big Squeeze: A Social and Political History of the Controversial Mammogram*. Ithaca, NY: ILR Press.

Ricoeur, Paul. 1984. *Time and Narrative*, vol. 1. Chicago: University of Chicago Press.

Ricoeur, Paul. 1988. *Time and Narrative*, vol. 3. Chicago: University of Chicago Press.

Ridgeway, Cecilia L., and Shelley J. Correll. 2004. "Unpacking the Gender System: A Theoretical Perspective on Gender Beliefs and Social Relations." *Gender & Society* 18 (4): 510–531. https://doi.org/10.1177/0891243204265269.

Rogers, Wendy A. 2019. "Analysing the Ethics of Breast Cancer Overdiagnosis: A Pathogenic Vulnerability." *Medicine, Health Care and Philosophy* 22 (1): 129–140. https://doi.org/10.1007/s11019-018-9852-z.

Rogers, Wendy A., Vikki A. Entwistle, and Stacy M. Carter. 2019. "Risk, Overdiagnosis and Ethical Justifications." *Health Care Analysis* 27 (4): 231–248. https://doi.org/10.1007/s10728-019-00369-7.

Rosenbaum, Lisa. 2014. "'Misfearing'—Culture, Identity, and Our Perceptions of Health Risks." *New England Journal of Medicine* 370 (7): 595–597. https://doi.org/10.1056/NEJMp1314638.

Rosich, Katherine J., and Janet R. Hankin. 2010. "Executive Summary: What Do We Know? Key Findings from 50 Years of Medical Sociology." *Journal of Health and Social Behavior* 51 (1) (supp.): S1–S9. https://doi.org/10.1177/0022146510383496.

Rothman, Barbara Katz. 1986. *The Tentative Pregnancy: How Amniocentesis Changes the Experience of Motherhood*. Auckland, NZ: Viking Penguin.

Rothman, Barbara Katz. 1991. *In Labor: Women and Power in the Birthplace*. New York: W. W. Norton.

Rozbroj, Tomas, Romi Haas, Denise O'Connor, Stacy M. Carter, Kirsten McCaffery, Rae Thomas, Jan Donovan, and Rachelle Buchbinder. 2021. "How Do People Understand Overtesting and Overdiagnosis? Systematic Review and Meta-Synthesis of Qualitative Research." *Social Science & Medicine* 285: 114255. https://doi.org/10.1016/j.socscimed.2021.114255.

Ruiz-Junco, Natalia. 2013. "Feeling Social Movements: Theoretical Contributions to Social Movement Research on Emotions." *Sociology Compass* 7 (1): 45–54. https://doi.org/10.1111/soc4.12006.

Ryan, Charlotte. 1991. *Prime Time Activism: Media Strategies for Grassroots Organizing*. Boston: South End Press.

References

Saldana, Johnny. 2013. *The Coding Manual for Qualitative Researchers*. London: Sage.

Sarda, Gita. 2009. *Artificially Maintained Scientific Controversies, the Construction of Maternal Choice and Caesarean Section Rates*. SSRN Scholarly Paper. ID 1592792. Rochester, NY: Social Science Research Network.

Scheff, Thomas J. 1963. "Decision Rules, Types of Error, and Their Consequences in Medical Diagnosis." *Behavioral Science* 8 (2): 97–107. https://doi.org/10.1002/bs.3830080202.

Schelling, Thomas. C. 1968. "The Life You Save May Be Your Own." In *Problems in Public Expenditure Analysis. Studies of Government Finance*, edited by Samuel B. Chase, 127–162. Washington, DC: The Brookings Institute.

Schneider, Joseph. 2005. *Donna Haraway: Live Theory*. New York: Continuum.

Schnittker, Jason. 2009. "Mirage of Health in the Era of Biomedicalization: Evaluating Change in the Threshold of Illness, 1972–1996." *Social Forces* 87 (4): 2155–2182. https://doi.org/10.1353/sof.0.0218.

Schroer, Markus. 2019. "Sociology of Attention: Fundamental Reflections on a Theoretical Program." In *The Oxford Handbook of Cognitive Sociology*, edited by Wayne H. Brekhus and Gabe Ignatow, 425–448. Oxford: Oxford University Press.

Schutz, Alfred. 1962. "On Multiple Realities." In *Collected Papers I: The Problem of Social Reality, Phaenomenologica*, edited by Maurice Natanson, 207–259. Dordrecht, Netherlands: Springer.

———. 1970. *On Phenomenology and Social Relations: Selected Writings*. Chicago: University of Chicago Press.

Schwalbe, Michael, Daphne Holden, Douglas Schrock, Sandra Godwin, Shealy Thompson, and Michele Wolkomir. 2000. "Generic Processes in the Reproduction of Inequality: An Interactionist Analysis." *Social Forces* 79 (2): 419–452. https://doi.org/10.1093/sf/79.2.419.

Schwartz, Lisa M., Steven Woloshin Jr., Floyd J. Fowler, and H. Gilbert Welch. 2004. "Enthusiasm for Cancer Screening in the United States." *JAMA* 291 (1): 71–78. https://doi.org/10.1001/jama.291.1.71.

"Shaheen & Blunt Introduce Bill to Make Breast Cancer Diagnostic Tests More Accessible & Affordable | U.S. Senator Jeanne Shaheen of New Hampshire." Accessed November 2, 2021. https://www.shaheen.senate.gov/news/press/shaheen-and-blunt-introduce-bill-to-make-breast-cancer-diagnostic-tests-more-accessible_affordable.

Shapiro, Sam, Philip Strax, and Louis Venet. 1971. "Periodic Breast Cancer Screening in Reducing Mortality from Breast Cancer." *Journal of the American Medical Association* 215 (11): 1777–1785. https://doi.org/10.1001/jama.1971.03180240027005.

Sharpe, Richard E., David C. Levin, Laurence Parker, and Vijay M. Rao. 2013. "The Effect of the Controversial US Preventive Services Task Force Recommendations on the Use of Screening Mammography." *Journal of the American College of Radiology: JACR* 10 (1): 21–24. https://doi.org/10.1016/j.jacr.2012.07.008.

Sheridan, Stacey L., Russell P. Harris, and Steven H. Woolf. 2004. "Shared Decision Making about Screening and Chemoprevention: A Suggested Approach from the U.S. Preventive Services Task Force." *American Journal of Preventive Medicine* 26 (1): 56–66. https://doi.org/10.1016/j.amepre.2003.09.011.

Shibutani, Tamotsu. 1955. "Reference Groups as Perspectives." *American Journal of Sociology* 60 (6): 562–569. https://doi.org/10.1086/221630.

Shim, Janet K. 2010. "Cultural Health Capital: A Theoretical Approach to Understanding Health Care Interactions and the Dynamics of Unequal Treatment." *Journal of Health and Social Behavior* 51 (1): 1–15. https://doi.org/10.1177/0022146509361185.

Silverman, Elaine, Steven Woloshin, Lisa M. Schwartz, Stephanie J. Byram, H. Gilbert Welch, and Baruch Fischhoff. 2001. "Women's Views on Breast Cancer Risk and Screening Mammography: A Qualitative Interview Study." *Medical Decision Making* 21 (3): 231–240. https://doi.org/10.1177/0272989X0102100308.

Simmel, Georg. 1908. *On Individuality and Social Forms*. Chicago: University of Chicago Press.

Simpson, Ruth. 1996. "Neither Clear nor Present: The Social Construction of Safety and Danger." *Sociological Forum* 11 (3): 549–562. https://doi.org/10.1007/BF02408392.

Siu, Albert L., and U.S. Preventive Services Task Force. 2016. "Screening for Breast Cancer: U.S. Preventive Services Task Force Recommendation Statement." *Annals of Internal Medicine* 164 (4): 279–296. https://doi.org/10.7326/M15-2886.

Sledge, Piper. 2021. *Bodies Unbound: Gender-Specific Cancer and Biolegitimacy*. New Brunswick, NJ: Rutgers University Press.

Small, Deborah. 2015. "On the Psychology of the Identifiable Victim Effect." In *Identified Versus Statistical Lives: An Interdisciplinary Perspective*, edited by I. Glenn Cohen, Norman Daniels, and Nir Eyal, 13–23. Oxford: Oxford University Press.

Snow, David, and Robert Benford. 1988. "Ideology, Frame Resonance and Participant Mobilization." *International Social Movement Research* 1: 197–218.

Snow, David, Robert Benford, Holly McCammon, Lyndi Hewitt, and Scott Fitzgerald. 2014. "The Emergence, Development, and Future of the Framing Perspective: 25+ Years since Frame Alignment." *Mobilization* 19 (1): 23–45. https://doi.org/10.17813/maiq.19.1.x74278226830m69l.

Solazzo, Alexa L., Bridget K. Gorman, and Justin T. Denney. 2017. "Cancer Screening Utilization among U.S. Women: How Mammogram and Pap Test Use Varies among Heterosexual, Lesbian, and Bisexual Women." *Population Research and Policy Review* 36 (3): 357–377. https://doi.org/10.1007/s11113-017-9425-5.

Spadea, Teresa, Silvia Bellini, Anton Kunst, Irina Stirbu, and Giuseppe Costa. 2010. "The Impact of Interventions to Improve Attendance in Female Cancer Screening among Lower Socioeconomic Groups: A Review." *Preventive Medicine* 50 (4): 159–164. https://doi.org/10.1016/j.ypmed.2010.01.007.

Sprague, Brian L., Kenyon C. Bolton, John L. Mace, Sally D. Herschorn, Ted A. James, Pamela M. Vacek, Donald L. Weaver, and Berta M. Geller. 2014. "Registry-Based Study of Trends in Breast Cancer Screening Mammography before and after the 2009 U.S. Preventive Services Task Force Recommendations." *Radiology* 270 (2): 354–361. https://doi.org/10.1148/radiol.13131063.

Squiers, Linda B., Debra J. Holden, Suzanne E. Dolina, Annice E. Kim, Carla M. Bann, and Jeanette M. Renaud. 2011. "The Public's Response to the U.S. Preventive Services Task Force's 2009 Recommendations on Mammography Screening." *American Journal of Preventive Medicine* 40 (5): 497–504. https://doi.org/10.1016/j.amepre.2010.12.027.

Stacey, Judith. 1988. "Can There Be A Feminist Ethnography?" *Women's Studies International Forum* 11 (1): 21–27. https://doi.org/10.1016/0277-5395(88)90004-0.

Steele, Whitney Randolph, Felicia Mebane, K. Viswanath, and Janice Solomon. 2005. "News Media Coverage of a Women's Health Controversy: How Newspapers and TV Outlets Covered a Recent Debate over Screening Mammography." *Women & Health* 41 (3): 83–97. https://doi.org/10.1300/J013v41n03_05.

Stefanek, Michael Edward. 2011. "Uninformed Compliance or Informed Choice? A Needed Shift in Our Approach to Cancer Screening." *JNCI: Journal of the National Cancer Institute* 103 (24): 1821–1826. https://doi.org/10.1093/jnci/djr474.

References

Stewart, Emily. 2020. "Anti-Maskers Explain Themselves." *Vox*, August 7. https://www.vox.com/the-goods/2020/8/7/21357400/anti-mask-protest-rallies-donald-trump-covid-19.

Stolberg, Sheryl Gay. 2002. "Guidelines by U.S. Urge Mammograms for Women at 40." *The New York Times*, February 22. https://www.nytimes.com/2002/02/22/us/guidelines-by-us-urge-mammograms-for-women-at-40.html.

Sulik, Gayle A. 2009. "Managing Biomedical Uncertainty: The Technoscientific Illness Identity." *Sociology of Health & Illness* 31 (7): 1059–1076. https://doi.org/10.1111/j.1467-9566.2009.01183.x.

———. 2010. *Pink Ribbon Blues: How Breast Cancer Culture Undermines Women's Health*. New York: Oxford University Press.

———. 2015. "How Should We Address Breast Cancer When Norms Continually Change?" *The Guardian*, October 20. https://www.theguardian.com/commentisfree/2015/oct/20/address-breast-cancer-norms-continually-change?CMP=share_btn_link.

"Surprise Medical Bills: New Protections for Consumers Take Effect in 2022." *KFF*. Accessed November 2, 2021. https://www.kff.org/private-insurance/fact-sheet/surprise-medical-bills-new-protections-for-consumers-take-effect-in-2022/.

Tabboni, Simonetta. 2001. "The Idea of Social Time in Norbert Elias." *Time & Society* 10 (1): 5–27. https://doi.org/10.1177/0961463X01010001001.

Tejeda, Silvia, Beti Thompson, Gloria D. Coronado, and Diane P. Martin. 2009. "Barriers and Facilitators Related to Mammography Use among Lower Educated Mexican Women in the USA." *Social Science & Medicine* 68 (5): 832–839. https://doi.org/10.1016/j.socscimed.2008.12.023.

Timmermans, Stefan, and Marc Berg. 2003. *The Gold Standard: The Challenge of Evidence-Based Medicine and Standardization in Health Care*. Philadelphia: Temple University Press.

Timmermans, Stefan, and Mara Buchbinder. 2010. "Patients-in-Waiting: Living between Sickness and Health in the Genomics Era." *Journal of Health and Social Behavior* 51 (4): 408–423. https://doi.org/10.1177/0022146510386794.

Timmermans, Stefan, and Hyeyoung Oh. 2010. "The Continued Social Transformation of the Medical Profession." *Journal of Health and Social Behavior* 51 (1) (supp.): S94–S106. https://doi.org/10.1177/0022146510383500.

Tosteson, Anna N. A., Dennis G. Fryback, Cristina S. Hammond, Lucy G. Hanna, Margaret R. Grove, Mary Brown, Qianfei Wang, Karen Lindfors, and Etta D. Pisano. 2014. "Consequences of False-Positive Screening Mammograms." *JAMA Internal Medicine* 174 (6): 954–961. https://doi.org/10.1001/jamainternmed.2014.981.

Trubetzkoy, Nikolai Sergeevich. 1969. *Principles of Phonology*. Berkeley: University of California Press.

Umberson, Debra, and Jennifer Karas Montez. 2010. "Social Relationships and Health: A Flashpoint for Health Policy." *Journal of Health and Social Behavior* 51 (1) (supp.): S54–S66. https://doi.org/10.1177/0022146510383501.

"U.S. Breast Cancer Statistics." 2019. *Breastcancer.org*. Accessed January 2, 2020. https://www.breastcancer.org/symptoms/understand_bc/statistics.

U.S. Preventive Services Task Force. 1989. *Guide to Clinical Preventive Services: Report of the U.S. Preventive Services Task Force*. Rockville, MD: Agency for Healthcare Research and Quality.

———. 2009. "Screening for Breast Cancer: U.S. Preventive Services Task Force Recommendation Statement." *Annals of Internal Medicine* 151: 716.

van Seijen, Maartje, Esther H. Lips, Alastair M. Thompson, Serena Nik-Zainal, Andrew Futreal, E. Shelley Hwang, Ellen Verschuur, Joanna Lane, Jos Jonkers, Daniel W. Rea, and Jelle Wesseling on behalf of the PRECISION team. 2019. "Ductal Carcinoma In Situ: To Treat or Not to Treat, That Is the Question." *British Journal of Cancer* 121 (4): 285–292. https://doi.org/10.1038/s41416-019-0478-6.

Ward, Jeremy K., and Patrick Peretti-Watel. 2020. "Understanding Vaccine Mistrust: From Perception Bias to Controversies." *Revue Francaise de Sociologie* 61 (2): 243–273. https://doi.org/10.3917/rfs.612.0243.

Weber, Max. 1949. *On the Methodology of the Social Sciences*. New York: The Free Press.

Wegwarth, Odette, and Gerd Gigerenzer. 2013. "Overdiagnosis and Overtreatment: Evaluation of What Physicians Tell Their Patients about Screening Harms." *JAMA Internal Medicine* 173 (22): 2086–2088. https://doi.org/10.1001/jamainternmed.2013.10363.

Welch, H. Gilbert. 2014. "Don't Slam Canada for Mammography Study." *CNN*, February 19. https://www.cnn.com/2014/02/19/opinion/welch-mammograms-canada/index.html.

Welch, H. Gilbert, Lisa M. Schwartz, and Steven Woloshin. 2011. *Overdiagnosed: Making People Sick in the Pursuit of Health*. Boston: Beacon Press.

Welch, H. Gilbert, Steven Woloshin, and Lisa M. Schwartz. 2008. "The Sea of Uncertainty Surrounding Ductal Carcinoma in Situ: The Price of Screening Mammography." *Journal of the National Cancer Institute* 100 (4): 228–229. https://doi.org/10.1093/jnci/djn013.

Wendland, Claire L. 2007. "The Vanishing Mother: Cesarean Section and 'Evidence-Based Obstetrics.'" *Medical Anthropology Quarterly* 21 (2): 218–233. https://doi.org/10.1525/maq.2007.21.2.218.

Werner, Anna. 2019. "Women Shocked by Cost of Mammograms: 'I Wasn't Expecting a Bill at All.'" *CBS News*, October 31. https://www.cbsnews.com/news/cost-of-mammograms-preventative-breast-exams-leave-women-with-unexpected-bills/.

Wharam, J. Frank, Bruce Landon, Fang Zhang, Xin Xu, Stephen Soumerai, and Dennis Ross-Degnan. 2015. "Mammography Rates 3 Years after the 2009 US Preventive Services Task Force Guidelines Changes." *Journal of Clinical Oncology: Official Journal of the American Society of Clinical Oncology* 33 (9): 1067–1074. https://doi.org/10.1200/JCO.2014.56.9848.

Wholey, Douglas, and Lawton Burns. 2000. "Tides of Change: The Evolution of Managed Care in the United States." In *Handbook of Medical Sociology*, fifth edition, edited by Chloe E. Bird, Peter Conrad, and Allen M. Fremont, 217–237. Saddle River, NJ: Prentice Hall.

Willis, Evan. 1998. "The 'New' Genetics and the Sociology of Medical Technology." *Journal of Sociology* 34 (2): 170–183. https://doi.org/10.1177/144078339803400205.

Wilt, Timothy J., Russell P. Harris, and Amir Qaseem. 2015. "Screening for Cancer: Advice for High-Value Care from the American College of Physicians." *Annals of Internal Medicine* 162 (10): 718. https://doi.org/10.7326/M14-2326.

Wright, Eric R., and Brea L. Perry. 2010. "Medical Sociology and Health Services Research: Past Accomplishments and Future Policy Challenges." *Journal of Health and Social Behavior* 51 (1) (supp.): S107–119. https://doi.org/10.1177/0022146510383504.

Xu, Xinling, Joshua R. Mann, James W. Hardin, Erin Gustafson, Suzanne W. McDermott, and Chelsea B. Deroche. 2017. "Adherence to US Preventive Services Task Force Recommendations for Breast and Cervical Cancer Screening for Women Who Have a Spinal Cord Injury." *Journal of Spinal Cord Medicine* 40 (1): 76–84. https://doi.org/10.1080/10790268.2016.1153293.

Xu, Xinling, Suzanne W. McDermott, Joshua R. Mann, James W. Hardin, Chelsea B. Deroche, Dianna D. Carroll, and Elizabeth A. Courtney-Long. 2017. "A Longitudinal Assessment of Adherence to Breast and Cervical Cancer Screening Recommendations among Women with and without Intellectual Disability." *Preventive Medicine* 100: 167–172. https://doi.org/10.1016/j.ypmed.2017.04.034.

Yu, Xue Qin. 2009. "Socioeconomic Disparities in Breast Cancer Survival: Relation to Stage at Diagnosis, Treatment and Race." *BMC Cancer* 9: 364. https://doi.org/10.1186/1471-2407-9-364.

Zerubavel, Eviatar. 1985. *Hidden Rhythms: Schedules and Calendars in Social Life*. Berkeley: University of California Press.

———. 1991. *The Fine Line: Making Distinctions in Everyday Life*. Chicago: University of Chicago Press.

———. 1993. "Horizons: On the Sociomental Foundations of Relevance." *Social Research* 60 (2): 397–413. http://www.jstor.org/stable/40970743.

———. 1997. *Social Mindscapes: An Invitation to Cognitive Sociology*. Cambridge, MA: Harvard University Press.

———. 2003. *Time Maps: Collective Memory and the Social Shape of the Past*. Chicago: University of Chicago Press.

———. 2011. *Ancestors and Relatives: Genealogy, Identity and Community*. New York: Oxford University Press.

———. 2015. *Hidden in Plain Sight: The Social Structure of Irrelevance*. New York: Oxford University Press.

———. 2018. *Taken for Granted: The Remarkable Power of the Unremarkable*. Princeton: Princeton University Press.

Index

Note: Italicized page numbers refer to tables or figures.

Access to Breast Cancer Diagnosis Act, 148
accountability, 23–24, 40–41, 93, 199, 211–212, 215
Affordable Care Act, 11, 116
alignment, autobiographical, 29, 73–84, 139–149, 187–193, 209, 215–220
alternatives, attentional, 21–23, 40, 59, 163, 202, 207–211. See also *diversity, attentional*
ambiguity, 48, 197, 199; value of, 212. See also confusion; uncertainty
ambivalence, 79; value of, 211–212. See also flexibility, mental
American Cancer Society, 4–13, 49, 50, 98, 100, 108, 115, 231n2 (ch. 1), 231n1 (ch. 4)
American College of Obstetrics and Gynecology, 5, *6*, 98
American College of Physicians, 5, *6*, 8
American College of Radiology, 5, *6*, 8–9, *12–13*, 48–49, 98, 231n2 (ch. 1)
anchors, attentional, 51, 73, 93, 98, 164, 202–203
Aronowitz, Robert, 1, 31–32, 43, 51, 60, 149, 161, 163, 168, 195, 231n1 (ch. 3), 232n1 (ch. 5)
asymmetry, attentional, 20–21, 24, 40–42, 54, 111, 128, 140, 188

Barad, Karen, 23–24, 30, 57, 93, 199, 212
battles, attentional: battles for attention, 93–95, 109–124, 207; battles over attention, 93–95, 97–109, 207; differentiation, 92, 95, 97–98; discrediting, 32, 92–97, 101–109, 127, 150, 174, 206; polarization, 32, 92, 96–101, 103, 105, 122; symmetrical analysis and, 24, 30, 204; value of analysis in terms of, 31–32, 92–95, 123, 206–207, 213
BCDDP. See Breast Cancer Detection Demonstration Project (BCDDP)

biases, attentional, 54, 101–109, 154–159; identified victim effect, 157–158; lead time bias, 172–174; over- and underattention, 54–55; type 1 and 2 errors, 26–27, 54–56. See also early detection: hegemonic cultural belief in
blind spots, cultural, 24. See also inattention
breast cancer: biology of, 46–47, 54–56, 165, 168–171 (see also overdiagnosis); fear of, 47, 60–63, 73–79, 141–146, 209 (see also screening paradox); gender and, 26, 62, 86–87, 199, 216 (see also gender); improvements in treatment of, 126, 175–177, 183–184, 204; prevalence statistics, 5–6. See also Ductal Carcinoma In-Situ (DCIS)
Breast Cancer Detection Demonstration Project (BCDDP), 7, *12*
Brekhus, Wayne, 41–42, 167, 196

Canadian National Breast Screening Study, 2, 8–9, *12*
Canadian Trials. See Canadian National Breast Screening Study
cascade of harms. See screening cascade
clinical medicine: emotion and, 101–104, 150–155, 157–161; norms of clinical attention and, 37–40, 44–45, 49–50, 101–104, 125–126, 137, 150–155, 157–159; Preventive Services Task Force composition and, 49–50, 101, 151, 203. See also individualism; victims, identified versus statistical
cognitive sociology, 3, 21–25, 27, 34–43, 196–197; attention and, 35–42, 196, 211–213; the sociology of time and, 166–168

253

communication, doctor-patient, 38–40, 68–72, 73, 84–89, 209–210; attentional deviance and, 87–89, 188, 193; attentional pauses, 210; conflicting patterns of attention and, 38–40; paternalism and, 60, 65
communities, attentional, 35–36; concepts of time and, 164–165, 166–168, 183–184; professions as, 37–40
conceptual models of cancer: biotemporality and, 165, 169–172; doctor/patient differences, 38, 88; lead time and, 172–174; as progressive, 47, 53–54, 204; projectivity and, 165, 172, 178. *See also* overdiagnosis
conflict, attentional. *See* battles, attentional
conflicts of interest, accusations of, 47–50, 84–85, 101–109, 231n1 (ch. 3)
confusion, conflicting mammography guidelines and, 25, 49, 61, 63–65, 80, 112–114
counterintuitiveness. *See* overdiagnosis: counterintuitiveness of

Davis, Murray, 36–37, 94
DCIS. *See* Ductal Carcinoma In-Situ (DCIS)
DeGloma, Thomas, 73, 189, 195
deviance, attentional, 45, 73, 87–89, 92, 186–187, 188, 193, 222
diffractive analysis: analytical symmetry and, 30, 199; exclusions and, 24, 33, 93, 212; intellectual generosity in, 24, 57
diversity, attentional, 35–40, 59, 84–90, 92–93, 207–209, 212, 227. *See also* alternatives, attentional
Ductal Carcinoma In-Situ (DCIS), 56, 131–134, 138, 153, 170, 178, 231n3 (ch. 1)

early detection: as foundational attention filter, 51, 57, 93, 203; hegemonic cultural belief in, 19–20, 50–57, 60–63, 72–79, 88–89, 110–112, 119, 131–133, 140–141, 163, 187–194, 201–202, 208–210; history of, 163, 168; overbelief in, 53–54, 131, 208; relationship to treatment, *57*, 58, 83, 118–119, 126, 163, 168–177
embodied experience, of mammograms, 86–87

emotion: anxiety of waiting for results, 134, 144–146, 191–193, 203, 217, 219; attentional roots of, 95, 97, 206–207; biasing effect of, 61–63, 103–104, 107–109, 154–159; clinical work and, 101–104, 151–154, 160–161; of guideline conflict, 1–3, 43, 95–97, 123; harms of screening and, 45, 133–136, 138–146, 203. *See also* fear; screening paradox
evidence-based medicine: critiques of, 18, 44–45, 101–102, 125–126, 150–153, 158–159; disparities and, 17–18, 158; epistemological authority of, 44, 48, 99–100, 103–104, 155–158; overuse and, 17, 18–19. *See also* victims, identified versus statistical
exclusions, attentional. *See* inattention

false-positive results. *See* overdiagnosis
fear: culture of, 16–19, 61, 76, 83, 89, 118; doctors', 16–19, 160–161; misfearing, 60–61, 75, 130; patients', 60–62, 73–79, 83, 141–143, 191–193, 209, 217. *See also* emotion; screening paradox
filter analysis, 24, 36–37, 42–43, 166–168, 195–196, 204, 211; early detection as attention filter, 50–58, 133, 201–203; foundational filters, 51, 57, 93, 203; professional attention filters, 37–40, 200; versus frame metaphor, 94
Fleck, Ludwik, 27
flexibility, mental: ambivalence and, 79, 211–212; attention and, 24, 31, 33, 40–41, 207, 210–213; dereification and, 40, 207, 211–213
forms, social, 36–37, 185. *See also* ideal types; *types, attentional*
framing: frame analysis, 93–95; framing contests, 94, 207

gender: breast cancer and, 26, 62, 199, 216; filter analysis and, 195–196; in medicine, 28, 62; patient perceptions of the mammography conflict and, 86–87, 216
Goffman, Erving, 22–23, 40, 93–94
guidelines for mammography: current, 5, *6*; history of debates, 5–13; international comparison, *14*

Index

Haraway, Donna, 23–24
harms of screening: anxious waiting as, 134, 138, 144–146, 191–193; competing definitions of, 4, 44–45, 55–56, 88, 130–146, 203, 217; counterintuitiveness of, 63–64, 107–108, 111, 119, 131–133, 140, 161; lack of attention to, relative to benefits, 20, 56, 73, 110–112, 116, 120–124, 135–136, 157; prior research on, 25, 130–131. *See also* overdiagnosis; overtreatment; screening cascade
healthcare: cultural differences in, 11–15, 19–20; disparities in, 16–18, 67, 81, 158, 222; managed care, 18–19, 196–197; overuse, 15–20, 196
Health Insurance Plan of Greater New York (HIP), 6–7, *12*
Hesse-Biber, Sharlene, 26, 28
HIP Trials. *See* Health Insurance Plan of Greater New York (HIP)

ideal types, 3, 36, 45, 202. *See also* forms, social; *types, attentional*
inattention: attentional asymmetry and, 40–42; benefits of analysis of, 30–31, 40, 84, 93, 199, 204, 211; early detection and, 53–55, 58, 133; filter metaphor and, 24, 42–43, 57–58, 94; sociology of, general definition, 22–24, 40–42; symmetrical analysis of, 40–42, 57, 199–200, 204, 211. See also *blind spots, cultural*; diffractive analysis: exclusions and
individualism, 38, 44–45, 89, 111–112, 132–133, 149, 157–159; personal anecdotes as data, 111–112, 136, 156–157. *See also* clinical medicine; victims, identified versus statistical
insurance: surprise bills for diagnostic mammograms, 146–148, 219–220; U.S. healthcare system and, 15, 18–19
irrelevance, 22–24, 36, 38–40, 55–56, 133, 136, 161–162, 171, 202–204. *See also* relevance, norms of

King, Samantha, 216
Klawiter, Maren, 10, 26
Kuhn, Thomas, 27, 35

lead time, 172–174
Lerner, Barron, 231n1 (intro)
Los Angeles Times, 4, 115–124, 226

marking, 22, 35–37, 41–42, 128–129, 168, 185; attention and, 41–42, 128–129
media: attentional battles and, 95, 109–115; bias, 49, 109, 113–114; coverage of mammography guidelines, 2–3, 11, 50, 63, 95, 115–123, 148, 226–227
medical knowledge, social construction of, 26–27
Mische, Ann, 165, 172
morality: gender and, 28, 62; of screening, 60, 62–63
mortality rates: as metric for evaluating screening, 100, 155, 177–179; lack of change in, 60, 149, 163, 169, 173, 178, 184
motherhood, 142–143
Mullaney, Jamie, 127–128

National Institutes of Health (NIH) Consensus Development Conferences, 7–9, *12*
National Medical Roundtable on Mammography, 7–9, *12*
New York Times, 4, 10, 113, 115–124, 226
NIH. *See* National Institutes of Health (NIH) Consensus Development Conferences
norms of attention: attentional weight and, 127; definition of, 3, 22, 34–36; discrediting of, in attentional battles, 92–93; temporality and, 166–168. *See also* clinical medicine: norms of clinical attention and; early detection: as foundational attention filter; inattention; *patterns of attention*; relevance, norms of; *types, attentional*
No Surprises Act, 148

overdiagnosis: counterfactuality of, 16–17, 55–56, 111–112, 133, 136, 157, 198; counterintuitiveness of, 16–17, 53–55, 63, 82–83, 107–111, 132–133; DCIS and, 56, 132–133, 134–135, 138, 143, 170, 178, 231n1 (ch. 3); definition of, 16–17; drivers of, 17–20; nonidentifiability and, 56, 157. *See also* harms of screening overtreatment, 4, 15–16, 26–27, 79, 82, 129–132, 143–144, 176. *See also* harms of screening

Pap test (Pap smear, cervical cancer screening), 71, 112–113, 145–146, 216–217
patterns of attention: as analytic focus, 24, 30–31, 34–43, 57, 93–94, 127–129, 199–200, 211; attentional dissonance and, 87, 209–210; in medical knowledge, 27, 30, 37–40, 127, 200–202; socially deviant, 45, 73, 87–89, 92, 186–188, 193, 222; sociology of attention and, 22–23, 34–37; sociotemporality and, 164–168, 184, 188–189, 206–207. *See also* norms of attention; *types, attentional*
Pink Ribbon Culture. *See* gender
population medicine. *See* evidence-based medicine
Prostate-Specific Antigen (PSA) Screening, 28, 31–32, 51, 60–61, 161, 205, 231n1 (ch. 3), 232n1 (ch. 5)
PSA. *See* Prostate-Specific Antigen (PSA) Screening

reification, of attention, 200–202, 207, 211–213; *See also* flexibility, mental: dereification and
relationships, attentional, 51, 93, 95, 202, 213
relevance, norms of, 3, 22–23, 35–42, 92, 127–128, 167, 200–203, 206, 207–211. *See also* irrelevance; norms of attention; clinical medicine: norms of clinical attention and
research methods: feminist, 158–159; of this study, 3–4, 215–227
risk(s): benefits of mammography and, prior research on, 25, 72–73; differing definitions of, 4, 82–83, 129–148, 150–159, 187–193, 203–204; legal, 19; social construction of, 28–29, 141–144, 187–193, 198

Scheff, Thomas, 26–27
Schutz, Alfred, 22, 40–42
screening, sociology of, 27–30, 198

screening cascade, 133–136, 192. *See also* harms of screening
screening paradox, 28–29, 60–63, 73, 75, 83, 89–90, 155, 209
Simmel, Georg, 3, 31, 36
Simpson, Ruth, 37, 54
statistical victims. *See* victims, identified versus statistical
Strax, Phillip, 6
Sulik, Gayle, 28, 88
survivor narratives. *See* screening paradox; victims, identified versus statistical: personal anecdotes and
Swedish Overview (Swedish Trials), 8–9, *12*
symmetrical analysis: of attention, 33, 40, 43, 57, 199–201, 204, 211; diffractive analysis and, 24, 57; sociology of screening and, 30

temporality: age, chronological versus biological, 166, 180–183; attention and, 164, 166–168, 183; biotemporality versus sociotemporality, 165, 168–172, 180–183; collective memory, 164–165; linear concepts of time, 165, 169–174; projectivity, 165, 172, 178; screening schedules and, 163, 165, 168–172, 174; sociology of time, 164–168; temporal conflict, 164–165; temporal norms, 164, 166, 189–190, 209; temporal patterns, 164; temporal strategies, 164, 168, 180, 206; turning points, 183–186
time, sociology of. *See* temporality
treatment, breast cancer: improvements in, 56–57, 118, 126, 175–177, 183–184, 204; significance relative to early detection, 56–57, 82–83, 118–119, 175–177, 179, 184, 204. *See also* overtreatment
types, attentional: definition of, 36–37; interventionism and skepticism as, 3–4, 30–32, 34, 44–50, *52*, 202; subtypes among patients (conscious interventionism, conscious skepticism, conflicted skepticism, default interventionism), 74–83, 139–146; value of analyzing, 30–32, 45, 202–206, 213. *See also* forms, social; ideal types; norms of attention; *patterns of attention*

Index

uncertainty, 18–19, 28–29, 48, 110, 197–200, 211–212; value of, 211–212. *See also* ambiguity; confusion

United States Preventive Services Task Force (USPSTF): critiques of, 2, 49–50, 66–67, 98–99, 101, 106–107, 116–118, 150–151, 203; mammography guidelines, 5, *6*, 8–13

USA Today, 4, 115–124, 226

USPSTF. *See* United States Preventive Services Task Force (USPSTF)

values: attentional weight and, 44, 50, 101–103, 105, 125–127, 137, 150–158, 206; clinical, 44, 50, 101–103, 125–126, 150–154. *See also* weighing, mental

victims, identified versus statistical, 149–162; personal anecdotes and, 111–112, 136, 157

Wall Street Journal, 4, 115–124, 226

Weber, Max, 3, 36, 45

weighing, mental, 125–129; in attentional battles, 98–105, 127, 206; attention and, 127–129; of clinical versus population-based evidence, 149–159; of the harms of screening, 131–137; of the harms of screening by patients, 140–146; language and, 137–138; sociotemporality and, 167; of treatment versus early detection, 175–177. *See also* values

Zerubavel, Eviatar, 22–23, 35–37, 41–42, 92, 128–129, 164–168

About the Author

Asia Friedman is an associate professor of sociology at the University of Delaware. Her first book, *Blind to Sameness: Sexpectations and the Social Construction of Male and Female Bodies*, won the Distinguished Book Award from the sex and gender section of the American Sociological Association in 2016. She is also the coeditor, with Anne Marie Champagne, of *Interpreting the Body: Between Meaning and Matter*.

Available titles in the Critical Issues in Health and Medicine series

Emily K. Abel, *Prelude to Hospice: Florence Wald, Dying People, and Their Families*

Emily K. Abel, *Suffering in the Land of Sunshine: A Los Angeles Illness Narrative*

Emily K. Abel, *Tuberculosis and the Politics of Exclusion: A History of Public Health and Migration to Los Angeles*

Marilyn Aguirre-Molina, Luisa N. Borrell, and William Vega, eds. *Health Issues in Latino Males: A Social and Structural Approach*

Anne-Emanuelle Birn and Theodore M. Brown, eds., *Comrades in Health: U.S. Health Internationalists, Abroad and at Home*

Karen Buhler-Wilkerson, *False Dawn: The Rise and Decline of Public Health Nursing*

Susan M. Chambré, *Fighting for Our Lives: New York's AIDS Community and the Politics of Disease*

Stephen M. Cherry, *Importing Care, Faithful Service: Filipino and Indian American Nurses at a Veterans Hospital*

Brittany Clair, *Carrying On: Another School of Thought on Pregnancy and Health*

James Colgrove, Gerald Markowitz, and David Rosner, eds., *The Contested Boundaries of American Public Health*

Elena Conis, Sandra Eder, and Aimee Medeiros, eds., *Pink and Blue: Gender, Culture, and the Health of Children*

Cynthia A. Connolly, *Children and Drug Safety: Balancing Risk and Protection in Twentieth-Century America*

Cynthia A. Connolly, *Saving Sickly Children: The Tuberculosis Preventorium in American Life, 1909–1970*

Brittany Cowgill, *Rest Uneasy: Sudden Infant Death Syndrome in Twentieth-Century America*

Patricia D'Antonio, *Nursing with a Message: Public Health Demonstration Projects in New York City*

Kerry Michael Dobransky, *Managing Madness in the Community: The Challenge of Contemporary Mental Health Care*

Tasha N. Dubriwny, *The Vulnerable Empowered Woman: Feminism, Postfeminism, and Women's Health*

Edward J. Eckenfels, *Doctors Serving People: Restoring Humanism to Medicine through Student Community Service*

Julie Fairman, *Making Room in the Clinic: Nurse Practitioners and the Evolution of Modern Health Care*

Jill A. Fisher, *Medical Research for Hire: The Political Economy of Pharmaceutical Clinical Trials*

Asia Friedman, *Mammography Wars: Analyzing Attention in Cultural and Medical Disputes*

Charlene Galarneau, *Communities of Health Care Justice*

Alyshia Gálvez, *Patient Citizens, Immigrant Mothers: Mexican Women, Public Prenatal Care and the Birth Weight Paradox*

Laura E. Gómez and Nancy López, eds., *Mapping "Race": Critical Approaches to Health Disparities Research*

Janet Greenlees, *When the Air Became Important: A Social History of the New England and Lancashire Textile Industries*

Gerald N. Grob and Howard H. Goldman, *The Dilemma of Federal Mental Health Policy: Radical Reform or Incremental Change?*

Gerald N. Grob and Allan V. Horwitz, *Diagnosis, Therapy, and Evidence: Conundrums in Modern American Medicine*

Rachel Grob, *Testing Baby: The Transformation of Newborn Screening, Parenting, and Policymaking*

Mark A. Hall and Sara Rosenbaum, eds., *The Health Care "Safety Net" in a Post-Reform World*

Laura L. Heinemann, *Transplanting Care: Shifting Commitments in Health and Care in the United States*

Rebecca J. Hester, *Embodied Politics: Indigenous Migrant Activism, Cultural Competency, and Health Promotion in California*

Laura D. Hirshbein, *American Melancholy: Constructions of Depression in the Twentieth Century*

Laura D. Hirshbein, *Smoking Privileges: Psychiatry, the Mentally Ill, and the Tobacco Industry in America*

Timothy Hoff, *Practice under Pressure: Primary Care Physicians and Their Medicine in the Twenty-first Century*

Beatrix Hoffman, Nancy Tomes, Rachel N. Grob, and Mark Schlesinger, eds., *Patients as Policy Actors*

Ruth Horowitz, *Deciding the Public Interest: Medical Licensing and Discipline*

Powel Kazanjian, *Frederick Novy and the Development of Bacteriology in American Medicine*

Claas Kirchhelle, *Pyrrhic Progress: The History of Antibiotics in Anglo-American Food Production*

Rebecca M. Kluchin, *Fit to Be Tied: Sterilization and Reproductive Rights in America, 1950–1980*

Jennifer Lisa Koslow, *Cultivating Health: Los Angeles Women and Public Health Reform*

Jennifer Lisa Koslow, *Exhibiting Health: Public Health Displays in the Progressive Era*

Susan C. Lawrence, *Privacy and the Past: Research, Law, Archives, Ethics*

Bonnie Lefkowitz, *Community Health Centers: A Movement and the People Who Made It Happen*

Ellen Leopold, *Under the Radar: Cancer and the Cold War*

Barbara L. Ley, *From Pink to Green: Disease Prevention and the Environmental Breast Cancer Movement*

Sonja Mackenzie, *Structural Intimacies: Sexual Stories in the Black AIDS Epidemic*

Stephen E. Mawdsley, *Selling Science: Polio and the Promise of Gamma Globulin*

Frank M. McClellan, *Healthcare and Human Dignity: Law Matters*

Michelle McClellan, *Lady Lushes: Gender, Alcohol, and Medicine in Modern America*

David Mechanic, *The Truth about Health Care: Why Reform Is Not Working in America*

Richard A. Meckel, *Classrooms and Clinics: Urban Schools and the Protection and Promotion of Child Health, 1870–1930*

Terry Mizrahi, *From Residency to Retirement: Physicians' Careers over a Professional Lifetime*

Manon Parry, *Broadcasting Birth Control: Mass Media and Family Planning*

Alyssa Picard, *Making the American Mouth: Dentists and Public Health in the Twentieth Century*

Heather Munro Prescott, *The Morning After: A History of Emergency Contraception in the United States*

Sarah B. Rodriguez, *The Love Surgeon: A Story of Trust, Harm, and the Limits of Medical Regulation*

David J. Rothman and David Blumenthal, eds., *Medical Professionalism in the New Information Age*

Andrew R. Ruis, *Eating to Learn, Learning to Eat: School Lunches and Nutrition Policy in the United States*

James A. Schafer Jr., *The Business of Private Medical Practice: Doctors, Specialization, and Urban Change in Philadelphia, 1900–1940*

Johanna Schoen, ed., *Abortion Care as Moral Work: Ethical Considerations of Maternal and Fetal Bodies*

David G. Schuster, *Neurasthenic Nation: America's Search for Health, Happiness, and Comfort, 1869–1920*

Karen Seccombe and Kim A. Hoffman, *Just Don't Get Sick: Access to Health Care in the Aftermath of Welfare Reform*

Leo B. Slater, *War and Disease: Biomedical Research on Malaria in the Twentieth Century*

Piper Sledge, *Bodies Unbound: Gender-Specific Cancer and Biolegitimacy*

Dena T. Smith, *Medicine over Mind: Mental Health Practice in the Biomedical Era*

Kylie M. Smith, *Talking Therapy: Knowledge and Power in American Psychiatric Nursing*

Matthew Smith, *An Alternative History of Hyperactivity: Food Additives and the Feingold Diet*

Paige Hall Smith, Bernice L. Hausman, and Miriam Labbok, *Beyond Health, Beyond Choice: Breastfeeding Constraints and Realities*

Susan L. Smith, *Toxic Exposures: Mustard Gas and the Health Consequences of World War II in the United States*

Rosemary A. Stevens, Charles E. Rosenberg, and Lawton R. Burns, eds., *History and Health Policy in the United States: Putting the Past Back In*

Marianne Sullivan, *Tainted Earth: Smelters, Public Health, and the Environment*

Courtney E. Thompson, *An Organ of Murder: Crime, Violence, and Phrenology in Nineteenth-Century America*

Barbra Mann Wall, *American Catholic Hospitals: A Century of Changing Markets and Missions*

Frances Ward, *The Door of Last Resort: Memoirs of a Nurse Practitioner*

Jean C. Whelan, *Nursing the Nation: Building the Nurse Labor Force*

Shannon Withycombe, *Lost: Miscarriage in Nineteenth-Century America*